T0362427

Cervical Myelopathy

Editor

MICHAEL G. FEHLINGS

NEUROSURGERY
CLINICS OF NORTH AMERICA

www.neurosurgery.theclinics.com

Consulting Editors
RUSSELL R. LONSER
DANIEL K. RESNICK

January 2018 • Volume 29 • Number 1

ELSEVIER

1600 John F. Kennedy Boulevard • Suite 1800 • Philadelphia, Pennsylvania, 19103-2899

http://www.theclinics.com

NEUROSURGERY CLINICS OF NORTH AMERICA Volume 29, Number 1
January 2018 ISSN 1042-3680, ISBN-13: 978-0-323-57065-7

Editor: Stacy Eastman
Developmental Editor: Laura Fisher

© 2018 Elsevier Inc. All rights reserved.

This periodical and the individual contributions contained in it are protected under copyright by Elsevier, and the following terms and conditions apply to their use:

Photocopying
Single photocopies of single articles may be made for personal use as allowed by national copyright laws. Permission of the Publisher and payment of a fee is required for all other photocopying, including multiple or systematic copying, copying for advertising or promotional purposes, resale, and all forms of document delivery. Special rates are available for educational institutions that wish to make photocopies for non-profit educational classroom use. For information on how to seek permission visit www.elsevier.com/permissions or call: (+44) 1865 843830 (UK)/(+1) 215 239 3804 (USA).

Derivative Works
Subscribers may reproduce tables of contents or prepare lists of articles including abstracts for internal circulation within their institutions. Permission of the Publisher is required for resale or distribution outside the institution. Permission of the Publisher is required for all other derivative works, including compilations and translations (please consult www.elsevier.com/permissions).

Electronic Storage or Usage
Permission of the Publisher is required to store or use electronically any material contained in this periodical, including any article or part of an article (please consult www.elsevier.com/permissions). Except as outlined above, no part of this publication may be reproduced, stored in a retrieval system or transmitted in any form or by any means, electronic, mechanical, photocopying, recording or otherwise, without prior written permission of the Publisher.

Notice
No responsibility is assumed by the Publisher for any injury and/or damage to persons or property as a matter of products liability, negligence or otherwise, or from any use or operation of any methods, products, instructions or ideas contained in the material herein. Because of rapid advances in the medical sciences, in particular, independent verification of diagnoses and drug dosages should be made.

Although all advertising material is expected to conform to ethical (medical) standards, inclusion in this publication does not constitute a guarantee or endorsement of the quality or value of such product or of the claims made of it by its manufacturer.

Neurosurgery Clinics of North America (ISSN 1042-3680) is published quarterly by Elsevier Inc., 360 Park Avenue South, New York, NY 10010-1710. Months of issue are January, April, July, and October. Business and Editorial Offices: 1600 John F. Kennedy Blvd., Suite 1800, Philadelphia, PA 19103-2899. Customer Service Office: 11830 Westline Industrial Drive, St. Louis, MO 63146. Periodicals postage paid at New York, NY, and additional mailing offices. Subscription prices are $417.00 per year (US individuals), $711.00 per year (US institutions), $449.00 per year (Canadian individuals), $884.00 per year (Canadian institutions), $505.00 per year (international individuals), $884.00 per year (international institutions), $100.00 per year (US students), and $255.00 per year (international and Canadian students). International air speed delivery is included in all *Clinics* subscription prices. All prices are subject to change without notice. **POSTMASTER:** Send address changes to *Neurosurgery Clinics of North America*, Elsevier Periodicals Customer Service, 11830 Westline Industrial Drive, St. Louis, MO 63146. **Customer Service: 1-800-654-2452 (US and Canada). From outside the US and Canada, call: 1-314-453-7041. Fax: 1-314-453-5170. E-mail: JournalsCustomerService-usa@elsevier.com (for print support) and journalsonlinesupport-usa@elsevier.com (for online support).**

Reprints. For copies of 100 or more, of articles in this publication, please contact the Commercial Reprints Department, Elsevier Inc., 360 Park Avenue South, New York, NY 10010-1710. Tel. 212-633-3874; Fax: 212-633-3820; E-mail: reprints@elsevier.com.

Neurosurgery Clinics of North America is covered in *MEDLINE/PubMed (Index Medicus), EMBASE/Excerpta Medica, and Current Contents/Clinical Medicine (CC/CM).*

Contributors

CONSULTING EDITORS

RUSSELL R. LONSER, MD
Professor and Chair, Department of Neurological Surgery, The Ohio State University Wexner Medical Center, Columbus, Ohio, USA

DANIEL K. RESNICK, MD, MS
Professor and Vice Chairman, Program Director, Department of Neurosurgery, University of Wisconsin School of Medicine and Public Health, Madison, Wisconsin, USA

EDITOR

MICHAEL G. FEHLINGS, MD, PhD, FRCSC, FACS
Vice Chair Research, Professor of Neurosurgery, Department of Surgery, Krembil Research Institute, University of Toronto, Gerry and Tootsie Halbert Chair in Neural Repair and Regeneration, Toronto Western Hospital, University Health Network, Toronto, Ontario, Canada

AUTHORS

FAHAD H. ABDULJABBAR, MBBS, FRCSC
Spine Fellow, Department of Orthopedic Surgery, McGill University Health Centre, Montreal, Quebec, Canada; Teaching Assistant, Division of Orthopedics, Department of Surgery, Faculty of Medicine, King Abdulaziz University Hospital, Jeddah, Saudi Arabia

MASARU ABIKO, MD
Department of Neurosurgery, Graduate School of Biomedical & Health Sciences, Hiroshima University, Hiroshima City, Hiroshima, Japan

FARHANA AKTER, MBBS, BSc, MSc, MRCS
Department of Clinical Neurosciences, Ann McLaren Laboratory of Regenerative Medicine, University of Cambridge, Cambridge, United Kingdom

ELSA V. AROCHO-QUINONES, MD
Resident, Department of Neurosurgery, Medical College of Wisconsin, Milwaukee, Wisconsin, USA

JETAN H. BADHIWALA, MD
Division of Neurosurgery, Department of Surgery, St. Michael's Hospital, University of Toronto, Toronto, Ontario, Canada

RAKAN BOKHARI, MBBS
Neurosurgery Resident, Department of Neurology and Neurosurgery, McGill University Health Centre, Montreal, Quebec, Canada; Division of Neurosurgery, Department of Surgery, Faculty of Medicine, King Abdulaziz University, Jeddah, Saudi Arabia

AVERY L. BUCHHOLZ, MD, MPH
Department of Neurological Surgery, University of Virginia Health System, Charlottesville, Virginia, USA

MATTHEW D. BUDDE, PhD
Associate Professor, Department of Neurosurgery, Medical College of Wisconsin, Milwaukee, Wisconsin, USA

THOMAS J. BUELL, MD
Department of Neurological Surgery, University of Virginia Health System, Charlottesville, Virginia, USA

MICHAEL G. FEHLINGS, MD, PhD, FRCSC, FACS
Vice Chair Research, Professor of Neurosurgery, Department of Surgery, Krembil Research Institute, University of Toronto, Gerry and Tootsie Halbert Chair in Neural Repair and Regeneration, Toronto Western Hospital, University Health Network, Toronto, Ontario, Canada

MARIO GANAU, MD, PhD, FACS
Department of Neurosurgery, Toronto Western Hospital, University Health Network, Toronto, Ontario, Canada

ZOHER GHOGAWALA, MD, FACS
Chairman, Professor, Department of Neurosurgery, Alan and Jacqueline Stuart Spine Center, Lahey Hospital & Medical Center, Tufts University School of Medicine, Burlington, Massachusetts, USA

JOHN GILLICK, MD
Fellow, Spine Division, Department of Neurological Surgery, Jack and Vickie Farber Institute for Neuroscience, Thomas Jefferson University, Philadelphia, Pennsylvania, USA

JUNYA HANAKITA, MD
Spinal Disorders Center, Fujieda Heisei Memorial Hospital, Fujieda, Shizuoka, Japan

JAMES S. HARROP, MD, FACS
Head, Division of Spine and Peripheral Nerve Surgery, Department of Neurological Surgery, Jack and Vickie Farber Institute for Neuroscience, Department of Orthopedic Surgery, Thomas Jefferson University Hospitals, Philadelphia, Pennsylvania, USA

YOSHITAKA HIRANO, MD
Spine Section, Department of Neurosurgery, Southern TOHOKU Research Institute for Neuroscience, Koriyama, Fukushima, Japan

LANGSTON T. HOLLY, MD, FAANS
Department of Neurosurgery, Ronald Reagan UCLA Medical Center, Santa Monica, California, USA

RANDY K. IDLER, MSc
Graduate Entry Medicine, University College Cork, Cork, Ireland

YASUNOBU ITOH, MD, PhD
Department of Neurosurgery, Tokyo General Hospital, Nakano-ku, Tokyo, Japan

MARK KOTTER, MD, MPhil, PhD
Department of Clinical Neurosciences, Ann McLaren Laboratory of Regenerative Medicine, University of Cambridge, Cambridge, United Kingdom

IZUMI KOYANAGI, MD
Director, Department of Neurosurgery, Hokkaido Neurosurgical Memorial Hospital, Sapporo, Japan

MICHAEL KRYSHTALSKYJ
University of Toronto, Toronto, Ontario, Canada

KAORU KURISU, MD, PhD
Department of Neurosurgery, Graduate School of Biomedical and Health Sciences, Hiroshima University, Hiroshima City, Hiroshima, Japan

SHEKAR N. KURPAD, MD, PhD
Sanford J Larson Professor and Chairman, Department of Neurosurgery, Medical College of Wisconsin, Director, Spinal Cord Injury Center, Froedtert Hospital, Milwaukee, Wisconsin, USA

ALLAN R. MARTIN, MD, PhD
Resident, Division of Neurosurgery, Departments of Surgery and Neurosurgery, Toronto Western Hospital, University of Toronto, Toronto, Ontario, Canada

MANABU MINAMI, MD
Spinal Disorders Center, Fujieda Heisei Memorial Hospital, Fujieda, Shizuoka, Japan

TAKAFUMI MITSUHARA, MD, PhD
Department of Neurosurgery, Graduate School of Biomedical and Health Sciences, Hiroshima University, Hiroshima City, Hiroshima, Japan

JUNICHI MIZUNO, MD, PhD
Department of Neurological Surgery, Aichi Medical University, Aichi Prefecture, Aichi; Head, Center for Minimally Invasive Spinal Surgery, Departments of Neurosurgery and Spine and Peripheral Nerve Surgery, Shin-Yurigaoka General Hospital, Kawasaki, Kanagawa; Department of Neurosurgery, Southern TOHOKU General Hospital, Iwanuma, Miyagi, Japan

KENTARO NAITO, MD
Department of Neurosurgery, Osaka City University, Graduate School of Medicine, Osaka, Japan

YUKOH OHARA, MD
Department of Spine and Peripheral Nerve Surgery, Center for Minimally Invasive Spinal Surgery, Shin-Yurigaoka General Hospital, Kawasaki, Kanagawa, Japan

KENJI OHATA, MD
Department of Neurosurgery, Osaka City University, Graduate School of Medicine, Osaka, Japan

LISA M. PALUBISKI, MSc
Graduate Entry Medicine, University College Cork, Cork, Ireland

JOHN C. QUINN, MD
Department of Neurological Surgery, University of Virginia Health System, Charlottesville, Virginia, USA

GEORGE RYMARCZUK, MD
Fellow, Spine Division, Department of Neurological Surgery, Jack and Vickie Farber Institute for Neuroscience, Thomas Jefferson University, Philadelphia, Pennsylvania, USA

CARLO SANTAGUIDA, MD, FRCSC
Assistant Professor, Department of Neurology and Neurosurgery, McGill University Health Centre, Montreal, Quebec, Canada

CHRISTOPHER I. SHAFFREY, MD
Department of Neurological Surgery, University of Virginia Health System, Charlottesville, Virginia, USA

FABRICE SMIELIAUSKAS, PhD
Assistant Professor, Health Services Research, The University of Chicago, Chicago, Illinois, USA

JUSTIN S. SMITH, MD, PhD
Department of Neurological Surgery, University of Virginia Health System, Charlottesville, Virginia, USA

GEOFFREY STRICSEK, MD
Resident, Department of Neurological Surgery, Jack and Vickie Farber Institute for Neuroscience, Thomas Jefferson University, Philadelphia, Pennsylvania, USA

TAKU SUGAWARA, MD, PhD
Department of Spinal Surgery, Research Institute for Brain and Blood Vessels-Akita, Akita City, Japan

NOBUAKI TADOKORO, MD, PhD
Department of Orthopedic Surgery, Kochi University of Technology, Kochi Medical School, Nankoku, Japan; Division of Neurosurgery, Department of Surgery, Krembil Research Institute, University of Toronto, Toronto, Ontario, Canada

TOSHIYUKI TAKAHASHI, MD
Spinal Disorders Center, Fujieda Heisei Memorial Hospital, Fujieda, Shizuoka, Japan

TOSHIHIRO TAKAMI, MD
Department of Neurosurgery, Osaka City University, Graduate School of Medicine, Osaka, Japan

MASAAKI TAKEDA, MD, PhD
Department of Neurosurgery, Graduate School of Biomedical and Health Sciences, Hiroshima University, Hiroshima City, Hiroshima, Japan

ALISSON R. TELES, MD
Spine Fellow, Department of Clinical Neurosciences, Neurosurgery, University of Calgary, Calgary, Alberta, Canada

LINDSAY TETREAULT, PhD
Division of Neurosurgery, Department of Surgery, Krembil Research Institute, University of Toronto, Department of Neurosurgery, Toronto Western Hospital, Toronto, Ontario, Canada; Graduate Entry Medicine, University College Cork, Cork, Ireland

MASATO TOMII, MD
Department of Neurosurgery, Southern TOHOKU General Hospital, Iwanuma, Miyagi, Japan

MICHAEL WEBER, MD, FRCSC
Assistant Professor, Department of Orthopedic Surgery, McGill University Health Centre, Montreal, Quebec, Canada

JEFFERSON R. WILSON, MD, PhD
Division of Neurosurgery, Department of Surgery, St. Michael's Hospital, University of Toronto, Toronto, Ontario, Canada

CHRISTOPHER D. WITIW, MD, MS
Resident, Division of Neurosurgery, Department of Surgery, University of Toronto, Toronto Western Hospital, Toronto, Ontario, Canada

TORU YAMAGATA, MD
Department of Neurosurgery, Osaka City General Hospital, Osaka, Japan

SATOSHI YAMAGUCHI, MD, PhD
Department of Neurosurgery, Graduate School of Biomedical and Health Sciences, Hiroshima University, Hiroshima City, Hiroshima, Japan

Contents

Preface: Current Knowledge in Degenerative Cervical Myelopathy xiii

Michael G. Fehlings

Epidemiology and Overview of the Clinical Spectrum of Degenerative Cervical Myelopathy 1

Satoshi Yamaguchi, Takafumi Mitsuhara, Masaru Abiko, Masaaki Takeda, and Kaoru Kurisu

Degenerative cervical spondylosis (DCM) is an umbrella term used to describe myelopathy caused by various degenerative changes in the cervical spine. This article outlines the spectrum of DCM and reviews the epidemiology of each factor composing DCM. The uniform term of DCM is expected to elucidate the epidemiology of myelopathy caused by degenerative changes of the cervical spine.

Pathobiology of Degenerative Cervical Myelopathy 13

Farhana Akter and Mark Kotter

Degenerative cervical myelopathy (DCM) is a common spinal cord disease caused by chronic mechanical compression of the spinal cord. The mechanism by which mechanical stress results in spinal cord injury is poorly understood. The most common mechanisms involved in the pathobiology of DCM include apoptosis, inflammation, and vascular changes leading to loss of neurons, axonal degeneration, and myelin changes. However, the exact pathophysiologic mechanisms of DCM are unclear. A better understanding of the pathogenesis of DCM is required for the development of treatments to improve outcomes. This article highlights the mechanisms of injury and pathology in DCM.

The Natural History of Degenerative Cervical Myelopathy 21

Jetan H. Badhiwala and Jefferson R. Wilson

Although degenerative cervical myelopathy (DCM) is the leading cause of spinal cord dysfunction among adults worldwide, little is known about its natural history. There is mounting evidence of the effectiveness of surgery for DCM in halting progression of symptoms and, in fact, in improving neurologic outcomes, functional status, and quality of life. However, surgical decision making relies on a weighing of the risks and benefits of alternative strategies. The authors reviewed the available literature pertaining to the natural course of DCM and the predictors of outcome of nonoperative approaches.

Imaging Evaluation of Degenerative Cervical Myelopathy: Current State of the Art and Future Directions 33

Allan R. Martin, Nobuaki Tadokoro, Lindsay Tetreault, Elsa V. Arocho-Quinones, Matthew D. Budde, Shekar N. Kurpad, and Michael G. Fehlings

Degenerative cervical myelopathy (DCM) is a common neurologic condition that is often treated with surgery. Imaging plays a central role in the management of DCM, including diagnosis, preoperative planning, postoperative assessment, and prognostication. Radiographs, computed tomography, and MRI offer unique and complementary assessments, and all have important uses in current clinical practice.

Emerging microstructural and functional MRI techniques have the potential to have a major impact, potentially transforming practice by offering earlier and more accurate diagnosis, monitoring for deterioration, and prediction of outcomes. In the future, it can be expected that imaging will play an even greater role in DCM management.

Pathophysiology of Calcification and Ossification of the Ligamentum Flavum in the Cervical Spine **47**

Toshiyuki Takahashi, Junya Hanakita, and Manabu Minami

Calcification of the ligamentum flavum (CLF) and ossification of the ligamentum flavum (OLF) in the cervical spine are differential diagnoses in patients with posterior extradural compressive lesions related to cervical degenerative disease. Preoperative computed tomography can facilitate the detection of characteristic findings and help one to distinguish between CLF and OLF. Although these are rare entities in the cervical spine, adequately timed surgical decompression is required in most patients who present with radiculomyelopathy.

Radiologic Evaluation of Ossification of the Posterior Longitudinal Ligament with Dural Ossification **55**

Junichi Mizuno

There are 3 basic radiologic patterns of dural ossification (DO). Although double-layer DO is most common, when examining neuroimaging of ossification of the posterior longitudinal ligament (OPLL), isolated DO or masse DO should be kept in mind. Bone window computed tomography (CT) is most sufficient in identifying any type of DO associated with OPLL. Sagittal reformation of CT has replaced polytomography. MRI is not optimal for the identification of DO and OPLL. Surgical approaches should be determined based on this important radiologic information to avoid an unexpected complication. Expansive laminoplasty is the procedure of choice when DO is predominant.

Ossification of the Ligaments in the Cervical Spine, Including Ossification of the Anterior Longitudinal Ligament, Ossification of the Posterior Longitudinal Ligament, and Ossification of the Ligamentum Flavum **63**

Yukoh Ohara

Ossification of the posterior longitudinal ligament (OPLL), ossification of the anterior longitudinal ligament (OALL), and ossification of the ligamentum flavum (OLF) sometimes are seen in the same patients, but the exact coexisting frequencies are not clear, especially in the cervical region. The most frequent combination is OPLL and OALL. Cervical OPLL can coexist with thoracic OLF but is rarely associated with cervical OLF. All of these ossifying diseases of the cervical spinal ligaments are influenced by dynamic factors of the spinal column. The most frequent levels in the cervical spine affected by OPLL, OALL, and OLF are different because of anatomic differences inherent to each ligament.

Importance of Sagittal Alignment of the Cervical Spine in the Management of Degenerative Cervical Myelopathy **69**

Thomas J. Buell, Avery L. Buchholz, John C. Quinn, Christopher I. Shaffrey, and Justin S. Smith

Cervical spine sagittal malalignment correlates with worse symptoms and outcomes in patients with degenerative cervical myelopathy (DCM) and should influence surgical management. An anterior versus posterior surgical approach may not significantly change outcomes in patients with preoperative lordosis; however, most studies suggest improved neurologic recovery among kyphotic patients after adequate correction of local sagittal alignment through an anterior or combined anteroposterior approach. There are no comprehensive guidelines for DCM management in the setting of cervical malalignment; therefore, surgical management should be tailored to individual patients and decisions made at the discretion of treating surgeons with attention to basic principles.

Anterior Cervical Option to Manage Degenerative Cervical Myelopathy 83

Zoher Ghogawala

Degenerative cervical myelopathy (DCM) is the most common cause of spinal cord dysfunction in the world. There are multiple types of anterior approaches for treating patients with DCM. Many strategies have been developed to reduce complications for multilevel anterior surgery. Posterior approaches are sometimes used to supplement more extensive anterior approaches. More recently, multilevel cervical arthroplasty has been used for this condition. More data will be available soon comparing anterior and posterior approaches with the goal of optimizing patient-related quality of life and reducing complications, which include dysphagia, weakness, and instrumentation failure in some cases.

Laminectomy with or Without Fusion to Manage Degenerative Cervical Myelopathy 91

Fahad H. Abduljabbar, Alisson R. Teles, Rakan Bokhari, Michael Weber, and Carlo Santaguida

Stand-alone cervical laminectomy for degenerative cervical myelopathy (DCM) has become increasingly rare because of risk of postlaminectomy kyphosis. This article discusses the biomechanics of cervical degeneration and how laminectomy effects spine stability and summarizes relevant clinical studies to help guide surgical decision making for the posterior treatment of DCM. Laminectomy and fusion remains a safe and efficacious treatment. Stand-alone laminectomy should be used only for a highly selected patient population with relative stiff lordotic cervical spines, using care to not disrupt facets and C2 and C7 muscle attachments.

History and Evolution of Laminoplasty 107

Yoshitaka Hirano, Yukoh Ohara, Junichi Mizuno, and Yasunobu Itoh

Techniques of expansive laminoplasty for degenerative cervical myelopathy and ossified posterior longitudinal ligament are described, focusing on the history of the surgical procedure. Laminectomy was the only approach for posterior decompression before Japanese orthopedic surgeons introduced laminoplasty from the 1970s to the 1980s to overcome the poor outcomes of laminectomy. Recent laminoplasty techniques offer less invasive maneuvers to the posterior cervical muscle structures to reduce axial neck pain and to obtain better functional outcome, but every operation is carried out based on the unchanged initial concept. Some recent attempts to improve the surgical results are also discussed.

Significant Predictors of Outcome Following Surgery for the Treatment of Degenerative Cervical Myelopathy: A Systematic Review of the Literature 115

Lindsay Tetreault, Lisa M. Palubiski, Michael Kryshtalskyj, Randy K. Idler, Allan R. Martin, Mario Ganau, Jefferson R. Wilson, Mark Kotter, and Michael G. Fehlings

This systematic review aims to summarize important clinical predictors of outcomes in patients undergoing surgery for the treatment of degenerative cervical

with C3-4 ACDF patients. The radiologic study of C3-4 ACDF patients shows that they had significant cervical lordosis, and cervical motion was dependent on the C3-4 segment, which accounted for 39.8% of C2-7 range of intervertebral motion (total motion). In C3-4 ACDF patients, not only static factors but also dynamic factors (instability) at the C3-4 level contributed to the major causes of degenerative cervical myelopathy.

Intraoperative Neurophysiologic Monitoring for Degenerative Cervical Myelopathy **159**

Masaaki Takeda, Satoshi Yamaguchi, Takafumi Mitsuhara, Masaru Abiko, and Kaoru Kurisu

Multimodal intraoperative neurophysiologic monitoring is a reliable tool for detecting intraoperative spine injury and is recommended during surgery for degenerative cervical myopathy (DCM). Somatosensory evoked potential (SEP) can be used to monitor spine and peripheral nerve injury during positioning in surgery for DCM. Compensation technique for transcranial evoked muscle action potentials (tcMEPs) should be adopted in intraoperative monitoring during surgery for DCM. Free-running electromyography is a useful real-time monitoring add-on modality in addition to SEP and tcMEP.

Health Economics and the Management of Degenerative Cervical Myelopathy **169**

Christopher D. Witiw, Fabrice Smieliauskas, and Michael G. Fehlings

Degenerative cervical myelopathy (DCM) is the leading cause of spinal cord impairment worldwide. Surgical intervention has been demonstrated to be effective and is becoming standard of care. Spine surgery, however, is costly, and value needs to be demonstrated. This article serves to summarize the key health economic concepts as they relate to the assessment of the value of surgery for DCM. This is followed by a discussion of current health economic research on DCM, which suggests that surgery is likely to be cost-effective. The article concludes with a summary of future questions that remain unanswered, such as which patient subgroups derive the most value from surgery and which surgical approaches are the most cost-effective.

Managing the Complex Patient with Degenerative Cervical Myelopathy: How to Handle the Aging Spine, the Obese Patient, and Individuals with Medical Comorbidities **177**

Geoffrey Stricsek, John Gillick, George Rymarczuk, and James S. Harrop

Degenerative cervical myelopathy (DCM) is the most common cause of nontraumatic spinal cord injury worldwide. Even relatively mild impairment in functional scores can significantly affect daily activities. Surgery is an effective treatment for DCM, but outcomes are dependent on more than technique and preoperative neurologic deficits.

Future Directions and New Technologies for the Management of Degenerative Cervical Myelopathy **185**

Mario Ganau, Langston T. Holly, Junichi Mizuno, and Michael G. Fehlings

The diagnosis and treatment of degenerative cervical myelopathy (DCM) has been evolving over the past 5 decades as a result of collaborations between clinicians and scientists. The most recent trends in basic and clinical research include advances in imaging, clinical diagnostic tools, molecular genetics, surgical techniques, and reparative/regenerative strategies. Spine surgeons are witnessing a fast-paced evolution, which is reshaping the management strategies available for an aging population that suffers increasingly from this degenerative condition.

NEUROSURGERY CLINICS OF NORTH AMERICA

FORTHCOMING ISSUE

April 2018
Neurocritical Care
Alejandro A. Rabinstein, *Editor*

RECENT ISSUES

October 2017
Intraoperative Imaging
J. Bradley Elder and Ganesh Rao, *Editors*

July 2017
Controversies in Spinal and Cranial Surgery
Russell R. Lonser and Daniel K. Resnick, *Editors*

April 2017
Subdural Hematomas
E. Sander Connolly Jr and Guy M. McKhann II, *Editors*

RELATED INTEREST

Neuroimaging Clinics, May 2015 (Vol. 25, Issue 2)
Spinal Infections
E. Turgut Tali, *Editor*
Available at: http://www.neuroimaging.theclinics.com

THE CLINICS ARE AVAILABLE ONLINE!
Access your subscription at:
www.theclinics.com

Preface

Current Knowledge in Degenerative Cervical Myelopathy

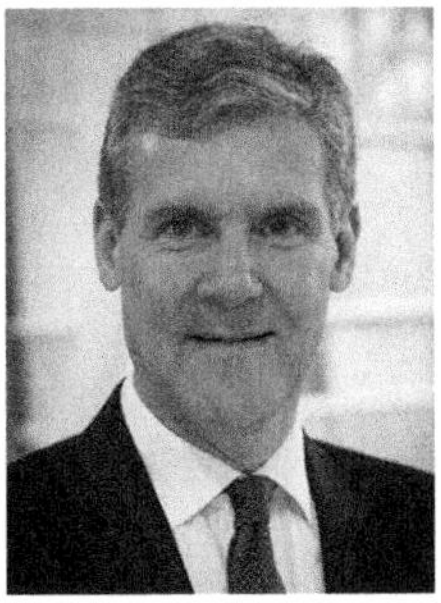

Michael G. Fehlings, MD, PhD, FRCSC
Editor

In 2015, my research group formally introduced the term *Degenerative Cervical Myelopathy* (DCM) to describe myelopathy caused by various degenerative changes in the cervical spine, including cervical spondylotic myelopathy and ossification of the posterior longitudinal ligament. DCM is the leading cause of spinal cord dysfunction in adults, resulting in motor and sensory dysfunction, and significantly affecting a patient's physical, psychological, and social well-being. The most common mechanisms involved in the pathobiology of DCM include apoptosis, inflammation, and vascular changes leading to loss of neurons, axonal degeneration, and myelin changes. The causes of DCM remain poorly understood, and the treatment of patients continues to be a significant health care challenge.

The multifactorial nature of DCM poses an inherent challenge to clinicians, as the diagnosis and prognosis for the disease can vary greatly depending on the patient. Furthermore, there remains a great deal of controversy regarding optimal management practices for DCM, especially when considering the use of surgical interventions. To address the knowledge gaps associated with DCM, I felt it was the perfect time to partner with *Neurosurgery Clinics of North America* and compile a special issue on the topic. This issue is meant to inform clinical practitioners and researchers on the current state of DCM care and research.

This DCM issue is a collection of 20 articles written by 46 researchers and surgeons with world-class expertise in the field. The compiled articles form three broad topic areas, which are meant to summarize current knowledge on the topic.

1. The first three articles describe the epidemiology, pathobiology, and natural history of DCM. A better understanding of the mechanisms of the disease builds the foundation for the following articles.
2. The focus then shifts to a discussion regarding the diagnosis of DCM. Here we explore the wide spectrum of causes of DCM and the specific tools and techniques used to diagnose patients, including radiographs, CT, and MR imaging.
3. Finally, the remaining twelve articles highlight the management of DCM in a variety of different scenarios dependent on disease severity and

neurosurgery.theclinics.com

Neurosurg Clin N Am 29 (2018) xiii–xiv
https://doi.org/10.1016/j.nec.2017.09.021
1042-3680/18/© 2017 Published by Elsevier Inc.

cause. There is mounting evidence regarding the effectiveness of surgery for DCM in halting the progression of symptoms; however, surgical decision making relies on a weighing of the risks and benefits of alternative strategies, which are thoroughly discussed here.

These articles complement work from the exciting field of DCM research, which has been very productive due to fruitful collaborations between researchers and clinicians. I have enjoyed serving as the editor for this issue, and it is my pleasure to share this work with you. I hope that the content compiled here will inform clinicians and lead to a deeper understanding of DCM, ultimately resulting in improved patient outcomes.

Michael G. Fehlings, MD, PhD, FRCSC
Department of Surgery
University of Toronto
Toronto Western Hospital
University Health Network
399 Bathurst Street
Toronto, Ontario M5T 2S8, Canada

E-mail address:
Michael.Fehlings@uhn.ca

Epidemiology and Overview of the Clinical Spectrum of Degenerative Cervical Myelopathy

Satoshi Yamaguchi, MD, PhD*,
Takafumi Mitsuhara, MD, PhD, Masaru Abiko, MD,
Masaaki Takeda, MD, PhD, Kaoru Kurisu, MD, PhD

KEYWORDS

• Myelopathy • Degeneration • Cervical spine • Spectrum • Epidemiology

KEY POINTS

- Compressive cervical myelopathy due to degeneration of the spine is a quite common disorder in adults, particularly in the elderly.
- The terminology to describe this condition has not been unified because degenerative pathologies arouse in the spine varies widely in each clinical case.
- This inconsistent terminology resulted in poor understanding of the epidemiology of this kind of myelopathy.
- Degenerative cervical myelopathy (DCM) has recently been proposed umbrella term to cover various myelopathic pathophysiologies caused by degeneration of the cervical spine.
- The novel term "DCM" is expected to elucidate the epidemiology of myelopathy caused by degenerative changes of the cervical spine.

INTRODUCTION

Cervical myelopathy stemming from degeneration of the cervical spine is a common cause of neurologic impairment in adults, particularly in the elderly. However, the epidemiology of this type of myelopathy has not been fully understood so far, probably due to inconsistent nomenclature. Degenerative cervical myelopathy (DCM) is a newly coined term to cover wide range of cervical degenerative pathologies causing myelopathy.[1] In this article, we outline this novel concept and its spectrum. Epidemiology of degenerative disorders related to DCM is also discussed.

DEGENERATIVE CERVICAL MYELOPATHY

Concept of Degenerative Cervical Myelopathy

"Degenerative cervical myelopathy" (DCM) is a recently proposed term to encompass compressive myelopathies caused by degenerative changes of the cervical spine.[1,2] Pathogeneses of DCM can be classified by the following conditions: cervical spondylotic myelopathy (CSM), nonosteoarthritic degeneration, and predisposing factors, such as congenital anomalies.[1] CSM is also an umbrella term used for various osteoarthritic changes causing cervical myelopathy. Nonosteoarthritic degeneration includes ligamentous pathologies that can be associated

Disclosure Statement: The authors have nothing to disclose regarding this article.
Department of Neurosurgery, Hiroshima University Graduate School of Biomedical and Health Sciences, Hiroshima City, Hiroshima, Japan
* Corresponding author. 1-2-3, Kasumi, Minami-ku, Hiroshima City, Hiroshima 7348551, Japan.
E-mail address: satjp02@gmail.com

Neurosurg Clin N Am 29 (2018) 1–12
https://doi.org/10.1016/j.nec.2017.09.001
1042-3680/18/© 2017 Elsevier Inc. All rights reserved.

with myelopathy. Representative congenital anomalies predisposing the patients to myelopathy are congenital canal stenosis, Down syndrome, and Klippel-Feil syndrome. To understand the concept of DCM, it might be easy to imagine a small umbrella of CSM is covered by a big umbrella of DCM. The big umbrella also comprises various pathogeneses such as nonosteoarthritic degeneration, congenital anomalies, and other predisposing factors (**Fig. 1**). Because DCM is a newly coined term, its epidemiology has scarcely been elucidated.[2] Nouri and colleagues[3] reviewed MR images of 458 patients with DCM and found that cervical spondylosis was most frequent cause of DCM with a frequency of 89.7%. Nearly 60% of spondylosis was accompanied by hypertrophy or enlargement of the ligamentum flavum (LF). Each of single-level discopathy, ossification of the posterior longitudinal ligament (OPLL), and spondylolisthesis had a prevalence with approximately 10%. More than 90% of OPLL was accompanied with spondylotic changes. Klippel-Feil syndrome was found in 2.0%. Multiple pathogeneses coexisted frequently in single cervical spine. These lesions might be found in the same spinal level or might be found in different spinal levels (**Fig. 2**).

Why Do We Need a Comprehensive Term?

Degenerative changes are theoretically possible to arise anywhere in the cervical spine because 7 vertebrae and intervertebral discs are continuously moving in a human's life. Even in a single vertebra, the spinal cord is surrounded by many components: the intervertebral disc, vertebral body, uncinated processes, facet joints, neural arch (lamina), posterior longitudinal ligament (PLL), and LF. Degenerative pathologies arose in any components of the vertebra may cause compressive myelopathy and such pathologies may arise in a single level or may coexist in multiple segments. Under the existence of multiple pathologies compressing the cervical cord in different spinal levels, it is often difficult to specify the lesion responsible for myelopathy. The responsible lesion may not always be single. In considerable numbers of the cases, the multiplicity of the responsible lesions makes the pathophysiology complicated.

When a physician sees a myelopathic patient with radiological evidence of multiple cervical spondylotic changes, there are several ways to describe this condition. From the semiologic perspective, you can describe the patient simply as cervical myelopathy. When the protruded disc seems to be the responsible lesion, the

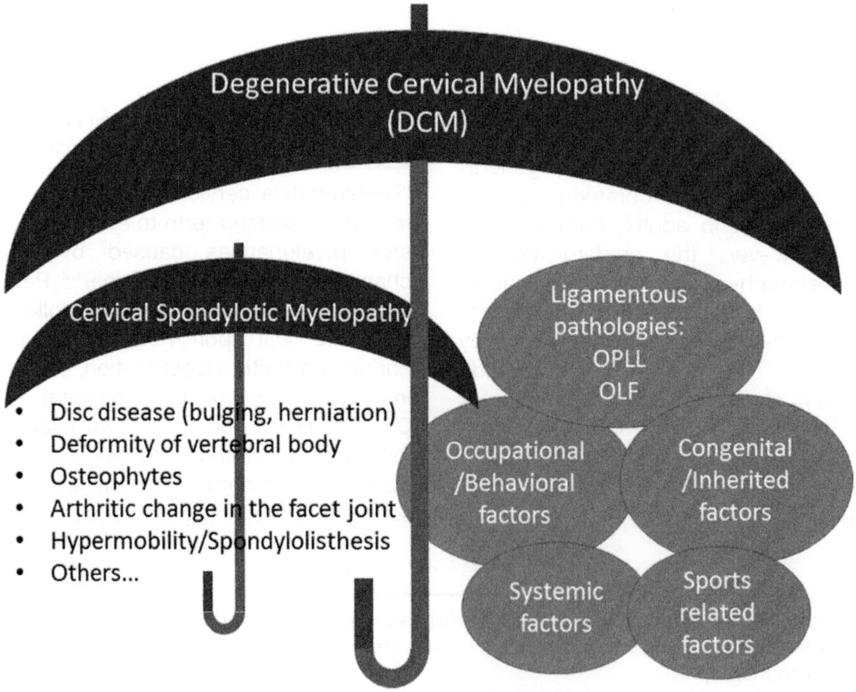

Fig. 1. Schematic drawing indicating the concept of DCM. The large umbrella of DCM covers its predisposing factors. The small umbrella of CSM is comprising various degenerative pathologies that arise in the cervical spine.

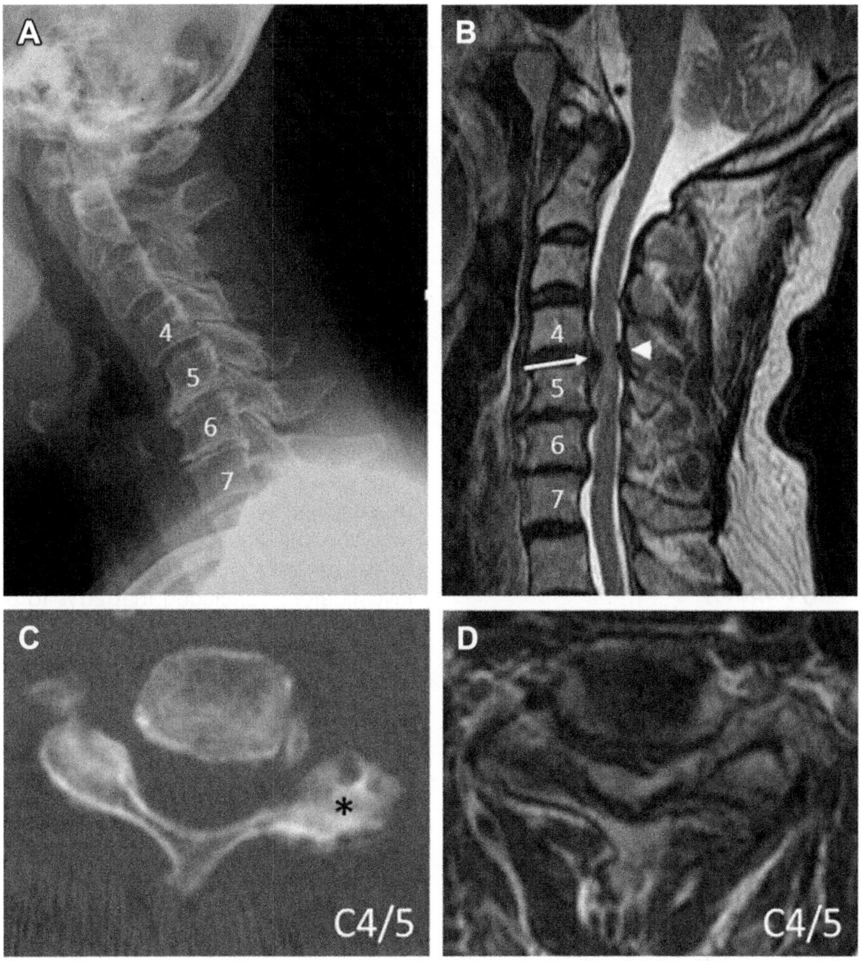

Fig. 2. An illustrative case of multiple pathogeneses found in single cervical column. This 81-year-old patient presented with progressive clumsiness and gait disturbance. (*A*) Lateral radiograph of the cervical spine in flexion posture showing slight anterior slippage of C4 vertebral body. Segments of C5/6 and C6/7 are rigid due to severe osteoarthritic changes. (*B*) Sagittal T2-weighted MRI showing the spinal cord is compressed at the C4/5 level. The cervical cord is compressed from the ventral side by a complex lesion of disc bulging and hypertrophic PLL (*arrow*). Enlarged LF is also compressing the spinal cord from the back side (*arrowhead*). (*C*) Axial CT image at C4/5 level showing hypertrophy of the right facet joint (*) due to severe osteoarthritic change. (*D*) Axial T2-weighted MRI showing circumferential compression of the spinal cord by multiple degenerative pathologies.

radiological diagnosis would be cervical disc herniation. If you can see some additional pathologies such as osteophytes and spondylolisthesis, the expression would be more comprehensive, like CSM. This kind of inconsistency would confuse not only the medical staff but also the patients. A uniform diagnostic term referring to a myelopathy caused by degenerative changes of the cervical spine would be practically significant.[1,4] Even in CSM, which is quite common among the general population, the exact epidemiology has not been established, probably due to inconsistent nomenclature. A uniform term would be useful from epidemiologic perspective.[5,6] In this regard, Nouri and colleagues[1] proposed a term "degenerative cervical myelopathy" (DCM), to comprise degenerative changes of the spine and predisposing factors.[4]

The Epidemiology of Degenerative Cervical Myelopathy

As is mentioned previously, DCM is a newly coined term in the field of spinal surgery and its epidemiology has not been elucidated. Therefore, we review the epidemiology of each component of DCM as follows: (1) cervical spondylosis and CSM; (2) ligamentous pathologies including OPLL and ossification of the LF (OLF); and (3) other predisposing factors: the occupation, congenital anomalies, and so forth. There might be debate if OPLL should be included in a spectrum of DCM because OPLL might not be purely a degenerative change. OPLL can be symptomatic at younger age and has been reported to be associated with genetic background, environmental factors, and the interaction with systemic pathologic condition, such as obesity and diabetes mellitus.[7,8] OPLL is distinct from other cervical degenerative disorders in that the ossification may progress unless it is surgically resected.[9] In this article, the authors take a position to support the original article regarding DCM that OPLL and OLF were included into the umbrella of DCM.[1]

THE EPIDEMIOLOGY OF DISORDERS RELATED TO DEGENERATIVE CERVICAL MYELOPATHY

Cervical Spondylosis and Cervical Spondylotic Myelopathy

The definition

Cervical spondylosis, or cervical osteoarthritis (OA), is an umbrella term to comprise various osteoarthritic changes arising in the cervical spine. CSM is defined as a myelopathy due to compression of the spinal cord by cervical spondylotic pathogeneses, and it is a common cause of spinal dysfunction usually seen in the elderly.[5,10–12] OA changes of the spine can be described as various radiological findings: disc bulging, disc herniations, loss of vertebral body height, osteophyte, arthritic change of the facet joint, and hypermobility/listhesis of the vertebral segment.[1,4,6] With regard to the terminology, we should differentiate the following words: cervical spondylosis and CSM. Cervical spondylosis (CS) is a condition showing deformities in the spinal column mainly due to the aging process. CS itself might be associated with cervical pain but it is neurologically asymptomatic. It is not until these structural changes compress the spinal cord that CS may cause myelopathy. CSM is a clinical symptomatic entity indicating myelopathy caused by CS.

The cascade of degenerative changes in the cervical spine

The cascade of spondylotic changes always starts from a degeneration of the intervertebral discs. Repetitive cervical motions in daily life make the nucleus pulposus dehydrated, fragmented, and finally collapsed. Degeneration of the disc will augment mechanical stress on the endplates of the adjacent vertebral bodies. The mechanical stress induces reactive bony changes, such as osteophytes, hypertrophic bone remodeling of the uncinated processes and facet joints, and enlargement of the PLL and LF. These reactive changes are originally intended to stabilize affected vertebral segment(s); however, such circumferential deformity may result in compression of the cervical cord (**Fig. 3**).[10,13–16] As are seen in the joints of other parts of the body, osteoarthritic changes of the cervical spine are common in the elderly population because of their aging process-related nature.[5,10,17] In a study examining 120 cervical spines removed from necropsy, osteoarthritis of the apophysial joints was seen in 65% of the specimens.[18] Moon and colleagues[19] investigated 460 radiograms of the cervical spine. The percentile incidences of CS in the seventh and eighth decades were 58.8% and 70.3%, respectively. However, it should be reminded that only a minority of patients with CS present with symptomatic myelopathy.[6,13] Karadimas and colleagues[20] systematically reviewed articles regarding natural history of CSM. The investigators concluded that 20% to 60% of patients showed neurologic decline over time without surgical intervention; however, the patterns of progression varied widely among the patients: some presented with steadily progressive neurologic symptoms, whereas others showed stepwise deterioration with interposed quiescent periods.[13,21]

Pathophysiology of cervical spondylotic myelopathy

The pathophysiology of CSM is multifactorial. Two major factors are static and dynamic insult on the spinal cord (**Fig. 4**). Static factor is persistent compression on the spinal cord by OA changes. From the ventral side, the spinal cord is compressed by degenerative discs (bulging or herniations), osteophytes, and hypertrophic PLL. From the dorsal side, hypertrophic facet joint(s) and enlarged LF are offending components to the spinal cord. When mechanical stresses surpass stabilization effect by spondylotic changes, the relevant spinal segment becomes unstable and hypermobile. Increased range of motion acts as a dynamic factor for the deterioration of myelopathy. Repetitive insult on the cord with spondylotic changes and buckling of the LF in flexion/extension motion may result in symptomatic myelopathy.[22] Circulatory disturbance is another factor of the pathophysiology of CSM. Microvasculopathy caused by repetitive compression of the spinal cord will result in irreversible ischemic changes, such as neuronal loss of the gray matter and demyelination of the white matter.[20,22–24]

Although the precise molecular mechanism contributing to the pathogenesis of CSM is incompletely understood, the pathophysiological

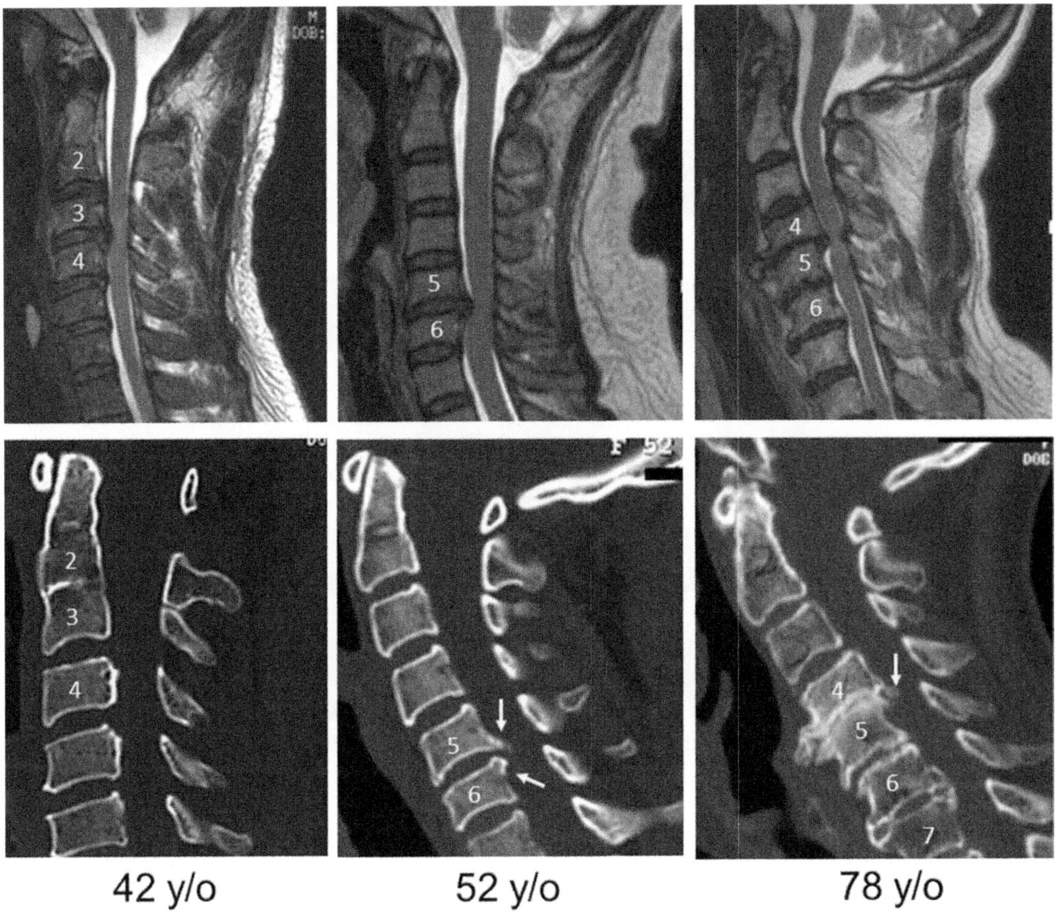

Fig. 3. Sagittal T2-weighted MRIs (*upper row*) and sagittal CT images (*lower row*) obtained from 3 different generations. Although all patients had cervical myelopathy due to segmental cervical canal stenosis, the compressive components are different from each other. In a 42-year-old patient (*left column*), disc bulging without osteophyte is the offending lesion. Congenital fusion of C2-3 might have affected the degenerative process of the C3/4 disc. In a 52-year-old patient (*center column*), disc bulging is accompanied with osteophyte formation (*arrows*). This complex lesion is compressing the cervical cord. In an elderly patient aged 78 years, the cervical cord is compressed at C4/5 level with osteophytes and a partially ossified PLL (*white arrow*). The intervertebral disc is almost collapsed. These examples illustrate well the chronologic steps of the degenerative cascade of the cervical spine.

phenomena triggered by the static and dynamic damages to the cervical cord have gradually been elucidated in experimental CSM models. Disruption of microvasculature leads to 2 pathologic conditions: reduction of the number of endothelial cells and inflammatory reaction. They may contribute synergically to the progression of the neurodegeneration of cervical myelopathy. Apoptosis in neuronal and oligodendroglial cells has been associated with the development of CSM as well. Axonal degeneration of the corticospinal tract distant from the site of injury can be explained by the ongoing oligodendrocytic apoptosis.[25,26] Even decompression surgery that is widely accepted as the gold standard treatment for CSM might be associated with neurologic decline. According to the study using a mouse compressive myelopathy model, decompression procedure was associated with reperfusion neural injury mediated by oxidative DNA damage in the ischemic cord. This reperfusion-related damage might be a molecular target to prevent postoperative neurologic decline in patients undergoing surgical treatment.[27,28]

The incidence and prevalence of cervical spondylotic myelopathy

The exact incidence and prevalence of CSM have been unclarified. There have been several articles reporting annual incidence of the CSM-related surgery and hospitalization. Kokubun and colleagues[29] surveyed surgical cases for CSM in a Japanese

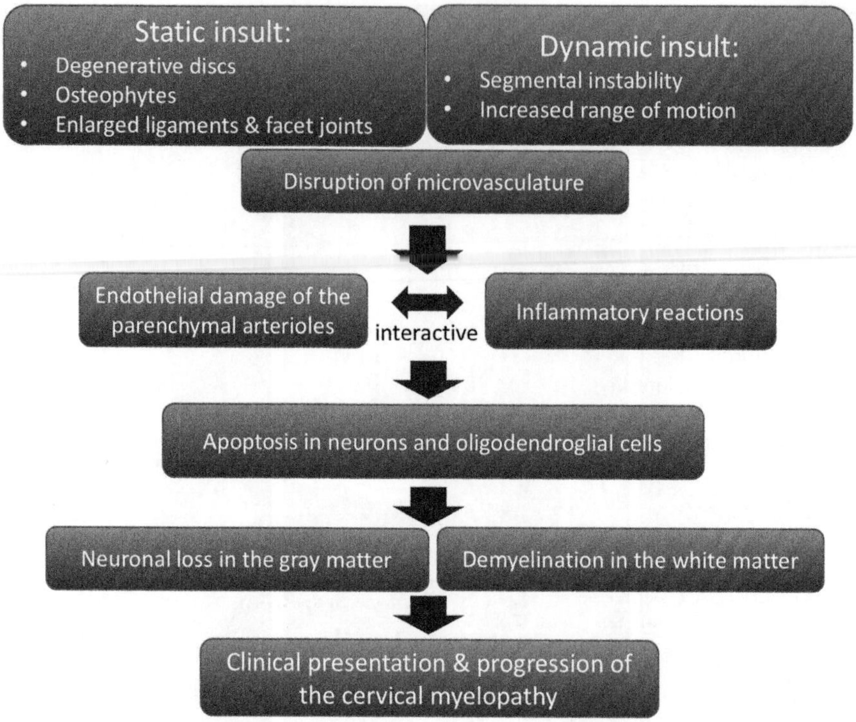

Fig. 4. A schematic drawing indicating the cascade of pathobiology of cervical spondylotic myelopathy.

northeastern prefecture that has a population of 2.26 million. The annual incidence of the cases operated on CSM was 5.7 per 100,000 residents. Boogaarts and Bartels[5] conducted a meta-analysis trying to elucidate the incidence and prevalence of CSM. However, they could not establish exact incidence and prevalence of CSM despite extensive review. Instead, they estimated annual incidence of surgical treatment for CSM with a rate of 1.6 per 100,000 inhabitants in the authors' referral region. Wu and colleagues[21] studied population-based epidemiologic investigation of CSM using a 12-year database of National Health Insurance Research in Taiwan. They showed the incidence of CSM-caused hospitalization was 4.04 per 100,000 person-years. Nouri and colleagues[1] estimated the incidence and prevalence by considering CSM to be a kind of nontraumatic form of spinal cord injury. With the provided rate of degenerative spinal diseases in all nontraumatic spinal cord injuries, they estimated the incidence and prevalence of DCM in the North American region are at a minimum of 41 and 605 per million, respectively.

Degenerative cervical spondylolisthesis

Degenerative spondylolisthesis is a pathologic condition that a vertebra translates anteriorly or posteriorly to the vertebra below. In flexion position, the spinal cord is compressed from the ventral side by the postero-superior edge of the lower adjacent vertebral body. In extension position, the dorsal side of the spinal cord might be compressed by the buckling of enlarged LF.[30–32] Although the incidence and prevalence of degenerative cervical spondylolisthesis (DCSL) still remain unclear, the distribution of the affected spinal segment has been reported in several articles. Jiang and colleagues[32] systematically reviewed the articles regarding DCSL. Among 102 patients, C4/5 (49.4%) was the most frequently affected site, followed by C3/4 (46%). Koakutsu and colleagues[30] examined radiographs obtained from the patients operated for cervical myelopathy. C4/5 and C3/4 slippage were found as a symptomatic level in 73% and 27% of the cases, respectively. Suzuki and colleagues[33] studied the prevalence of cervical spondylolisthesis in patients with neck pain or radiculopathy using upright cervical kinetic MR images. Grade 1 with 2 to 3-mm slippage of the vertebral body and grade 2 with more than 3 mm of slippage were observed with a prevalence of 16.4% and 3.4% of all patients, respectively. The most prevalent levels were C4/5 and C5/6. These results showed that DCSL tended to be found mainly in C3/4 and C4/5. This tendency is probably because DCSL arises secondarily after the primary cervical spondylotic changes of lower cervical spine.

Ligamentous Pathologies

Ossification of the posterior longitudinal ligament

OPLL is a ligamentous disorder characterized by an ectopic bone formation in the PLL and it is a well-known pathogenic factor of cervical myelopathy.[34,35] Presentation of myelopathy in patients with cervical OPLL is induced by static factors, dynamic factors, or a combination of both. A static factor is a space-occupying effect of the ossified ligament on the spinal cord. When a certain spinal segment becomes rigid by OPLL bridging vertebral bodies, the adjacent spinal segments would compensate the range of motion of the cervical spine. Such a hypermobile segment can be a dynamic factor causing myelopathy.[36] Matsunaga and colleagues[37] prospectively studied a cohort of 450 patients with OPLL. During a mean follow-up term with 17.6 years, 146 patients (32.4%) were surgically treated for OPLL. Among 323 patients without myelopathy at the first examination, 55 patients (17%) developed myelopathy during the follow-up period. Risk factors of the evolution of myelopathy were higher space-occupying ratio of ossified ligament in the spinal canal (>60%) and increased range of motion. These results support the idea that not only the static factor but dynamic factor is significantly associated with the presentation of myelopathy in patients with OPLL. Japanese orthopedic doctors have played a leading role in the epidemiologic study of OPLL. According to the review studies by Matsunaga and Sakou,[7] the prevalence of OPLL in the general Japanese population was 1.9% to 4.3% among the population older than 30 years. Radiograph-based surveys in Asian countries reported that the prevalence of OPLL in Korea, Taiwan, Philippines, and Singapore were 0.6%, 2.1% to 3.0%, 1.5%, and 0.8%, respectively.[7,38–44] In Western countries, those rates of the United States, West Germany, and Italy were 0.1% to 1.3%, 0.1%, and 1.7%, respectively.[45–49] A computed tomography (CT)-based survey by Fujimori and colleagues[50] reported higher prevalence of cervical OPLL than those of radiograph-based studies. In the San Francisco area, overall prevalence of cervical OPLL was 2.2%. The rates of ethnicity-based prevalence were 1.3% in Caucasian Americans, 4.8% in Asian Americans, 1.9% in Hispanic Americans, 2.1% in African Americans, and 3.2% in Native Americans. Asian Americans had significantly higher prevalence of cervical OPLL than Caucasian Americans. Ossified ligaments might be found in other spinal segments in patients with cervical OPLL. According to CT-based studies, OLF was found in 56.2% to 64.6% of the patients with cervical OPLL, mainly in the thoracic spine.[34,35]

Ossification of the ligamentum flavum

OLF in the cervical spine is rarely identified compared with its thoracic counterpart and its pathogenesis and epidemiology have not been established.[51] Guo and colleagues[52] evaluated whole spinal MR images obtained from 1736 southern Chinese volunteers. OLF was identified in 66 (3.8%) and only 4 individuals (0.2%) had cervical OLFs. Al-Jarallah and colleagues[53] surveyed the prevalence of OLF on MR images obtained from 102 individuals of the Arab population in Kuwait. They identified a total of 26 segments of OLF and reported that the prevalence of OLF was 18.6% in the sample population. Among all OLFs, 57.7% of OLFs were found in the cervical spine.

Other Predisposing Factors to Degeneration of the Cervical Spine

Occupational, behavioral, congenital/inherited, systemic, and sports-related factors have been associated with degeneration of the cervical spine.[10,54,55]

Occupational and behavioral factors

Mahbub and colleagues[56] surveyed the prevalence of CS using cervical spine radiographs obtained from 98 coolies in a city of Bangladesh. The result showed a considerably higher prevalence of CS with a rate of 39.8% in coolies even though more than half of the subjects were relatively young at younger than 40 years. Higher prevalence of spondylosis was significantly associated with longer duration of the occupation. Petren-Mallmin and Linder[57] compared cervical MR images taken at 5-year interval from asymptomatic young military high-performance aircraft pilots and a middle-aged control group without pilot experience. A significant reduction in the signal intensity of the intervertebral discs was observed in young pilots. The result suggested increased risk of premature degeneration of the intervertebral discs in young military pilots. In coolies and aircraft pilots, repetitive stress and/or heavy loads on the neck were considered predisposing factors to premature degeneration of their cervical spine.[56,57] Involuntary movement disorders, such as cervical dystonia, athetoid cerebral palsy, and torticollis, have been raised as a predisposing factor to premature CS. Osteoarthritic changes in patients with involuntary movements are different from those of the healthy population. Flexion/extension stress in the healthy population is likely to cause spondylosis at the C5/6 level, whereas in patients with involuntary movement disorders, mechanical stress by lateral bending and axial rotation is likely to cause degeneration at the C3/4 and C4/5 levels.[58,59]

Congenital and inherited factors

Congenital disorders such as congenital cervical stenosis (CCS), Klippel-Fiel syndrome (KFS), and Down syndrome have been associated with the predisposing factor to CS.[60–62] CCS is a disorder showing inherently narrow spinal canal without osteoarthritic change. CCS has lower neural arch and flat-shaped spinal canal in the axial plane and it can be morphometrically defined by several parameters.[62] Pavlov and colleagues[63] proposed the ratio known as the Torg-Pavlov method: CCS is indicated when the ratio of the sagittal diameter of the cervical canal to that the corresponding vertebral body is less than 0.8. According to Bajwa and colleagues,[64] sagittal canal diameter less than 13 mm and interpedicular distance less than 23 mm are strongly correlated with CCS. Narrow spinal canal directly means a reduction of the space available for the cord, and is considered as a predisposing factor to the development of myelopathy and spinal cord injury.[65,66] With regard to the prevalence of CCS, a skeletal specimen–based study indicated that cervical stenosis was present in 4.9% of the adult population.[67] Jenkins and colleagues[62] studied 1000 cervical MRIs and reported overall prevalence of CCS with 6.8%.

Down syndrome has been associated with the predisposing factor to CSM. Atlantoaxial subluxation due to the laxity of the transverse ligament and hypoplasia of the neural arch of the atlas may result in cervical myelopathy in patients with Down syndrome.[68,69] KFS is characterized by congenital cervical fusion and this syndrome has been raised as a predisposing factor to cervical myelopathy. Spondylotic change and compensatory hypermobility in the segment adjacent to the fused vertebrae tend to cause spinal cord compression and resultant myelopathy.[1,70] The prevalence of congenital cervical fusion (CCF), including KFS, in the general population has been estimated at 0.71%.[11] Among a global cohort of patients with cervical myelopathy, the prevalence of CCF was reported to be 3.9%.[70] Increased risk of disc degeneration was suggested in patients with generalized joint laxity including Ehlers-Danlos syndrome.[60] Besides the previously mentioned syndromes, McKay and colleagues[68] raised the following genetic syndromes as a predisposing factor to spinal instability and/or cervical stenosis: Larsen syndrome, 22q11.2 deletion syndrome, pseudoachondroplasia, Morquio syndrome, Goldenhar syndrome, spondyloepiphyseal dysplasia congenita, Kniest dysplasia, and the chin-on-chest deformity of fibrodysplasia ossificans progressive.

Systemic factors

Spondylosis in a different spinal region may act as a predisposing factor to degenerative change in the cervical spine. Okada and colleagues[71] studied an association between the progression of cervical disc degeneration and that of lumbar disc degeneration by evaluating MRIs of the patients with lumbar disc herniation and healthy volunteers. The prevalence of cervical disc degeneration was significantly higher in the lumbar disc herniation group compared with the control (98% vs 88.5%). Schairer and colleagues[72] conducted a retrospective cohort study to assess the concomitance of CS and thoracolumbar spinal deformity on the database obtained from 47,560 patients. The prevalence of CS in patients with thoracolumbar spinal deformity was significantly higher than overall patients (31.0% vs 13.1%). The presence of musculoskeletal disorder outside of the spine has also been associated with higher risk of CS. Radcliff and colleagues[73] conducted a prospective case-control study to compare the incidence of undiagnosed cervical myelopathy in patients with hip fractures and age-matched controls who underwent total hip arthroplasty. The incidence of myelopathy was significantly higher in patients with hip fracture (18%) than in the control group (0%). Sonnesen and colleagues[74] compared osseous changes in the upper cervical spine between patients with and without osteoarthriticlike changes in the temporomandibular joint with obstructive sleep apnea. Cervical spondylotic changes were found more frequently in patients with temporomandibular joint disorders than without those disorders. The investigators suggested a possible biomechanical relationship between the temporomandibular joint and upper cervical spine.

Sports-related factors

Elite athletes of American football have been associated with increased incidence of cervical disc disease.[75] In contact sports like American football, the cervical spine is susceptible not only to overuse injuries but also to direct axial loading impact, especially in flexion/extension posture. These repetitive minor and occasional strong impacts on the cervical spine promote osteoarthritic and ligamentous degeneration and may promote spondylosis.[76] The presence of degenerative changes and resultant spinal canal stenosis has been associated with the risk of cervical cord injury.[77–80] Jonasson and colleagues[81] conducted a survey using a questionnaire regarding the frequency of joint pain in 75 male athletes. The athletes included divers, weight-lifters, wrestlers, orienteers, and ice-hockey players. The annual frequency of cervical pain during the reference week and year was 35% and 55%, respectively. Athletes reporting the highest frequency of the cervical pain were wrestlers and ice-hockey players. Villavicencio and colleagues[82] studied the incidence of cervical pain in triathletes. The lifetime incidence of neck pain was 48.3%, and 21.4% of the pain was related to intervertebral disc involvement. Neck pain and the number of previous sports-related injuries were strongly correlated. A strong tendency toward neck pain was observed in athletes with overuse injuries. It may be concluded that contact sports players and certain elite athletes may be predisposed to degeneration of the cervical spine. However, it is still unclear that these specific populations are actually prone to present with cervical myelopathy in the future.

SUMMARY

DCM is an umbrella term to describe myelopathy caused by various degenerative changes in the cervical spine. The authors outlined the spectrum of DCM and reviewed the epidemiology of each factor composing DCM. The epidemiology of DCM might be close to that of CSM because 90% of DCM is derived from cervical spondylosis; however, the epidemiology of CSM itself has not been fully understood. OPLL is also a common predisposing factor of DCM. The prevalence of OPLL varies widely among the regions and human races. Premature spondylosis is associated with some specific occupations, such as coolies and fighter aircraft pilots. Involuntary movement disorders involving the neck might accelerate degenerative process of the cervical spine. Congenital syndromes are also factors to predispose the patients to early onset of spinal osteoarthritic changes. Congenital canal stenosis, KFS, and Down syndrome have been associated with CS. Systemic factors like concomitant thoracolumbar spondylosis and sports-related factors in elite athletes have also been raised as predisposing factors for CS. The uniform term of DCM is expected to elucidate the epidemiology of myelopathy caused by degenerative changes of the cervical spine.

REFERENCES

1. Nouri A, Tetreault L, Singh A, et al. Degenerative cervical myelopathy: epidemiology, genetics, and pathogenesis. Spine (Phila Pa 1976) 2015;40(12): E675–93.
2. Davies BM, McHugh M, Elgheriani A, et al. The reporting of study and population characteristics in degenerative cervical myelopathy: a systematic review. PLoS One 2017;12(3):e0172564.
3. Nouri A, Martin A, Tetreault L, et al. MRI analysis of the combined prospectively collected AOSpine North America and International Data: the prevalence and spectrum of pathologies in a global cohort of patients with degenerative cervical myelopathy. Spine (Phila Pa 1976) 2017;42(14): 1058–67.
4. Tetreault L, Goldstein CL, Arnold P, et al. Degenerative cervical myelopathy: a spectrum of related disorders affecting the aging spine. Neurosurgery 2015;77(Suppl 4):S51–67.
5. Boogaarts HD, Bartels RH. Prevalence of cervical spondylotic myelopathy. Eur Spine J 2015; 24(Suppl 2):139–41.
6. Fehlings MG, Tetreault LA, Wilson JR, et al. Cervical spondylotic myelopathy: current state of the art and future directions. Spine (Phila Pa 1976) 2013; 38(22 Suppl 1):S1–8.
7. Matsunaga S, Sakou T. Ossification of the posterior longitudinal ligament of the cervical spine: etiology and natural history. Spine (Phila Pa 1976) 2012; 37(5):E309–14.
8. Stetler WR, La Marca F, Park P. The genetics of ossification of the posterior longitudinal ligament. Neurosurg Focus 2011;30(3):E7.
9. Xing D, Wang J, Ma JX, et al. Qualitative evidence from a systematic review of prognostic predictors for surgical outcomes following cervical ossification of the posterior longitudinal ligament. J Clin Neurosci 2013;20(5):625–33.
10. Baron EM, Young WF. Cervical spondylotic myelopathy: a brief review of its pathophysiology, clinical course, and diagnosis. Neurosurgery 2007; 60(1 Supp1 1):S35–41.
11. Brown MW, Templeton AW, Hodges FJ 3rd. The incidence of acquired and congenital fusions in the cervical spine. Am J Roentgenol Radium Ther Nucl Med 1964;92:1255–9.
12. Northover JR, Wild JB, Braybrooke J, et al. The epidemiology of cervical spondylotic myelopathy. Skeletal Radiol 2012;41(12):1543–6.
13. Joaquim AF, Ghizoni E, Tedeschi H, et al. Management of degenerative cervical myelopathy: an update. Rev Assoc Med Bras (1992) 2016;62(9): 886–94.
14. Kumaresan S, Yoganandan N, Pintar FA, et al. Contribution of disc degeneration to osteophyte formation in the cervical spine: a biomechanical investigation. J Orthop Res 2001;19(5):977–84.
15. Mattei TA, Goulart CR, Milano JB, et al. Cervical spondylotic myelopathy: pathophysiology, diagnosis,

and surgical techniques. ISRN Neurol 2011;2011: 463729.
16. Miyazaki M, Hong SW, Yoon SH, et al. Kinematic analysis of the relationship between the grade of disc degeneration and motion unit of the cervical spine. Spine (Phila Pa 1976) 2008;33(2):187–93.
17. Shedid D, Benzel EC. Cervical spondylosis anatomy: pathophysiology and biomechanics. Neurosurgery 2007;60(1 Supp1 1):S7–13.
18. Holt S, Yates PO. Cervical spondylosis and nerve root lesions. Incidence at routine necropsy. J Bone Joint Surg Br 1966;48(3):407–23.
19. Moon MS, Yoon MG, Park BK, et al. Age-related incidence of cervical spondylosis in residents of Jeju Island. Asian Spine J 2016;10(5):857–68.
20. Karadimas SK, Erwin WM, Ely CG, et al. Pathophysiology and natural history of cervical spondylotic myelopathy. Spine (Phila Pa 1976) 2013;38(22 Suppl 1):S21–36.
21. Wu JC, Ko CC, Yen YS, et al. Epidemiology of cervical spondylotic myelopathy and its risk of causing spinal cord injury: a national cohort study. Neurosurg Focus 2013;35(1):E10.
22. Lebl DR, Hughes A, Cammisa FP Jr, et al. Cervical spondylotic myelopathy: pathophysiology, clinical presentation, and treatment. HSS J 2011;7(2):170–8.
23. Mizuno J, Nakagawa H, Inoue T, et al. Clinicopathological study of "snake-eye appearance" in compressive myelopathy of the cervical spinal cord. J Neurosurg 2003;99(2 Suppl):162–8.
24. Mizuno J, Nakagawa H, Chang HS, et al. Postmortem study of the spinal cord showing snake-eyes appearance due to damage by ossification of the posterior longitudinal ligament and kyphotic deformity. Spinal Cord 2005;43(8):503–7.
25. Karadimas SK, Gatzounis G, Fehlings MG. Pathobiology of cervical spondylotic myelopathy. Eur Spine J 2015;24(Suppl 2):132–8.
26. Yu WR, Liu T, Kiehl TR, et al. Human neuropathological and animal model evidence supporting a role for Fas-mediated apoptosis and inflammation in cervical spondylotic myelopathy. Brain 2011;134(Pt 5):1277–92.
27. Karadimas SK, Laliberte AM, Tetreault L, et al. Riluzole blocks perioperative ischemia-reperfusion injury and enhances postdecompression outcomes in cervical spondylotic myelopathy. Sci Transl Med 2015;7(316):316ra194.
28. Vidal PM, Karadimas SK, Ulndreaj A, et al. Delayed decompression exacerbates ischemia-reperfusion injury in cervical compressive myelopathy. JCI Insight 2017;2(11) [pii:92512].
29. Kokubun S, Sato T, Ishii Y, et al. Cervical myelopathy in the Japanese. Clin Orthop Relat Res 1996;(323): 129–38.
30. Koakutsu T, Nakajo J, Morozumi N, et al. Cervical myelopathy due to degenerative spondylolisthesis. Ups J Med Sci 2011;116(2):129–32.
31. Park MS, Moon SH, Lee HM, et al. The natural history of degenerative spondylolisthesis of the cervical spine with 2- to 7-year follow-up. Spine (Phila Pa 1976) 2013;38(4):E205–10.
32. Jiang SD, Jiang LS, Dai LY. Degenerative cervical spondylolisthesis: a systematic review. Int Orthop 2011;35(6):869–75.
33. Suzuki A, Daubs MD, Inoue H, et al. Prevalence and motion characteristics of degenerative cervical spondylolisthesis in the symptomatic adult. Spine (Phila Pa 1976) 2013;38(17):E1115–20.
34. Hirai T, Yoshii T, Iwanami A, et al. Prevalence and distribution of ossified lesions in the whole spine of patients with cervical ossification of the posterior longitudinal ligament a multicenter study (JOSL CT study). PLoS One 2016;11(8):e0160117.
35. Kawaguchi Y, Nakano M, Yasuda T, et al. Characteristics of ossification of the spinal ligament; incidence of ossification of the ligamentum flavum in patients with cervical ossification of the posterior longitudinal ligament. Analysis of the whole spine using multidetector CT. J Orthop Sci 2016;21(4):439–45.
36. Azuma Y, Kato Y, Taguchi T. Etiology of cervical myelopathy induced by ossification of the posterior longitudinal ligament: determining the responsible level of OPLL myelopathy by correlating static compression and dynamic factors. J Spinal Disord Tech 2010;23(3):166–9.
37. Matsunaga S, Sakou T, Taketomi E, et al. Clinical course of patients with ossification of the posterior longitudinal ligament: a minimum 10-year cohort study. J Neurosurg 2004;100(3 Suppl Spine):245–8.
38. Yamauchi H. Epidemiological and pathological study of ossification of the posterior longitudinal ligament of the cervical spine. Investigation Committee 1977 report on the ossification of the spinal ligaments of the Japanese Ministry of Public Health and Welfare. Tokyo: Springer-Verlag; 1978. p. 21–5 [in Japanese].
39. Kim TJ, Bae KW, Uhm WS, et al. Prevalence of ossification of the posterior longitudinal ligament of the cervical spine. Joint Bone Spine 2008;75(4):471–4.
40. Kurokawa T. Prevalence of ossification of the posterior longitudinal ligament of the cervical spine in Taiwan, Hong Kong, and Singapore. Investigation Committee 1977 report on the ossification of the spinal ligaments of the Japanese Ministry of Public Health and Welfare. Tokyo: Springer-Verlag; 1978. p. 8–9 [in Japanese].
41. Liu KC. Epidemiological study on ossification of the posterior longitudinal ligament (OPLL) in the cervical spine–comparison of the prevalence between Japanese and Taiwanese. Nihon Seikeigeka Gakkai Zasshi 1990;64(5):401–8 [in Japanese].
42. Yamaura I, Kamikozuru M, Shinomiya K. Therapeutic modalities and epidemiological study of ossification of the posterior longitudinal ligament of the cervical

spine. Investigation Committee 1977 report on the ossification of the spinal ligaments of the Japanese Ministry of Public Health and Welfare. Tokyo: Springer-Verlag; 1978. p. 18–20 [in Japanese].
43. Tezuka S. Epidemiological study of ossification of the posterior longitudinal ligament of the cervical spine in Taiwan. Investigation Committee 1977 report on the ossification of the spinal ligaments of the Japanese Ministry of Public Health and Welfare. Tokyo: Springer-Verlag; 1980. p. 19–23 [in Japanese].
44. Lee T, Chacha PB, Khoo J. Ossification of posterior longitudinal ligament of the cervical spine in non-Japanese Asians. Surg Neurol 1991;35(1):40–4.
45. Yamauchi H. Radiological examination by plain film of the cervical spine in West Germany. Investigation Committee 1978 report on the ossification of the spinal ligaments of the Japanese Ministry of Public Health and Welfare. Tokyo: Springer-Verlag; 1979. p. 22–3 [in Japanese].
46. Terayama K, Ohtsuka Y. Epidemiological study of ossification of the posterior longitudinal ligament on Bologna in Italy. Investigation Committee 1983 report on the ossification of the spinal ligaments of the Japanese Ministry of Public Health and Welfare. Tokyo: Springer-Verlag; 1984. p. 55–62 [in Japanese].
47. Izawa K. Comparative radiographic study on the incidence of ossification of the cervical spine among Japanese, Koreans, Americans, and Germans. J Jpn Ortop Assoc 1980;54:461–74 [in Japanese].
48. Firooznia H, Benjamin VM, Pinto RS, et al. Calcification and ossification of posterior longitudinal ligament of spine: its role in secondary narrowing of spinal canal and cord compression. N Y State J Med 1982;82(8):1193–8.
49. Ijiri K, Sakou T, Taketomi E. Epidemiological study of ossification of posterior longitudinal ligament in Utah. Investigation Committee 1995 report on the ossification of the spinal ligaments of the Japanese Ministry of Public Health and Welfare. Tokyo: Springer-Verlag; 1996. p. 24–5 [in Japanese].
50. Fujimori T, Le H, Hu SS, et al. Ossification of the posterior longitudinal ligament of the cervical spine in 3161 patients: a CT-based study. Spine (Phila Pa 1976) 2015;40(7):E394–403.
51. Inoue H, Seichi A, Kimura A, et al. Multiple-level ossification of the ligamentum flavum in the cervical spine combined with calcification of the cervical ligamentum flavum and posterior atlanto-axial membrane. Eur Spine J 2013;22(Suppl 3):S416–20.
52. Guo JJ, Luk KD, Karppinen J, et al. Prevalence, distribution, and morphology of ossification of the ligamentum flavum: a population study of one thousand seven hundred thirty-six magnetic resonance imaging scans. Spine (Phila Pa 1976) 2010;35(1):51–6.
53. Al-Jarallah K, Al-Saeed O, Shehab D, et al. Ossification of ligamentum flavum in Middle East Arabs: a hospital-based study. Med Princ Pract 2012;21(6):529–33.
54. Olive PM, Whitecloud TS 3rd, Bennett JT. Lower cervical spondylosis and myelopathy in adults with Down's syndrome. Spine (Phila Pa 1976) 1988;13(7):781–4.
55. Patel AA, Spiker WR, Daubs M, et al. Evidence of an inherited predisposition for cervical spondylotic myelopathy. Spine (Phila Pa 1976) 2012;37(1):26–9.
56. Mahbub MH, Laskar MS, Seikh FA, et al. Prevalence of cervical spondylosis and musculoskeletal symptoms among coolies in a city of Bangladesh. J Occup Health 2006;48(1):69–73.
57. Petren-Mallmin M, Linder J. Cervical spine degeneration in fighter pilots and controls: a 5-yr follow-up study. Aviat Space Environ Med 2001;72(5):443–6.
58. Chen PL, Wang PY. Spondylotic myelopathy in patients with cervical dystonia. J Chin Med Assoc 2012;75(2):81–3.
59. Wong AS, Massicotte EM, Fehlings MG. Surgical treatment of cervical myeloradiculopathy associated with movement disorders: indications, technique, and clinical outcome. J Spinal Disord Tech 2005;18(Suppl):S107–14.
60. Lee SM, Oh SC, Yeom JS, et al. The impact of generalized joint laxity (GJL) on the posterior neck pain, cervical disc herniation, and cervical disc degeneration in the cervical spine. Spine J 2016;16(12):1453–8.
61. Nouri A, Tetreault L, Zamorano JJ, et al. Prevalence of Klippel-Feil syndrome in a surgical series of patients with cervical spondylotic myelopathy: analysis of the prospective, multicenter AOSpine North America Study. Global Spine J 2015;5(4):294–9.
62. Jenkins TJ, Mai HT, Burgmeier RJ, et al. The triangle model of congenital cervical stenosis. Spine (Phila Pa 1976) 2016;41(5):E242–7.
63. Pavlov H, Torg JS, Robie B, et al. Cervical spinal stenosis: determination with vertebral body ratio method. Radiology 1987;164(3):771–5.
64. Bajwa NS, Toy JO, Young EY, et al. Establishment of parameters for congenital stenosis of the cervical spine: an anatomic descriptive analysis of 1,066 cadaveric specimens. Eur Spine J 2012;21(12):2467–74.
65. Horne PH, Lampe LP, Nguyen JT, et al. A novel radiographic indicator of developmental cervical stenosis. J Bone Joint Surg Am 2016;98(14):1206–14.
66. Singh A, Tetreault L, Fehlings MG, et al. Risk factors for development of cervical spondylotic myelopathy: results of a systematic review. Evid Based Spine Care J 2012;3(3):35–42.

67. Lee MJ, Cassinelli EH, Riew KD. Prevalence of cervical spine stenosis. Anatomic study in cadavers. J Bone Joint Surg Am 2007;89(2):376–80.
68. McKay SD, Al-Omari A, Tomlinson LA, et al. Review of cervical spine anomalies in genetic syndromes. Spine (Phila Pa 1976) 2012;37(5):E269–77.
69. Matsunaga S, Imakiire T, Koga H, et al. Occult spinal canal stenosis due to C-1 hypoplasia in children with Down syndrome. J Neurosurg 2007;107(6 Suppl): 457–9.
70. Nouri A, Martin AR, Lange SF, et al. Congenital cervical fusion as a risk factor for development of degenerative cervical myelopathy. World Neurosurg 2017;100:531–9.
71. Okada E, Matsumoto M, Fujiwara H, et al. Disc degeneration of cervical spine on MRI in patients with lumbar disc herniation: comparison study with asymptomatic volunteers. Eur Spine J 2011;20(4): 585–91.
72. Schairer WW, Carrer A, Lu M, et al. The increased prevalence of cervical spondylosis in patients with adult thoracolumbar spinal deformity. J Spinal Disord Tech 2014;27(8):E305–8.
73. Radcliff KE, Curry EP, Trimba R, et al. High incidence of undiagnosed cervical myelopathy in patients with hip fracture compared with controls. J Orthop Trauma 2016;30(4):189–93.
74. Sonnesen L, Petersson A, Wiese M, et al. Osseous osteoarthritic-like changes and joint mobility of the temporomandibular joints and upper cervical spine: is there a relation? Oral Surg Oral Med Oral Pathol Oral Radiol 2017;123(2): 273–9.
75. Albright JP, Moses JM, Feldick HG, et al. Nonfatal cervical spine injuries in interscholastic football. JAMA 1976;236(11):1243–5.
76. Tempel ZJ, Bost JW, Norwig JA, et al. Significance of T2 hyperintensity on magnetic resonance imaging after cervical cord injury and return to play in professional athletes. Neurosurgery 2015;77(1):23–30 [discussion: 30–1].
77. Torg JS, Guille JT, Jaffe S. Injuries to the cervical spine in American football players. J Bone Joint Surg Am 2002;84-A(1):112–22.
78. Torg JS, Naranja RJ Jr, Pavlov H, et al. The relationship of developmental narrowing of the cervical spinal canal to reversible and irreversible injury of the cervical spinal cord in football players. J Bone Joint Surg Am 1996;78(9): 1308–14.
79. Ladd AL, Scranton PE. Congenital cervical stenosis presenting as transient quadriplegia in athletes. Report of two cases. J Bone Joint Surg Am 1986; 68(9):1371–4.
80. Maroon JC, El-Kadi H, Abla AA, et al. Cervical neurapraxia in elite athletes: evaluation and surgical treatment. Report of five cases. J Neurosurg Spine 2007;6(4):356–63.
81. Jonasson P, Halldin K, Karlsson J, et al. Prevalence of joint-related pain in the extremities and spine in five groups of top athletes. Knee Surg Sports Traumatol Arthrosc 2011;19(9):1540–6.
82. Villavicencio AT, Burneikiene S, Hernandez TD, et al. Back and neck pain in triathletes. Neurosurg Focus 2006;21(4):E7.

Pathobiology of Degenerative Cervical Myelopathy

Farhana Akter, MBBS, BSc, MSc, MRCS*,
Mark Kotter, MD, MPhil, PhD

KEYWORDS

• Degenerative cervical myelopathy • Pathobiology • Chronic spinal cord compression • Cell loss • Axon degeneration • Myelin changes

KEY POINTS

- Degenerative cervical myelopathy (DCM) is caused by mechanical stress.
- The pathobiology of DCM includes inflammation, apoptosis and vascular changes.
- A full understanding of the mechanisms of injury is currently lacking.

INTRODUCTION

Degenerative cervical myelopathy (DCM) is caused by mechanical compression of the spinal cord. However, the mechanism by which mechanical stress results in spinal cord injury is poorly understood. Furthermore, there is a poor correlation between disease severity and degree of compression measured by static MRI scanning[1,2] DCM is thought to be composed of a static and dynamic component. Static factors include developmental canal stenosis, bulging of the intervertebral disc posterior margin, and hypertrophy of the ligamentum flavum. Dynamic factors include invagination of the ligamentum flavum[3] and shearing and tethering of the spinal cord as a result of neck movements. The most common mechanisms involved in the pathobiology of DCM include apoptosis of cells, an inflammatory response, and vascular changes leading to axon degeneration, myelin changes, and cell loss. However, the exact pathophysiologic mechanisms of DCM are unclear. As a result, surgery is the only available treatment of DCM. Surgery can halt disease progression and enable a degree of recovery[4,5]; however, most patients have long-term disability. A better understanding of the pathogenesis of DCM is required for the development of treatments to improve outcomes. In this article, the authors discuss the pathophysiology of DCM and recent advances in our understanding of the disease.

PATHOBIOLOGY OF DEGENERATIVE CERVICAL MYELOPATHY

Human Studies

Histopathologic studies of human DCM suggest that the disease is progressive in nature and mainly affects white matter tracts. Wallerian degeneration of motor axons in the lateral corticospinal tract is one of the major signs of early disease.[6] Clinically, patients present with signs of corticospinal tract damage, including spastic gait. DCM also affects the central gray matter and posterior column leading to symptoms of impaired sensation, proprioception, and sphincter disturbance.[7]

Disclosure Statement: The authors confirm that they have no commercial or financial conflicts of interest.
Department of Clinical Neurosciences, Ann McLaren Laboratory of Regenerative Medicine, University of Cambridge, West Forvie Building, Forvie Site Box 213, Hills Road, Cambridge CB2 0SZ, UK
* Corresponding author.
E-mail address: farhanaakter@doctors.org.uk

Neurosurg Clin N Am 29 (2018) 13–19
https://doi.org/10.1016/j.nec.2017.09.015
1042-3680/18/© 2017 Elsevier Inc. All rights reserved.

Animal Studies

Preclinical animal studies have highlighted that a range of mechanisms of injury are involved in the pathogenesis of DCM following compression (**Fig. 1**). The most common pathogenesis observed is loss of neurons following compression. Other cells affected include oligodendrocytes, astrocytes, and microglia. Mechanisms of injury include apoptosis of cells, inflammation, and vascular changes.

Cellular Changes

Neuron loss

Neurons are vulnerable to spinal cord compression. Degeneration of neurons and axons are a prominent feature in human postmortem studies and can cause significant atrophy of the spinal cord. Studies have shown loss of neurons in patients with DCM, particularly in the anterior horn.[8] In addition, segmental loss of interneurons occurs[9] as well as loss of lower motor neurons in the anterior horns.[8,9] These findings have been echoed in animal studies, with the greatest cell loss in the gray matter of the ventral horns at the focus of the lesion.[10–14]

Oligodendrocyte loss

Oligodendrocytes make and maintain myelin sheaths. The loss of oligodendrocytes results in demyelination and impaired axon function and survival.[15] Several studies have demonstrated the loss of oligodendrocytes in chronic compression models. Most published studies were performed in the Tiptoe-walking-Yoshimura (Twy/Twy) mice model, and these studies demonstrated apoptosis of oligodendrocytes in the compressed group. Studies in rats have also shown evidence of oligodendrocyte apoptosis using Terminal deoxynucleotidyl transferase dUTP nick end labeling (TUNEL) staining[16] More importantly, postmortem samples of human individuals affected by DCM demonstrated clear evidence of demyelination.[17]

Astrogliosis

Astrogliosis (also known as astrocytosis or reactive astrocytosis) is an abnormal increase in the number of astrocytes. Reactive astrocytes are characterized by high-level expression of glial fibrillary acidic protein (GFAP), an intermediate filament protein. Several articles have demonstrated increased expression of GFAP in compressed groups compared with control Twy/Twy mice[8,18] This finding has also been reported in rats,[19]

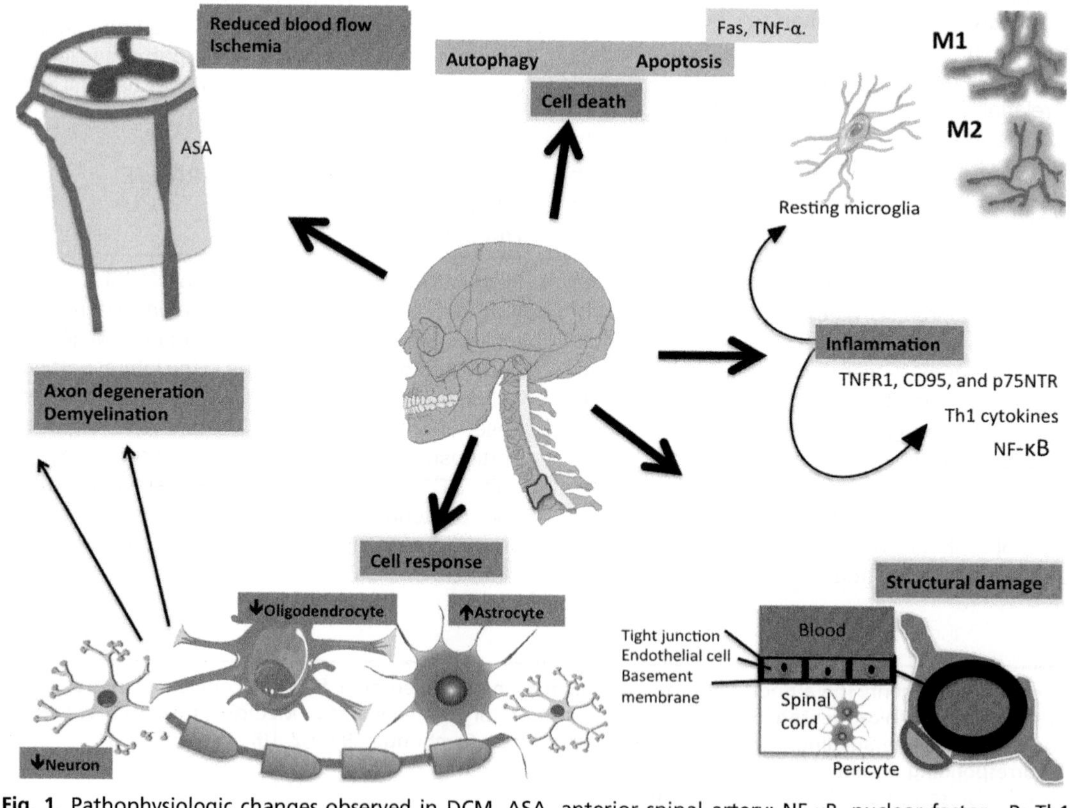

Fig. 1. Pathophysiologic changes observed in DCM. ASA, anterior spinal artery; NF-κB, nuclear factor–κB; Th1, T-helper 1; TNF-α, tumor necrosis factor–α; TNFR1, tumor necrosis factor receptor 1.

dogs,[20] and rabbits.[13,21] In contrast, Dhillon and colleagues[10] found reduced levels of astrocytes at the lesion center following compression but increased levels above and below the site of compression. Astrogliosis minimizes and repairs the initial damage but eventually has detrimental effects. It is not currently known which signaling pathways and molecular mediators trigger and modulate reactive astrocytes and scar formation. An understanding of these processes is essential to understand the pathogenesis of DCM and how astrocyte activity can be targeted to harness their potential use as therapeutic treatments for DCM.

Mechanisms of Injury

Inflammation

The role of the innate inflammatory response in DCM has been investigated in several studies. In human postmortem tissue, increased numbers of activated macrophages at the compressed sites have been demonstrated up to 4 years after the onset of symptoms.[8] In preclinical models, an increase in microglia was reported in compressed cords,[10,19] which increased with worsening cord compression.[22] Microglia have been identified in both gray and white matter, particularly the anterior horn, anterior column, and lateral column of the spinal cord.[22] Increasing cord compression correlated with increased numbers of activated microglia.[22] Activated microglia may display either a proinflammatory M1 phenotype or an antiinflammatory M2 phenotype, which may lead to detrimental or beneficial roles in the nervous system. The M1 phenotype results from exposure to T-helper 1 (Th1) cytokines, such as interferon gamma, tumor necrosis factor-alpha (TNF-α), and interleukin (IL)-6. The M2 phenotype results from exposure to activated via T-helper 2 cytokines, such as IL-4, IL-10, and IL-13. Microglia numbers may also be increased via a Fas-mediated process. Fas (First apoptotic signal) is a transmembrane receptor of the tumor necrosis factor (TNF) receptor superfamily. Fas is a receptor that is involved in the mechanism of cell death, and it plays an important role in mediating neural apoptosis. Yu and colleagues[8] demonstrated an increase in Iba1-positive microglia/macrophages in the compressed lesion center, which was reduced by functionally blocking the Fas ligand. Markers of the M1 phenotype, TNF-α and CD86, are present in chronically compressed spinal cords[23] and are increased in severe compression compared with moderate compression. There is also an upregulation of cysteine-rich protein 61, which is an inducer of M1 macrophages, in the compressed cords. Arginase-1 and CD163 expression, an indicator of M2 macrophage transition, did not significantly differ between the severe and moderate compression groups or in the control groups.[23] Other studies, however, have shown that with an increased duration of compression, although there is an increase in the M1 phenotype, the M2 phenotype predominates.[22] It is important to fully characterize the M1/M2 phenotypes to understand whether they represent destructive or regenerative phenotypes and, consequently, which response can be modulated to promote recovery.

Compression also leads to an increase in Th1 cytokines in the Twy/Twy mouse model, which results in neuronal loss.[22] Chronic compression leads to overexpression of TNF receptor 1 (TNFR1), CD95, and p75 neurotrophin receptor (P75NTR)[24]; microarray analysis revealed higher levels of chemokine signals that were responsible for these upregulated inflammatory markers.[23] The nuclear factor–κB pathway is a prototypical proinflammatory signaling pathway and activation of this pathway in DCM has been observed.[25] From the available studies, it seems that the inflammatory pathway and proinflammatory mediators have been poorly investigated. Many of the studies have been performed on the Twy/Twy model, in which compression occurs at C2-C3 as a consequence of spontaneous ossification. In contrast, human spinal cord compression mostly occurs between C3 and C7. Published studies have made no attempt to inhibit other secondary injury mechanisms in order to characterize the true extent of the inflammation. Furthermore, individual cytokine and interleukin responses to antiinflammatory agents have not been investigated.

Apoptosis

Apoptosis is the process of programmed cell death that can be initiated by intrinsic (mitochondrial) and extrinsic pathways. The intrinsic pathway is initiated by mitochondrial dysfunction. *Bcl-2* (B-cell lymphoma 2) and Bax (bcl-2-like protein 4), which are antiapoptotic and proapoptotic proteins, respectively, modulate the intrinsic pathway. One study demonstrated increased expression of Bcl-2 in Twy/Twy mice.[8] The second well-established apoptotic pathway involves signaling by cell surface death receptors. These death receptors are members of the TNFR family and include TNFR1, Fas, FasL (First apoptotic signal ligand), p75, and DR3 (death receptor 3).

Apoptosis as a mechanism of cellular injury has been investigated in several animal models of DCM. Studies in the Twy/Twy model showed increased apoptosis in neurons and oligodendrocytes.[24,26] The presence of apoptotic markers is increased in the presence of severe compression.[27] Apoptosis in this model can occur via the Fas pathway[18] and is mediated by an increase in Fas/FasL interaction activating caspase.[8] The caspase family of cysteine proteases regulates the execution of the mammalian apoptotic cell death program. Although the Fas-mediated apoptosis studies did investigate caspase activation, this should be investigated further by investigating the upstream and downstream components of the caspase apoptotic pathway. Preventing the activation of Fas-mediated cell death using neutralization of endogenous FasL is a highly relevant neuroprotective approach.[8] Currently, the available data do not fully delineate the full extent of apoptosis-mediated injury in DCM nor its interaction with other mechanisms of injury.

Vascular changes

Vascular changes following chronic cord compression have been investigated in several animal studies. Early studies in dogs by Gooding and colleagues[28] demonstrated that vascular insufficiency combined with maximum compression led to more widespread myelin changes in the white matter compared with compression alone. Vascular insufficiency was induced by ligating the bilateral lateral spinal arteries at C3, followed by anterior spinal artery (ASA) ligation at C1 and vertebral artery ligation proximal to C6. In addition, vascular insufficiency can also cause glial fibrosis and necrosis.[20] These early studies were useful in the development of our understanding of the potential pathologic changes in DCM; however, there was no quantitative analysis of the histopathologic changes or statistical confirmation of the extent of the myelin changes and no confirmation of the presence of demyelination. Furthermore, these studies are difficult to replicate and prone to selection and detection bias, with no evidence of randomization or blinding.

Recently, further studies have attempted to correlate vascular morphology with function scores. Microscopic computed tomography has been used to demonstrate the reduction of ASA[29,30] and ARA diameter[30] following chronic cord compression. There is also an initial reduction of the vascular network following compression, which improves with an increased duration of compression.[30] This process of reduction in vascular diameter and network is associated with an initial reduction in the Basso Beattie Bresnahan score followed by recovery with an increased duration of compression. Cheng and colleagues[30] assessed somatosensory evoked potentials (SEPs) and found a reduction of amplitude at day 28 following compression, which improved with an increased duration of compression. Initially, latency was also prolonged but subsequently improved at day 70. However, motor function and SEP did not fully return to the baseline. SEPs are presynaptic and postsynaptic responses that reflect sequential activation of neural structures along the somatosensory pathways. Several characteristics of SEPs can be measured, including peak latencies, component amplitudes, and waveform morphology. SEPs correlate well with postoperative recovery in patients with DCM.[31] The SEP responses by amplitude and latency could represent an indicator for the extent of ultrastructural damage of the spinal cord after chronic compressive injuries.[32] The aforementioned studies did not investigate the effects of changes in vascular diameter on ischemic changes or hypoxic changes. Furthermore, the extent to which the reduced diameter of the ARA/ASA reduces blood flow was not assessed in the aforementioned studies.

Several articles have assessed spinal cord blood flow at compressed sites.[32,33] Kurokawa and colleagues[32] used a microsphere technique to assess spinal cord blood flow and demonstrated a reduced blood flow at the compressed site. However, no histologic or functional data were generated in this study. An alternative technique used to assess blood flow is the hydrogen clearance method, used by Harkey and colleagues[33] and Al-Mefty and colleagues.[34] Both groups demonstrated a reduction in blood flow immediately following compression, which continued to decrease as the duration of compression increased.

Axon degeneration

Progressive axonal loss results in atrophy of lateral and posterior funiculi.[17] Axonal degeneration following injury takes place both toward the proximal cell body (retrograde degeneration) and toward the distal axon terminal (Wallerian or orthograde degeneration). Axonal degeneration occurs at the site of compression[35] and also at sites cranial and caudal to the compression site.[36] Compression also leads to Wallerian degeneration of the caudal axons of corticospinal tracts,[16] in the anterior horn[37] and in the lateral funiculi, caudal to the site of compression[38]

Neurofilaments are important structural components of axons.[39] Klironomos and colleagues[13] demonstrated a loss of cellular levels of neurofilaments in myelopathic rabbits. Neurofilament integrity is also important for the plasticity of neuronal processes. However, other components of the neuronal cytoskeleton, including actin filaments and microtubules, were not analyzed. The investigators also described decreased levels of the calcium-binding protein, S-100, which is thought to be transported along the axon in DCM. However, this protein has been found in many cells, including astrocytes and Schwann cells, suggesting that this may not be specific to neurones. Studies using spinal cord injury models have reported increased levels of S-100 protein[40,41]; therefore, the link between this protein and DCM and its time profile needs to be characterized. Cheung and colleagues[42] used an imaging technique to demonstrate the presence of axonal degeneration (AD). Diffusion tensor imaging was used to confirm compression of the spinal cord at C5-C6 with evidence of decreased diffusivity (AD) near the center of the lesion. AD is reduced in axonal injury and, therefore, could represent axon loss in compressed spinal cords.[43] There was also evidence of reduced fractional anisotropy at the compressed site, which suggests that there is reduced microstructural integrity.[42] There was increased diffusivity near the lesion center,[42] which could be a result of changes in axon diameter or density.[43]

Myelin damage

Changes in the myelin sheath have been described in several articles investigating the pathophysiology of DCM. Primary demyelination is usually due to a direct insult targeted at the oligodendrocyte. Secondary demyelination (or Wallerian degeneration) is the process of myelin degeneration as a consequence of primary axonal loss. Demyelination is best demonstrated by the presence of nude axons, using electron microscopy.[44] Without the demonstration of nude axons, it is difficult to determine whether demyelination is present. Unfortunately, many of the techniques used, such as Luxol fast blue staining, cannot be used when high resolution of fibers is required.[45,46] Only limited studies exist that have investigated DCM with electron microscopy.[17] These studies demonstrate evidence of demyelination. Moreover, the most effective method to demonstrate secondary demyelination is by determining whether remyelination has taken place, by identifying abnormally thin myelin sheaths.[46] Ito and colleagues[17] show evidence of remyelination in DCM. However, to what extent demyelination and remyelination occurs in DCM remains elusive.

Another technique that can be used to detect the presence of axon degeneration or demyelination is electrophysiology. The amplitude of SEP studies represents axon density, and the latency of SEP is often prolonged in demyelination.[47] Several studies have investigated electrophysiologic changes in patients with DCM. The evaluation of posterior column function in DCM by Somatosensory Evoked Potential found that SSEP abnormalities correlated well with radiological evidence of cord compression.[31,48] Motor evoked potentials are more sensitive than SSEPS for the detection of CSM and are thought to correlate with Upper motor neuron signs.[48] Delays in central motor conduction time indicates demyelination in individuals with subclinical myelopathy and of myelopathic patients with varied degrees of cord compression.[49] Demyelination, therefore, is very likely to be an important factor in DCM.

SUMMARY

There is a paucity of data describing the pathophysiology of DCM and the physiology of recovery following decompression. It is imperative to delineate intrinsic and extrinsic mechanisms of cell death associated with DCM, including upstream and downstream regulators of these pathways. A full understanding of the inflammatory and proinflammatory pathways, including the microglial response, innate immune response, cytokine, and interleukin profile is also currently lacking. Current animal models do not fully recapitulate the disease. Efforts to develop a novel mouse model that develops lesions at C5-C6 and the use of these models to induce spinal cord compression more reflective of the human condition are warranted.

REFERENCES

1. Lebl DR, Hughes A, Cammisa FP, et al. Cervical spondylotic myelopathy: pathophysiology, clinical presentation, and treatment. HSS J 2011;7(2):170–8.
2. Boden SD, McCowin PR, Davis DO, et al. Abnormal magnetic-resonance scans of the cervical spine in asymptomatic subjects. A prospective investigation. J Bone Joint Surg Am 1990;72:1178–84.
3. Nishida N, Kato Y, Imajo Y, et al. Biomechanical analysis of cervical spondylotic myelopathy: the influence of dynamic factors and morphometry of the spinal cord. J Spinal Cord Med 2012;35(4):256–61.
4. Fehlings MG, Barry S, Kopjar B, et al. Anterior versus posterior surgical approaches to treat cervical spondylotic myelopathy: outcomes of the prospective multicenter AOSpine North America CSM study in 264 patients. Spine 2013;38:2247–52.
5. Fehlings MG, Ibrahim A, Tetreault L, et al. Global perspective on the outcomes of surgical decompression in patients with cervical spondylotic myelopathy. Spine 2015;40:1322–8.
6. McMinn RMH. Last's anatomy. Regional and applied. Hong Kong: Elsevier; 1998.
7. Lunsford LD, Bissonette DJ, Zorub DS. Anterior surgery for cervical disc disease. Part 2: treatment of cervical spondylotic myelopathy in 32 cases. J Neurosurg 1980;53(1):12–9.

8. Yu WR, Liu T, Kiehl TR, et al. Human neuropathological and animal model evidence supporting a role for Fas-mediated apoptosis and inflammation in cervical spondylotic myelopathy. Brain 2011;134(Pt 5):1277–92.
9. Ogino H, Tada K, Okada K, et al. Canal diameter, anteroposterior compression ratio, and spondylotic myelopathy of the cervical spine. Spine (Phila Pa 1976) 1983;8(1):1–15.
10. Dhillon RS, Parker J, Syed YA, et al. Axonal plasticity underpins the functional recovery following surgical decompression in a rat model of cervical spondylotic myelopathy. Acta Neuropathol Commun 2016;4(1):89.
11. Kanchiku T, Taguchi T, Kaneko K, et al. A new rabbit model for the study on cervical compressive myelopathy. J Orthop Res 2001;19(4):605–13.
12. Jiang H, Wang J, Xu B, et al. A model of acute central cervical spinal cord injury syndrome combined with chronic injury in goats. Eur Spine J 2017;26(1):56–63.
13. Klironomos G, Karadimas S, Mavrakis A, et al. New experimental rabbit animal model for cervical spondylotic myelopathy. Spinal Cord 2011;49(11):1097–102.
14. Yoshizumi T, Murata H, Yamamoto S, et al. Granulocyte colony-stimulating factor improves motor function in rats developing compression myelopathy spine. Spine (Phila Pa 1976) 2016;41(23):1380–7.
15. Franklin RJ, Ffrench-Constant C. Remyelination in the CNS: from biology to therapy. Nat Rev Neurosci 2008;9:839–55.
16. Karadimas SK, Moon ES, Yu WR, et al. A novel experimental model of cervical spondylotic myelopathy (CSM) to facilitate translational research. Neurobiol Dis 2013;54:43–58.
17. Ito T, Oyanagi K, Takahashi H, et al. Cervical spondylotic myelopathy. Clinicopathologic study on the progression pattern and thin myelinated fibers of the lesions of seven patients examined during complete autopsy. Spine (Phila Pa 1976) 1996;21:827–33.
18. Yu WR, Baptiste DC, Liu T, et al. Molecular mechanisms of spinal cord dysfunction and cell death in the spinal hyperostotic mouse: implications for the pathophysiology of human cervical spondylotic myelopathy. Neurobiol Dis 2009;33(2):149–63.
19. Moon ES, Karadimas SK, Yu WR, et al. Riluzole attenuates neuropathic pain and enhances functional recovery in a rodent model of cervical spondylotic myelopathy. Neurobiol Dis 2014;62:394–406.
20. Hukuda S, Wilson CB. Experimental cervical myelopathy- effects of compression and ischemia on canine cervical cord. J Neurosurg 1972;37(6):631.
21. Ozawa H, Jian Wu Z, Tanaka Y, et al. Morphologic change and astrocyte response to unilateral spinal cord compression in rabbits. J Neurotrauma 2004;21(7):944–55.
22. Hirai T, Uchida K, Nakajima H, et al. The prevalence and phenotype of activated microglia/macrophages within the spinal cord of the hyperostotic mouse (Twy/Twy) changes in response to chronic progressive spinal cord compression: implications for human cervical compressive myelopathy. PLoS One 2013;8(5):e64528.
23. Takano M, Kawabata S, Komaki Y, et al. Inflammatory cascades mediate synapse elimination in spinal cord compression. J Neuroinflammation 2014;11:40.
24. Uchida K, Nakajima H, Watanabe S, et al. Apoptosis of neurons and oligodendrocytes in the spinal cord of spinal hyperostotic mouse (Twy/Twy): possible pathomechanism of human cervical compressive myelopathy. Eur Spine J 2012;21(3):490–7.
25. Karadimas SK, Klironomos G, Papachristou DJ, et al. Immunohistochemical profile of NF-kappaB/p50, NF-kappaB/p65, MMP-9, MMP-2, and u-PA in experimental cervical spondylotic myelopathy. Spine (Phila Pa 1976) 2013;38(1):4–10.
26. Yamaura I, Yone K, Nakahara S, et al. Mechanism of destructive pathologic changes in the spinal cord under chronic mechanical compression. Spine (Phila Pa 1976) 2002;27(1):21–6.
27. Inukai T, Uchida K, Nakajima H, et al. Tumor necrosis factor-alpha and its receptors contribute to apoptosis of oligodendrocytes in the spinal cord of spinal hyperostotic mouse (Twy/Twy) sustaining chronic mechanical compression. Spine 2009;34(26):2848–57.
28. Gooding MR, Wilson CB, Hoff JT. Experimental cervical myelopathy- effects of ischemia and compression of canine cervical spinal cord. J Neurosurg 1975;43(1):9–17.
29. Long HQ, Xie WH, Chen WL, et al. Value of micro-CT for monitoring spinal microvascular changes after chronic spinal cord compression. Int J Mol Sci 2014;15(7):12061–73.
30. Cheng X, Long H, Chen W, et al. Three-dimensional alteration of cervical anterior spinal artery and anterior radicular artery in rat model of chronic spinal cord compression by micro-CT. Neurosci Lett 2015;606:106–12.
31. Lo Y. How has electrophysiology changed the management of cervical spondylotic myelopathy? Eur J Neurol 2008;15(8):781–6.
32. Kurokawa R, Murata H, Ogino M, et al. Altered blood flow distribution in the rat spinal cord under chronic compression. Spine (Phila Pa 1976) 2011;36(13):1006–9.
33. Harkey HL, al-Mefty O, Marawi I, et al. Experimental chronic compressive cervical myelopathy: effects of decompression. J Neurosurg 1995;83(2):336–41.
34. Al-Mefty O, Harkey HL, Marawai I, et al. Experimental chronic compressive cervical myelopathy. J Neurosurg 1993;79(4):550–61.

35. Kubota M, Kobayashi S, Nonoyama T, et al. Development of a chronic cervical cord compression model in rat: changes in the neurological behaviors and radiological and pathological findings. J Neurotrauma 2011;28(3):459–67.
36. Prange T, Carr EA, Stick JA, et al. Cervical vertebral canal endoscopy in a horse with cervical vertebral stenotic myelopathy. Equine Vet J 2012;44(1):116–9.
37. Yamamoto S, Kurokawa R, Kim P. Cilostazol, a selective type III phosphodiesterase inhibitor: prevention of cervical myelopathy in a rat chronic compression model. J Neurosurg Spine 2014;20(1):93–101.
38. Penny C, Macrae A, Hagen R, et al. Compressive cervical myelopathy in young Texel and Beltex sheep. J Vet Intern Med 2007;21(2):322–7.
39. Wang H, Wu M, Zhan C, et al. Neurofilament proteins in axonal regeneration and neurodegenerative diseases. Neural Regen Res 2012;7(8):620–6.
40. Cao F, Yang XF, Liu WG, et al. Elevation of neuron-specific enolase and S-100beta protein level in experimental acute spinal cord injury. J Clin Neurosci 2008;15:541–4.
41. Kwon BK, Stammers AM, Belanger LM, et al. Cerebrospinal fluid inflammatory cytokines and biomarkers of injury severity in acute human spinal cord injury. J Neurotrauma 2010;27(4):669–82.
42. Cheung MM, Li DT, Hui ES, et al. In vivo diffusion tensor imaging of chronic spinal cord compression in rat model. Conf Proc IEEE Eng Med Biol Soc 2009;2009:2715–8.
43. Aung WY, Mar S, Benzinger TL. Diffusion tensor MRI as a biomarker in axonal and myelin damage. Imaging Med 2013;5:427–40.
44. Rowland LP, Pedley TA. Merritt's neurology. Philadelphia: USA. Wolters Kluwer Lippincott Williams & Wilkins; 2010.
45. Pistorio AL, Hendry SH, Wang X. A modified technique for high-resolution staining of myelin. J Neurosci Methods 2006;15:135–46.
46. Blakemore WF. Pattern of remyelination in the CNS. Nature 1974;249:577–8.
47. Mallik A, Weir AI. Nerve conduction studies: essentials and pitfalls in practice. J Neurol Neurosurg Psychiatry 2005;76(Suppl 2):ii23–31.
48. Restuccia D, Di Lazzaro V, Lo Monaco M, et al. Somatosensory evoked potentials in the diagnosis of cervical spondylotic myelopathy. Electromyogr Clin Neurophysiol 1992;32(7–8):389–95.
49. Lo YL, Chan LL, Lim W, et al. Systematic correlation of transcranial magnetic stimulation and magnetic resonance imaging in cervical spondylotic myelopathy. Spine (Phila Pa 1976) 2004;29(10):1137–45.

The Natural History of Degenerative Cervical Myelopathy

Jetan H. Badhiwala, MD, Jefferson R. Wilson, MD, PhD*

KEYWORDS

• Cervical spondylotic myelopathy • Degenerative cervical myelopathy • Natural history • Outcomes • Spine surgery • Spinal cord

KEY POINTS

- The natural history of degenerative cervical myelopathy (DCM) is mixed, but generally consists of stepwise neurologic decline, with variable periods of quiescence.
- The contemporary literature indicates 20% to 62% of patients with DCM will deteriorate at 3 to 6 years of follow-up, as assessed by the modified Japanese Orthopedic Association scale.
- Nonoperative treatment modalities for DCM include cervical traction, cervical collar, analgesics, physical therapy, bedrest, avoidance of risk activities and environments (eg, slippery floors), and spinal injections.
- Multiple studies have explored the prognostic value of several demographic, clinical, and radiological characteristics, but none appear to reliably predict the risk of neurologic deterioration associated with use of conservative strategies for the treatment of DCM.
- Further prospective studies evaluating the course of disease, particularly mild DCM, are needed.

INTRODUCTION

Degenerative cervical myelopathy (DCM) is a spinal condition that results in chronic, nontraumatic compression of the cervical spinal cord. It is the leading cause of spinal cord dysfunction among adults worldwide.[1] This clinicopathologic entity encompasses osteoarthritic degeneration (ie, cervical spondylosis) and ligamentous aberrations (ie, ossification of the posterior longitudinal ligament, hypertrophy of the ligamentum flavum). The issues of quality, value, and cost are moving to the forefront of health care policy making, and spine surgery is no exception. With increasing scrutiny, there is a need for us to provide evidence backing the value of the interventions we perform. The value of surgery for DCM, as with any intervention for any disease, is measured against the yardstick of the natural history of the condition; that is, the outcome that results in the absence of any intervention. In the case of DCM, this is equivalent to nonoperative management, or observation. Traditionally, DCM has been considered a progressive disease, with the role of surgery being to halt progression of neurologic dysfunction and further disability. More recent evidence indicates surgical intervention for DCM is actually associated with improvement in function and quality of life.[2,3] Nonetheless, more data are needed on the outcomes of nonoperative treatment of DCM for these data to be interpreted meaningfully. Serial clinical follow-up rather than surgery is sometimes recommended in cases of mild DCM, particularly if there is concomitant neck pain or radiculopathy, which

The authors have no conflicts of interest to disclose.
Division of Neurosurgery, Department of Surgery, St. Michael's Hospital, University of Toronto, 30 Bond Street, Toronto, Ontario M5B 1W8, Canada
* Corresponding author.
E-mail address: wilsonjeff@smh.ca

Neurosurg Clin N Am 29 (2018) 21–32
https://doi.org/10.1016/j.nec.2017.09.002
1042-3680/18/© 2017 Elsevier Inc. All rights reserved.

neurosurgery.theclinics.com

are thought to possibly benefit from nonoperative treatment modalities like analgesics, physiotherapy, spinal injections, and/or orthoses. Herein, we provide a narrative review of the natural history of DCM. We summarize the neurologic, functional, and quality-of-life outcomes of nonoperative management, and also the predictors of said outcomes. We also examine the course of nonmyelopathic patients with radiological evidence of cervical spinal cord compression.

NATURAL HISTORY

Table 1 provides a summary of studies providing longitudinal data on the progression and outcome of DCM treated nonsurgically.

Neurologic Outcome

Cervical spondylosis was first clearly defined in 1948 by Brain and colleagues.[4] Early on, DCM was thought of as a disease causing a variable degree of disability, but one in which the natural tendency was toward a state of arrest or stability.[5] Lees and Turner[6] provided one of the first accounts of the natural history of DCM. This was a retrospective study of 44 patients with clinical evidence of myelopathy followed at St. Bartholomew's Hospital in London, England. The investigators observed and described the course of DCM to contain long or shorter periods of exacerbation, with interspersed long periods of quiescence, without new or worsening symptoms. Exacerbations often left patients worse than they were previously. Few patients deteriorated gradually over several years. At last follow-up, 2 patients (4.5%) had no disability, 3 (6.8%) mild disability, 21 (47.7%) moderate disability, and 18 (40.9%) severe disability. No relation between age and prognosis was found. Despite the seemingly poor outcomes, the investigators concluded that when it came to management of DCM, "a very conservative approach should be the rule," although they acknowledged the need for prospective studies.

The contemporary literature would suggest anywhere between 20% and 62% of patients with DCM will deteriorate neurologically within 3 to 6 months.[7] **Fig. 1** provides a graph of rates of deterioration at varying lengths of follow-up with conservative treatment of DCM, as evaluated by the Japanese Orthopedic Association (JOA) or modified JOA (mJOA) scale or Nurick grade. Kadanka and colleagues[8–12] conducted the only randomized controlled trial (RCT) on the topic. From 1993 to 1998, 68 patients with mild or moderate DCM (mJOA score $\geq$12) were randomized to conservative or operative treatment. Surgery consisted of anterior decompression in 22 patients, corpectomy in 6 patients, and laminoplasty in 5 patients. Conservative strategies included cervical collar, anti-inflammatory medications, and intermittent bedrest for patients with pain, discouragement from participation in high-risk activities, and avoidance of risky environments (eg, physical overloading, movement on slippery surfaces, manipulation therapies, or prolonged flexion of the head). No significant difference was observed in mean mJOA score within or between the conservative and surgical cohorts over a 36-month period. At the 3-year mark, 24.1% of the surgical cohort had improved 2 or more points on the mJOA scale, not significantly different from the corresponding proportion in the conservative cohort (23.3%). At the 10-year mark, mean mJOA score was 15.0 in conservatively and 14.0 in surgically treated patients.

A cause for concern in patients with cervical spinal cord compression, whether symptomatic or not, is the development or exacerbation of myelopathic symptoms secondary to even minor trauma, especially mechanisms involving hyperextension of the neck. In a cohort of 199 patients with asymptomatic cervical spinal cord compression, Bednarik and colleagues[13] reported 14 patients suffered a traumatic event to the head, spine, trunk, or shoulder region over a median follow-up of 44 months. Of these patients, 1 (7.1%) developed myelopathy. By contrast, 44 (23.8%) of 185 patients who experienced no trauma developed myelopathy, suggesting the risk of myelopathy after minor trauma to be low. Nonetheless, another study seemed to suggest the opposite. Katoh and colleagues[14] retrospectively assessed the influence of trauma in a group of 118 patients with ossification of the posterior longitudinal ligament. Twenty-seven patients sustained minor trauma to the spine. Of 8 patients with preexisting myelopathy, 7 (87.5%) deteriorated neurologically. Of 19 patients who were previously asymptomatic, 13 (68.4%) developed myelopathy.

Functional Ability

The current literature suggests a progressive decline in patients' ability to participate in activities of daily living over time.[7]

In their RCT of conservative versus operative therapy for mild or moderate DCM, Kadanka and colleagues[8–12] evaluated patients' ability to perform activities of daily living (eg, buttoning shirts, brushing hair and teeth, putting shoes on, walking, running, going up and down stairs) by video recording. Blinded observers rated patients' functional abilities as follows: excellent (+3), very good (+2), slightly better (+1), no change (0), slightly worse (−1), much worse (−2), or poor (−3). In the conservative group, the number of patients with declining scores gradually increased during follow-up from 6.3% at 1 year to 20.9% at 2 years and 27.3% at 3 years. No such change was observed in operative patients, in whom the distribution of scores remained relatively stable over time. A significant difference between groups favoring conservative over operative treatment was observed at 6 months, but not at 12, 24, or 36 months. The investigators also performed a timed 10-m walk test, measured as the time (in seconds) taken to walk as fast as possible (without running) on a 10-m track. Patients in the conservative group had relatively stable performance on this test over 36 months, scoring a mean of 7.4 seconds at baseline and 7.5 seconds at baseline. A small, but significant, difference was observed between groups, favoring the nonoperative cohort (7.5 vs 9.4 seconds) at 3 years. However, walk times were comparable between surgical (7.3 seconds) and conservative (7.1 seconds) cohorts at 10-year follow-up.

Sampath and colleagues[15] conducted a prospective study on patients with subacute DCM, defined by at least 8 weeks of symptoms. Patients were seen by a Cervical Spine Research Society surgeon and prescribed either medical or surgical therapy. A total of 23 patients received conservative treatment, including a combination of pharmacotherapy, home exercise, physical therapy, bedrest, cervical traction, and neck bracing. By contrast, 20 patients underwent surgery. At a mean follow-up of 29.8 months, the surgical group demonstrated significant improvements in overall functional status as well as work and social activities. Conservatively treated patients, too, exhibited functional improvements, but this did not reach statistical significance. Additionally, surgical patients experienced no change in the number of activities that worsened their symptoms from before to after treatment, whereas the number of activities that exacerbated symptoms in the medical cohort increased from baseline to follow-up (+0.63). Neither treatment had a significant effect on employment status.

Patient-Reported Outcomes

As discussed previously, Kadanka and colleagues[8–12] had 2 blinded physicians evaluate patients' functional ability based on video recording. Using the same scale, patients were also asked to rate their own abilities. A significant difference in patients' self-evaluation comparing surgically and conservatively treated cohorts was observed only at 6-month follow-up, and not at 1, 2, 3, or 10 years. At 6 months, 60.6% of patients undergoing surgery rated their abilities as improved and 24.2% as worse, compared with 20.0% and 34.3%, respectively, in the conservative group. At 10-year follow-up, 56.0% of patients in the conservative group rated their function as worse, compared with 45.5% in the surgical group ($P = .47$). No change in patients' self-rating of their functional abilities was observed for patients treated conservatively over time, with 34.3% rating their function unfavorably at 6 months and 36.7% at 36 months. By contrast, those treated with surgery were found to rate their abilities less favorably with time. At 3-year follow-up, only 20% of patients rated their abilities as improved, whereas 55% viewed their functional abilities unfavorably. Interestingly, this is the opposite of the trend seen in physicians' rating of patients' functional abilities based on video recording, as discussed previously, in which patients in the conservative group were felt to have declining function over time, whereas no change was observed in the surgical cohort. This suggests the observation of worsening patient self-report of function may be due to the phenomenon of "response shift," wherein patients' conceptualization of their quality of life "shifts" following a change, establishing a new baseline in their minds. On the other hand, patients treated conservatively may have become accustomed to their day-to-day difficulties, reflected as stability in their self-ratings of function. Findings from other studies, too, have suggested patients with DCM do not expect substantial improvement, and are generally satisfied with stability.[15]

Sampath and colleagues[15] prospectively evaluated 23 patients treated conservatively and 20 patients treated by surgery for subacute DCM. In this study, patient satisfaction was based on a on 5-point scale: (1) very satisfied; (2) satisfied; (3) neither satisfied nor dissatisfied; (4) dissatisfied; (5) very dissatisfied. At follow-up, satisfaction ratings were higher in the surgical group (1.95) than the conservative cohort (2.35), although not statistically significant. The investigators also evaluated pain scores using a 6-point scale, ranging from 0 (no pain) to 5 (excruciating pain). Both surgical (−0.98) and conservative cohorts (−0.61) had improved pain scores at follow-up, but in the operative group, this difference was statistically significant.

Need for Surgery

Conversion to surgery in natural history cohorts indicates failure of conservative treatment modalities. In their systematic review, Karadimas and

Table 1
Summary of studies evaluating the outcomes of nonoperative treatment of degenerative cervical myelopathy

Author (Year)	N	Study Design	Eligibility Criteria	Conservative Treatment	Baseline Characteristics	Follow-up	Neurologic Outcomes	Surgery	Predictors
Symptomatic									
Lees and Turner[6] 1963	44	Retrospective cohort	• Radiological and myelographic evidence of cervical spondylosis with signs of cord damage • Extensor plantar responses • No reasonable doubt that myelopathy was due to cervical spondylosis	• Clinical follow-up	• 28 M, 16 F • Age 31–40 y: 8 41–50 y: 11 51–60 y: 15 61–70 y: 9 71–80 y: 1	• ≥ 5 y: 26	• NR	• 8 (18.2%)	
Roberts[42] 1966	28	Retrospective cohort	• DCM diagnosed by myelography	• Bedrest, cervical collar (plastic or metal frame)	• 21 M, 7 F • Mean age: 54.2 y.	• Mean: 3 y	• NR	• 1 (4%)	
Barnes and Saunders[22] 1984	45	Retrospective cohort	• Myelopathy with evidence of corticospinal tract dysfunction, with or without sensory involvement or radiculopathy • Plain radiological changes of cervical spondylosis • Myelographic evidence of a complete or partial block to the flow of contrast medium in the cervical spine • No other reasonable diagnosis	• Clinical follow-up • Cervical collar (n = 15)	• 32 M, 12 F • Mean age: 65 y • Mean symptom duration: 1.2 y.	• Mean: 8.2 y	• Nurick grade Improved (≥1): 9 (20%) Unchanged: 30 (66.7%) Worse (≥1): 6 (13.3%)	• NR	• Sex (female) • Cervical mobility

Nakamura et al,[43] 1998	64	Retrospective cohort	• DCM treated conservatively • Motor disability in the upper or lower limbs, or both (JOA)	• Cervical traction, brace, plaster bed holding head and trunk	• 46 M, 18 F • Mean age: 52 y. • Mean symptom duration: 24 mo.	• Mean: 74 mo	• Upper limb JOA score Improved: 31 (55%) Unchanged: 25 (45%) Worse: 0 • Lower limb JOA score Improved: 35 (57%) Unchanged: 24 (39%) Worse: 2 (3%)	19 (29.7%)	• Degree of disability before treatment • Age, symptom duration (not significant)
Bednarik and Kadanka et al,[8–12] (1999–2011)	33	Randomized trial	• Clinical signs and symptoms of cervical cord dysfunction • MRI showing monosegmental or multisegmental cord compression caused by spondylosis • Age < 75 y • mJOA ≥ 12 (mild or moderate DCM)	• Cervical collar, anti-inflammatory medications and intermittent bedrest for patients with pain, discouragement from participation in high-risk activities, and avoidance of risky environments	• 26 M, 7 F • Median age: 54 y. • Median symptom duration: 1.0 y. • Median mJOA: 15	• 6, 12, 24, 36 mo	• mJOA (6 mo) Improved/unchanged: 24 (72.7%) Worse: 9 (27.3%) • mJOA (1 y) Improved/unchanged: 28 (84.9%) Worse: 5 (15.2%) • mJOA (2 y), n = 32 Improved/unchanged: 21 (65.6%) Worse: 11 (34.4%) • mJOA (3 y), n = 30 Improved/unchanged: 22 (73.3%) Worse: 8 (26.7%)	• NR	• Spinal transverse area • Age • CMCT

(continued on next page)

Table 1
(continued)

Author (Year)	N	Study Design	Eligibility Criteria	Conservative Treatment	Baseline Characteristics	Follow-up	Neurologic Outcomes	Surgery	Predictors
Matsumoto et al,[33] 2000	52	Retrospective cohort	• Cervical compressive myelopathy based on neurologic examination and MR findings • JOA $\geq$ 10	• Cervical brace • Restriction of daily activities • Cervical traction (n = 3)	• 39 M, 13 F • Mean age: 55 y. • Mean JOA: 14.0 • Mean symptom duration: 7 mo.	• Mean: 3 y	• Improvement in JOA score or JOA score $\geq$ 15: 36 (69%) • Mean change in JOA score: +0.4	• 10 (19.2%)	
Sampath et al,[15] (2000)	23	Prospective cohort	• Symptom duration $\geq$ 8 wk • One or more physical examination findings of myelopathy	• Pharmacologic therapy • Steroids • Bedrest • Home exercise • Cervical traction • Neck bracing • Spinal injection	• NR	• Mean: 29.8 mo	• Mean change in number of symptoms: +0.42	• NR	
Matsumoto et al,[36] (2001)	27	Retrospective cohort	• Mild to moderate DCM (JOA 10) • Cervical soft disc herniation • Able to walk without cane	• Cervical bracing • Restriction of daily activities • Physical therapy (n = 4)	• 20 M, 7 F • Mean age: 44.4 y. • Mean JOA: 13.8	• Mean: 3.9 y	• NR	• 10 (37.0%)	

Yoshimatsu et al,[35] 2001	69	Retrospective cohort	• DCM based on clinical signs and presence of compression of the spinal cord by MRI	• Conservative treatment • "Rigorous" conservative treatment (cervical traction for 3–4 h daily for 1–3 mo, orthosis)	• 35 M, 34 F • Mean age: 67 y.	• Mean: 29 mo	• JOA Improved: 16 (23%) Unchanged: 10 (14%) Worse: 43 (62%)	• 22 (31.9%)	
Shimomura et al,[37] 2007; Sumi et al,[34] 2012	56	Prospective cohort	• Mild DCM (JOA ≥ 13)	• Cervical traction 8 h/d for 2 wk	• 38 M, 18 F • Mean age: 55.1 y. • Mean JOA: 14.6	• Mean: 35.6 mo[37] and 78.9 mo[34]	• 3 y JOA < 13: 11 (19.6%) • 6.5 y JOA < 13 with a decrease of ≥ 2: 14 (25.5%) Decrease in JOA ≥ 2: 17 (30.9%)	• 3 y: 9 (16.1%) • 6.5 y: 12 (21.8%)	• Circumferential spinal cord compression
Oshima et al,[16] (2012)	45	Retrospective cohort	• Motor JOA scores ≥ 3 in both upper and lower limbs • Cervical spinal cord compression with T2 signal on MRI • No disc herniation or OPLL	• Clinical follow-up	• 27 M, 18 F • Mean age: 59 y.	• Mean: 78 mo	• NR	• 18 (40%)	• Total cervical ROM, segmental kyphosis at level of maximal compression, local slip

Abbreviations: CMCT, central motor conduction time; DCM, degenerative cervical myelopathy; F, female; JOA, Japanese Orthopedic Association; M, male; mJOA, modified JOA; NR, not reported; ROM, range of motion.

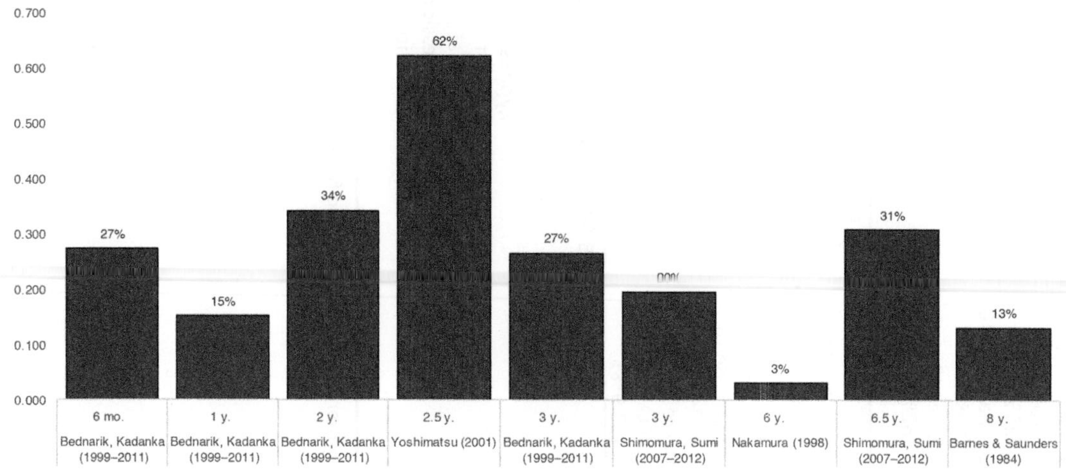

Fig. 1. Bar graph summary of rates of neurologic deterioration, as measured by the JOA or mJOA scale or Nurick grade, by duration of follow-up and study.

colleagues[7] found the reported rate of operation after failed nonoperative management to range from 4% to 40% during a follow-up period of 3 to 7 years. Oshima and colleagues[16] retrospectively evaluated 45 patients with DCM treated nonoperatively. All patients had JOA scores of 3 or greater in both upper and lower limbs and presence of increased signal on T2-weighted MRI (T2WI). The authors performed a Kaplan-Meier survival analysis with conversion to surgery due to neurologic deterioration as the endpoint, which revealed that 82% and 56% of patients did not require surgery at 5 and 10 years after initial conservative treatment, respectively.

Mortality

In their 10-year follow-up, Kadanka and colleagues[11] examined overall survival and constructed Kaplan-Meier curves for patients with mild or moderate DCM randomized to surgery or conservative treatment. No difference was observed in mortality. Ten patients treated operatively and 7 in the conservative group died during study follow-up, all of natural causes.

PREDICTORS OF OUTCOME

Predictors of surgical outcome in DCM have been relatively well studied; among these are age, symptom duration, baseline severity of myelopathy, presence of psychiatric comorbidities, smoking status, cervical curvature, T2 signal on MRI, and diameter of the spinal canal.[17–20] The complementary identification of factors associated with improvement (or worsening) in the setting of nonoperative treatment would permit selective targeting of spinal decompression to those patients with DCM who are most likely to benefit from surgery, but who would otherwise deteriorate with a conservative strategy. Nonetheless, compared with surgery, fewer studies have evaluated demographic, clinical, and radiological factors associated with outcomes in patients who are treated nonoperatively. The quality of evidence from these studies is generally poor and few definitive conclusions can be drawn.[7]

With regard to evidence derived from RCTs, Kadanka and colleagues[10] investigated the relation of clinical, electrophysiological, and imaging parameters to clinical outcome in patients with mild or moderate DCM randomized to surgery or conservative therapy. In patients treated conservatively, older age, larger transverse area of the spinal cord, higher Pavlov index, and normal values of central motor conduction time to the upper extremities were associated with positive response to treatment, defined as no change or improvement in mJOA score. The Pavlov index is the ratio of the anteroposterior (AP) diameter of the spinal canal to the AP diameter of the vertebral body from measurement on lateral cervical spine radiograph, with higher values suggesting a congenitally wider spinal canal.[21] On the other hand, greater clinical severity of DCM, as indicated by lower mJOA score, and smaller transverse area of the spinal cord predicted response to surgical decompression.

Barnes and Saunders[22] retrospectively evaluated 45 patients with DCM treated conservatively over a mean follow-up of 8.2 years. Patients were separated into those who had improved at least 1 Nurick grade (9; 20%), remained unchanged (30; 66.7%), or had deteriorated (6; 13.3%) at least 1 Nurick grade over the course of follow-up. The group that deteriorated was more likely to be female. Moreover, greater range of neck and head movement was associated with neurologic deterioration. Dynamic changes, that is, movement of the spinal cord against protruding osteophytes within the canal during flexion and extension, is thought to be an important mechanism in the pathogenesis of DCM.[23–25] This provides the rationale for external collar immobilization as a nonoperative treatment modality, to remove the dynamic factor. Multiple investigators have reported less frequent neurologic deterioration with cervical collar use, although these were generally low-quality, early studies.[6,26–28] Other studies have also implicated dynamic factors in the efficacy (or lack thereof) of conservative therapy for DCM. Oshima and colleagues[16] performed a Kaplan-Meier survival analysis for conversion to surgery due to neurologic deterioration after conservative treatment for DCM. Cox proportional hazards analysis revealed total cervical range of motion $\geq$50°, segmental kyphosis at the maximum compression segment, and local slip of 2 mm or more to be significant adverse prognostic factors, predicting need for surgery. Likewise, significant postoperative mobility has been also associated with poorer outcomes and recurrence of DCM after surgery.[29–31]

Static imaging parameters, too, have been studied and implicated as predictors of the natural course of DCM. Importantly, increased signal intensity (ISI) on T2WI is often considered an indication to operate, as it may reflect myelomalacia or gliosis, and spell the beginning of irreversible damage to the spinal cord.[18,32] However, the available evidence would indicate the presence of ISI on T2WI does not increase or decrease the probability of deterioration with conservative management.[33–35] Matsumoto and colleagues[33] retrospectively evaluated 52 patients with mild DCM who underwent conservative treatment with a cervical brace. An area of ISI on T2WI was absent in 18 patients (34.6%), present focally in 24 (46.2%), and present at multiple segments in 10 (19.2%). No difference in achievement of satisfactory outcome, defined as an improvement in JOA score or a JOA score $\geq$15, was seen in those without ISI (78%), with focal ISI (63%), or with multisegmental ISI (70%). Thirty-nine patients underwent follow-up MRI at an average interval of 28 months. Of 28 patients with areas of ISI on T2WI at baseline who underwent follow-up MRI, the area of ISI had regressed in 5 (18%). Mean JOA score in these 5 patients improved from 13.4 before treatment to 16.4 at follow-up, with a satisfactory outcome being reached in all 5 (100%). Of 23 patients in whom ISI had not regressed, satisfactory outcome was still achieved in 16 (70%).

The extent of compression on MRI, as measured by transverse area of the spinal cord at the site of maximal compression, has generally not been associated with outcome in patients treated nonsurgically,[33,34,36] apart from in 1 study.[10] Nonetheless, there is some circumferential compression that may portend worse outcomes. Shimomura and colleagues[37] conducted a prospective cohort study in 56 patients with mild DCM (JOA $\geq$13) treated conservatively with cervical traction. At a mean follow-up of 35.6 months, 11 patients (19.6%) had deteriorated to moderate or severe forms of myelopathy (JOA <13). Age, gender, follow-up period, developmental or dynamic canal factors on plain lateral radiographs, and presence of T2 signal within the cord were not important prognostic factors. Only circumferential spinal cord compression was found to predict a deteriorating clinical condition, with 10 of 33 patients with circumferential compression having a worse neurologic outcome.

It is thought the natural history of DCM may differ depending on the etiology of cervical spinal cord compression. Soft disc herniations causing myelopathy, for example, frequently regress on follow-up MRI.[38,39] Indeed, some investigators have observed neurologic deficits, too, to follow a more benign course in the case of soft disc herniations. Matsumoto and colleagues[36] retrospectively compared outcomes in 27 patients with mild DCM secondary to soft disc herniations. Seventeen patients underwent conservative treatment, and the remaining 10 ultimately underwent decompressive surgery, either because of neurologic deterioration or because their disability remained unchanged (preoperative JOA $\leq$14). JOA scores were comparable in both groups at baseline (13.6 vs 14.1), and significantly higher in conservatively treated patients at 3 (14.9 vs 12.9) and 6 months (15.6 vs 12.1), but not at final follow-up (16.2 vs 16.0). Patient satisfaction was comparable: 77% in the conservative cohort and 90% in the surgical group. In 59% of patients, there was spontaneous regression of the disc herniation with resolution of neurologic symptoms. Diffuse-type disc herniations (as assessed on sagittal plane MRIs) were found to be more likely to regress on follow-up MRI examination than more focal herniations (78% vs 37%, respectively). In addition, paramedian rather than median disc herniations were more frequently seen in patients requiring surgery. The investigators reasoned that disc herniations that migrate diffusely into the epidural space may be more susceptible to breakdown by inflammatory mediators. Moreover, because the spinal canal is narrower and the spinal cord is tethered by the nerve roots and dentate ligaments laterally, the spinal cord may be more susceptible to compression by a paramedian disc herniation. On a similar note, Sumi and colleagues[34] distinguished MRI findings into 2 categories based on the shape of the lateral aspect of the spinal cord at the level of maximal compression: (1) "ovoid," with a round and convex corner at both sides; and (2) "angular-edged," with an acute angle lateral corner at 1 or both sides. Angular-edged deformity was found to correlate with greater risk of neurologic worsening in patients with DCM treated conservatively, with 36% of patients deteriorating, as compared with those with an ovoid deformity (5%).

Although we often evaluate surgery for DCM as a single, homogeneous intervention, the outcome of surgery is impacted by several factors, including likely the surgical technique used (ie, Anterior cervical discectomy and fusion vs laminoplasty vs laminectomy alone vs laminectomy with instrumented fusion). Similarly, there are many different conservative treatment modalities for DCM, each with its own efficacy, although likely similar. Among these are traction,[37,40] collar,[6,26–28] analgesics, physical therapy, bedrest, avoidance of risk activities (eg, contact sports) and environments (eg, slippery floors),[37] and spinal injections. At the present time, it is unclear which specific modality of nonoperative treatment is most or least effective.[41] Yoshimatsu and colleagues[35] examined 69 patients who underwent conservative treatment of DCM. Neurologic function was evaluated by the JOA. Age, AP diameter of the spinal canal, presence of ISI on MRI, and number of intervertebral discs compressing the spine were not found to predict either improved or worsened neurologic function on logistic regression. However, the rate of improvement was found to be higher in those who underwent "rigorous" conservative therapy, which included cervical traction for 3 to 4 hours per day for 1 to 3 months combined with cervical orthosis, drug therapy, and exercise therapy. Of patients receiving rigorous conservative therapy, 38% improved, 14% remained unchanged, and 49% worsened in neurologic function, as compared with 6%, 16%, and 78%, respectively, in those receiving "nonrigorous" conservative treatment. In addition, longer duration of symptoms was found to predict deterioration, and shorter duration of symptoms, improvement. The investigators conclude the probability of symptomatic improvement in mild DCM may be maximized by implementing intense conservative therapy early in the disease course.

SUMMARY

There remains a paucity of high-quality evidence regarding the natural course of DCM. Rates of deterioration with nonoperative strategies may reach upward of 50% at 3 to 6 years. Nonoperative care is not recommended for patients with moderate or severe DCM, in which conservative approaches carry significant risk of neurologic deterioration and outcomes are inferior to those of surgery. For patients with mild DCM, there is low evidence to suggest nonoperative management may have a role. The single RCT on the topic failed to find a difference in outcomes between mildly myelopathic patients treated surgically and those managed nonoperatively. However, the outcomes of surgery in this study appeared to be subpar. The most recent and robust evidence, coming from the AOSpine Cervical Spondylotic Myelopathy North America[2] and International[3] studies, has found surgical decompression to not only halt progression of myelopathy, but result in improvement in neurologic outcomes, functional status, and quality of life. This, together with the seemingly unpredictable risk of neurologic decline with conservative treatment, should be clearly communicated to patients. Depending on patient preference, it would not be unreasonable to start with a "wait-and-see" approach in those with mild, nonprogressive DCM. This could include immobilization with a cervical orthosis. Patients should be counseled on the risk of exacerbation of symptoms with even minor trauma. No demographic, clinical, radiological, or electrophysiological characteristics appear to predict the risk of neurologic deterioration reliably. Therefore, clinicians should exercise vigilance if the nonoperative route is chosen, and patients should receive close clinical follow-up. Progression of neurologic deficits should trigger prompt surgery.

There remains a need for prospective studies evaluating the natural course of mild DCM. As evidence of the efficacy of surgery continues to mount, however, a randomized trial is unlikely to be feasible, owing to ethical concern over randomizing patients who could potentially benefit from surgical intervention to conservative therapy, the merits of which are uncertain. A prospective cohort study of patients with mild DCM is hence perhaps the best we will be able to achieve to address this important question.

REFERENCES

1. Nurick S. The pathogenesis of the spinal cord disorder associated with cervical spondylosis. Brain 1972;95(1):87–100.

2. Fehlings MG, Wilson JR, Kopjar B, et al. Efficacy and safety of surgical decompression in patients with cervical spondylotic myelopathy: results of the AO-Spine North America prospective multi-center study. J Bone Joint Surg Am 2013;95(18):1651–8.
3. Fehlings MG, Ibrahim A, Tetreault L, et al. A global perspective on the outcomes of surgical decompression in patients with cervical spondylotic myelopathy: results from the prospective multicenter AOSpine international study on 479 patients. Spine (Phila Pa 1976) 2015;40(17):1322–8.
4. Brain WR, Knight GC, Bull JW. Discussion of rupture of the intervertebral disc in the cervical region. Proc R Soc Med 1948;41(8):509–16.
5. Brain WR, Knight GC, Bull JW. Diseases of the nervous system. London: Oxford University Press; 1962.
6. Lees F, Turner JW. Natural history and prognosis of cervical spondylosis. Br Med J 1963;2(5373): 1607–10.
7. Karadimas SK, Erwin WM, Ely CG, et al. Pathophysiology and natural history of cervical spondylotic myelopathy. Spine (Phila Pa 1976) 2013;38(22 Suppl 1):S21–36.
8. Kadanka Z, Bednarik J, Vohanka S, et al. Conservative treatment versus surgery in spondylotic cervical myelopathy: a prospective randomised study. Eur Spine J 2000;9(6):538–44.
9. Kadanka Z, Mares M, Bednanik J, et al. Approaches to spondylotic cervical myelopathy: conservative versus surgical results in a 3-year follow-up study. Spine (Phila Pa 1976) 2002;27(20):2205–10 [discussion: 2210–2211].
10. Kadanka Z, Mares M, Bednarik J, et al. Predictive factors for mild forms of spondylotic cervical myelopathy treated conservatively or surgically. Eur J Neurol 2005;12(1):16–24.
11. Kadanka Z, Bednarik J, Novotny O, et al. Cervical spondylotic myelopathy: conservative versus surgical treatment after 10 years. Eur Spine J 2011; 20(9):1533–8.
12. Bednarik J, Kadanka Z, Vohanka S, et al. The value of somatosensory- and motor-evoked potentials in predicting and monitoring the effect of therapy in spondylotic cervical myelopathy. Prospective randomized study. Spine (Phila Pa 1976) 1999;24(15): 1593–8.
13. Bednarik J, Sladkova D, Kadanka Z, et al. Are subjects with spondylotic cervical cord encroachment at increased risk of cervical spinal cord injury after minor trauma? J Neurol Neurosurg Psychiatry 2011;82(7):779–81.
14. Katoh S, Ikata T, Hirai N, et al. Influence of minor trauma to the neck on the neurological outcome in patients with ossification of the posterior longitudinal ligament (OPLL) of the cervical spine. Paraplegia 1995;33(6):330–3.
15. Sampath P, Bendebba M, Davis JD, et al. Outcome of patients treated for cervical myelopathy. A prospective, multicenter study with independent clinical review. Spine (Phila Pa 1976) 2000;25(6):670–6.
16. Oshima Y, Seichi A, Takeshita K, et al. Natural course and prognostic factors in patients with mild cervical spondylotic myelopathy with increased signal intensity on T2-weighted magnetic resonance imaging. Spine (Phila Pa 1976) 2012;37(22):1909–13.
17. Suri A, Chabbra RP, Mehta VS, et al. Effect of intramedullary signal changes on the surgical outcome of patients with cervical spondylotic myelopathy. Spine J 2003;3(1):33–45.
18. Takahashi M, Yamashita Y, Sakamoto Y, et al. Chronic cervical cord compression: clinical significance of increased signal intensity on MR images. Radiology 1989;173(1):219–24.
19. Naderi S, Ozgen S, Pamir MN, et al. Cervical spondylotic myelopathy: surgical results and factors affecting prognosis. Neurosurgery 1998;43(1):43–9 [discussion: 49–50].
20. Tetreault L, Kopjar B, Cote P, et al. A clinical prediction rule for functional outcomes in patients undergoing surgery for degenerative cervical myelopathy: analysis of an international prospective multicenter data set of 757 subjects. J Bone Joint Surg Am 2015;97(24):2038–46.
21. Pavlov H, Torg JS, Robie B, et al. Cervical spinal stenosis: determination with vertebral body ratio method. Radiology 1987;164(3):771–5.
22. Barnes MP, Saunders M. The effect of cervical mobility on the natural history of cervical spondylotic myelopathy. J Neurol Neurosurg Psychiatry 1984; 47(1):17–20.
23. Adams CB, Logue V. Studies in cervical spondylotic myelopathy. II. The movement and contour of the spine in relation to the neural complications of cervical spondylosis. Brain 1971;94(3):568–86.
24. Adams CB, Logue V. Studies in cervical spondylotic myelopathy. I. Movement of the cervical roots, dura and cord, and their relation to the course of the extrathecal roots. Brain 1971;94(3):557–68.
25. Fukui K, Kataoka O, Sho T, et al. Pathomechanism, pathogenesis, and results of treatment in cervical spondylotic myelopathy caused by dynamic canal stenosis. Spine (Phila Pa 1976) 1990; 15(11):1148–52.
26. Clarke E, Robinson PK. Cervical myelopathy: a complication of cervical spondylosis. Brain 1956; 79(3):483–510.
27. Campbell AM, Phillips DG. Cervical disk lesions with neurological disorder. Differential diagnosis, treatment, and prognosis. Br Med J 1960; 2(5197):481–5.
28. LaRocca H. Cervical spondylotic myelopathy: natural history. Spine (Phila Pa 1976) 1988;13(7):854–5.

29. Yoshii N, Nakahara S. Mobility of the cervical spine after anterior interbody fusion for spondylotic myelopathy—a radiographic study. Clin Biomech (Bristol, Avon) 1988;3(1):19–26.
30. Adams CB, Logue V. Studies in cervical spondylotic myelopathy. 3. Some functional effects of operations for cervical spondylotic myelopathy. Brain 1971; 94(3):587–94.
31. Gonzalez-Feria L, Peraita-Peraita P. Cervical spondylotic myelopathy: a cooperative study. Clin Neurol Neurosurg 1975;78(1):19–33.
32. Mehalic TF, Pezzuti RT, Applebaum BI. Magnetic resonance imaging and cervical spondylotic myelopathy. Neurosurgery 1990;26(2):217–26 [discussion: 226–217].
33. Matsumoto M, Toyama Y, Ishikawa M, et al. Increased signal intensity of the spinal cord on magnetic resonance images in cervical compressive myelopathy. Does it predict the outcome of conservative treatment? Spine (Phila Pa 1976) 2000;25(6): 677–82.
34. Sumi M, Miyamoto H, Suzuki T, et al. Prospective cohort study of mild cervical spondylotic myelopathy without surgical treatment. J Neurosurg Spine 2012;16(1):8–14.
35. Yoshimatsu H, Nagata K, Goto H, et al. Conservative treatment for cervical spondylotic myelopathy. Prediction of treatment effects by multivariate analysis. Spine J 2001;1(4):269–73.
36. Matsumoto M, Chiba K, Ishikawa M, et al. Relationships between outcomes of conservative treatment and magnetic resonance imaging findings in patients with mild cervical myelopathy caused by soft disc herniations. Spine (Phila Pa 1976) 2001; 26(14):1592–8.
37. Shimomura T, Sumi M, Nishida K, et al. Prognostic factors for deterioration of patients with cervical spondylotic myelopathy after nonsurgical treatment. Spine (Phila Pa 1976) 2007;32(22):2474–9.
38. Mochida K, Komori H, Okawa A, et al. Regression of cervical disc herniation observed on magnetic resonance images. Spine (Phila Pa 1976) 1998;23(9): 990–5 [discussion: 996-997].
39. Bush K, Chaudhuri R, Hillier S, et al. The pathomorphologic changes that accompany the resolution of cervical radiculopathy. A prospective study with repeat magnetic resonance imaging. Spine (Phila Pa 1976) 1997;22(2):183–6 [discussion: 187].
40. Borden JN. Good samaritan cervical traction. Clin Orthop Relat Res 1975;(113):162–3.
41. Rhee JM, Shamji MF, Erwin WM, et al. Nonoperative management of cervical myelopathy: a systematic review. Spine (Phila Pa 1976) 2013;38(22 Suppl 1): S55–67.
42. Roberts AH. Myelopathy due to cervical spondylosis treated by collar immobilization. Neurology 1966;16: 951–4.
43. Nakamura K, Kurokawa T, Hoshino Y, et al. Conservative treatment for cervical spondylotic myelopathy: achievement and sustainability of a level of "no disability". J Spinal Disord 1998; 11(2):175–9.

Imaging Evaluation of Degenerative Cervical Myelopathy

Current State of the Art and Future Directions

Allan R. Martin, MD, PhD[a,*], Nobuaki Tadokoro, MD, PhD[b,c], Lindsay Tetreault, PhD[c,d], Elsa V. Arocho-Quinones, MD[e], Matthew D. Budde, PhD[e], Shekar N. Kurpad, MD, PhD[f], Michael G. Fehlings, MD, PhD, FRCSC[c]

KEYWORDS

• Magnetic resonance imaging • MRI • Spine • Degenerative cervical myelopathy

KEY POINTS

- Radiographs, CT, and MRI offer unique and complementary assessments, and all have important uses in current clinical practice.
- Several microstructural and functional MRI techniques can reveal detailed information about changes in the spinal cord and brain, including diffusion tensor imaging, myelin imaging, atrophy measures, and functional MRI.
- These emerging MRI techniques have the potential to transform clinical practice by offering earlier and more accurate diagnosis, monitoring of disease progression and treatment effects, and prediction of outcomes.

INTRODUCTION

Degenerative Cervical Myelopathy

Degenerative cervical myelopathy (DCM) is a spectrum of disorders that involve extrinsic spinal cord compression leading to neurologic dysfunction, including intervertebral disk herniation, cervical spondylotic myelopathy (CSM), and ossified posterior longitudinal ligament (OPLL).[1] These pathologies variably involve degeneration of the intervertebral disks, hypertrophy and/or ossification of the spinal ligaments, and remodeling (flattening and widening) of the vertebrae.[1] These changes lead to compression of the spinal cord and result in ischemia, dynamic (motion-related) injury, and inflammation that injure the gray and white matter of the cervical spinal cord. The

Disclosure Statement: The authors have nothing to disclose.

[a] Division of Neurosurgery, Department of Surgery, University of Toronto, 8 Queen Victoria Street, Toronto, Ontario M4J1E9, Canada; [b] Department of Orthopedic Surgery, Kochi University, Kochi Medical School, Kohasu Oko-chou, Nankoku 783-8505, Japan; [c] Division of Neurosurgery, Department of Surgery, Krembil Research Institute, University of Toronto, 60 Leonard Avenue, Toronto, Ontario M5T 2S8, Canada; [d] Graduate Entry Medicine, University College Cork, College Road, Cork T12 YN60, Ireland; [e] Department of Neurosurgery, Medical College of Wisconsin, W. Wisconsin Avenue, Milwaukee, WI 53226, USA; [f] Department of Neurosurgery, Medical College of Wisconsin, Spinal Cord Injury Center, Froedtert Hospital, W. Wisconsin Avenue, Milwaukee, WI 53226, USA
* Corresponding author.
E-mail address: allan.martin@utoronto.ca

Neurosurg Clin N Am 29 (2018) 33–45
https://doi.org/10.1016/j.nec.2017.09.003
1042-3680/18/© 2017 Elsevier Inc. All rights reserved.

neurosurgery.theclinics.com

most common level of compression is C5-6, but compression often occurs at multiple levels in the region between C3 and C7.[2] The prevalence of symptomatic DCM is poorly characterized due to a lack of large population-based studies and challenges with accurate diagnosis; however, estimates suggest that it is the most common cause of myelopathy in adults.[3,4]

Clinical Management of Degenerative Cervical Myelopathy

When DCM symptoms arise, they typically begin with subtle fine motor dysfunction of the hands, imbalance when walking, and numbness of the hands. As myelopathic impairment worsens, marked loss of hand dexterity, gait dysfunction, severe hand numbness, bladder incontinence, and focal weakness of the upper extremities commonly occur. Clinical practice guidelines recommend surgery for moderate to severe cases,[5] but the optimal treatment of mild CSM is unclear because some patients experience long-term stability whereas others deteriorate.[6] For individuals with minimal deficits, the decision to undergo surgery is difficult, because the risks and benefits are closely balanced. Due to this uncertainty, surgery is often delayed until the onset of more substantial neurologic deficits, but these are only partially reversible with surgery.[7] Thus, prediction or early detection of neurologic decline could substantially improve patient outcomes. Unfortunately, efforts to identify clinical and imaging predictors have shown weak performance.[8]

The Role of Imaging in Degenerative Cervical Myelopathy

The field of medical imaging has rapidly evolved over the past 50 years, and several of these advances have led to major changes in the clinical management of DCM. Imaging currently plays several critical roles in managing DCM patients, including diagnosis, planning surgical treatment, prognostication, and postoperative assessment. Although MRI can be considered the gold standard imaging investigation, providing the most important clinical information for each of these purposes, radiographs and CT continue to be useful, contributing unique and complementary information. This article reviews each of these imaging modalities and describe their strengths, limitations, and clinical utility for the aforementioned clinical uses (**Table 1**), followed by a discussion of emerging spinal cord imaging techniques and their implications for the future of clinical management of DCM.

A SUMMARY OF CURRENT IMAGING TECHNIQUES

Radiographs

Radiographs, also known as plain films or x-rays, are based on the differential tissue absorption of electromagnetic radiation in the x-ray spectrum (3×10^{16} to 3×10^{19}). Despite their simplicity and numerous limitations, radiographs provide versatile 2-D views of the spine that display several important features and can identify many sources of pathology. Due to the high calcium and mineral

Table 1
Strengths and limitations of current imaging techniques

	Radiographs	CT	MRI	Quantitative MRI
Strengths	• Alignment (physiologic) • Osteophytes • Spondylosis • OPLL, ossified ligamentum flavum • Bony lesions • Versatile projections/angles • Instability (flexion/extension)	• 3-D • Detailed bony anatomy/lesions • Spondylosis • OPLL, ossified ligamentum flavum • Screw planning • Bone quality	• 3D • Detailed soft tissue anatomy • Spinal cord compression • Disks • Ligaments • Microhemorrhage • Intramedullary signal change (T1-weighted, T2-weighted)	• Spinal cord tissue changes (microstructure) • May improve diagnosis, monitoring for progression, outcome prediction
Limitations	• 2-D • Minimal soft tissue view	• Supine • Limited soft tissue view	• Supine • Limited bony anatomy • Spinal cord tissue changes	• Complex techniques (acquisition and analysis) • Limited by noise, wide range of normal

composition of bones, radiography offers excellent contrast between the vertebrae and surrounding structures. Plain films of the spine offer several advantages over other imaging techniques, particularly because they can be taken with the patient and x-ray machine in almost any position, allowing assessment of spinal alignment and instability under physiologic conditions.

CT

CT is a modality that is also based on x-ray absorption, but it can perform high-resolution cross-sectional imaging and provide 3-D views of the anatomy. Similar to radiographs, CT provides an excellent view of bony structures, albeit with the limitation that the subject is in the supine position. CT is widely available, fast (studies can usually be completed in under 10 minutes), and easy to access, allowing primary care physicians to order these investigations without long wait times. The view of soft tissues offered by CT is poor, however, and not sufficient to identify spinal cord compression in individuals with suspected DCM. CT myelography is an invasive technique in which contrast dye is injected into the lumbar cistern prior to CT imaging, providing excellent visualization of the contour of the spinal cord and potentially compressive surrounding structures. CT myelography, however, involves risks and is an uncomfortable or painful procedure, and in the current era it is rarely performed in patients who can undergo MRI. CT, in general, also has the major drawback of involving much higher doses of ionizing radiation (100× that of a plain film) and should therefore be used sparingly, particularly in younger individuals.

MRI

MRI is among the most elegant technologies that mankind has developed, built on complex physics and intricate engineering. This imaging technique involves the manipulation of the magnetic spins of protons within water molecules (although other variations have been used in a research context). Placing a subject in a strong magnetic field causes the spins of water protons to align parallel or antiparallel to the field, with a slight imbalance creating a net magnetization. These protons are then excited with radiofrequency electromagnetic radiation, specifically at the frequency at which water protons precess (wobble on their axis), known as the Larmor frequency. This can be used to coerce the net magnetization into a direction perpendicular to the main magnetic field, while causing protons to precess in phase with each other. At this point, these in-phase protons have a maximal electromagnetic signal that can be read by induction coils, but the signal quickly decays due to spin-spin dephasing (known as T2 decay), which combines with the dephasing effects of local magnetic field inhomogeneity (collectively known as T2* decay). The spins also return to a state of equilibrium parallel to the main magnetic field, restoring the original net magnetization (known as T1 recovery). Different tissues have unique T1, T2, and T2* properties and thus offer the opportunity to create images that show brilliant contrast between structures. Various MRI sequences have been devised that produce images with T1-weighted, T2-weighted, and T2*-weighted contrast, each highlighting different anatomic and pathologic features. Furthermore, several methods of nulling specific tissues or regions are available, such as fat suppression with short-tau inversion recovery, which allows inspection of the spinal ligaments that tend to be surrounded by a small amount of fat. As a result, MRI provides noninvasive imaging of the spinal cord and surrounding tissues with unprecedented detail, playing a central role in clinical management of DCM.

CURRENT USES OF IMAGING IN DEGENERATIVE CERVICAL MYELOPATHY

Diagnosis

The diagnosis of DCM is typically made using a combination of clinical and imaging findings that identify it as the most likely cause of symptoms, while ruling out other pathologies. More specifically, diagnosis requires 1 or more symptoms (hand clumsiness, gait imbalance, numbness, weakness, and bladder dysfunction) and signs (fine motor dysfunction of the hands, hyperreflexia, gait ataxia, sensory deficits, and focal weakness) that localize to the cervical spinal cord, combined with the presence of spinal cord compression on MRI. This may seem straightforward, but DCM is a surprisingly complex condition that involves multiple mechanisms of tissue injury, and its diagnosis is frequently challenging, particularly in mild cases. First, mild symptoms are often intermittent and subjective, creating uncertainty about their relevance. Clinical examination is also subjective and varies between practitioners, and the diagnosis of mild DCM is often based on subtle hyperreflexia or gait ataxia. Furthermore, imaging criteria for spinal cord compression vary widely between studies, and a clear consensus of what constitutes compression does not exist. This is complicated by the fact that mild compression of the spinal cord due to bulging disks, osteophytes, or ligaments is present in a large number of healthy, asymptomatic individuals, particularly in the cervical region. Estimates of the prevalence of asymptomatic cervical spinal cord compression range from 8% to 57%, making it far more common than DCM.[9–14] In addition, spinal cord compression may not be evident on supine imaging because it is positional or dynamic in nature. For example, if a patient tends to be kyphotic when upright, the spinal cord may be compressed anteriorly as it is pressed up against the vertebral bodies, bulging disks, osteophytes, or OPLL. Therefore, correct diagnosis of DCM often requires expert judgment to combine clinical and imaging findings.

Radiographs and CT can show the degree of bony canal stenosis, but they do not show the spinal cord and are thus not sufficient for diagnosis of DCM. MRI is the most useful imaging investigation for DCM diagnosis, because it clearly shows the outline of the spinal cord and nerve roots in relation to surrounding cerebrospinal fluid (CSF). T2-weighted images have the greatest contrast between cord and CSF, but T1-weighted or other image types may also show good contrast. Any deformation of the spinal cord from its normal shape, such as flattening, indentation, torsion, or circumferential narrowing due to adjacent tissues (eg, a bulging disk), should be considered a type of compression that may or may not cause neurologic dysfunction.[14] Cases of dynamic compression may require flexion/extension MRI to diagnose, which is an approach that is gaining popularity.[15] Certain older studies suggested that T2-weighted signal hyperintensity within the spinal cord was necessary to identify tissue injury and diagnose DCM,[16] but more recent large studies have found that this hyperintensity is only present in approximately 60% of all DCM patients and in fewer than half of patients with mild DCM.[17] When MRI is not possible due to metallic implants (eg, pacemaker) or severe claustrophobia, CT myelography remains a useful option to identify spinal cord compression, although in cases of severe stenosis, a complete block of CSF may prevent diffusion of the contrast agent rostrally, leading to incomplete imaging of the upper cervical cord that may also be compressed.

Surgical Planning

Many individuals with DCM are treated surgically, which may be performed using an anterior, posterior, or combined surgical approach and may or may not include instrumentation, such as fixation or arthroplasty. A complete discussion of the available surgical treatment options is beyond the scope of this article, but imaging provides the bulk of information that influences the surgical approach and the number of levels that require decompression. The authors advocate that radiographs, CT, and MRI all provide useful information for surgical planning and should all be obtained, whenever possible, prior to surgical treatment of DCM.

Radiographs can identify and characterize numerous elements that are important for surgical planning, including spinal alignment, osteophytes, spondylosis, and OPLL. The alignment of the spine is best assessed under load-bearing conditions (which is impossible with standard CT and MRI scanners), with the patient standing, sitting, and in postures of flexion or extension. Thus, radiographs are an essential part of surgical planning for DCM, because they can reveal abnormal alignment in the sagittal plane in terms of kyphosis, hyperlordosis, spondylolisthesis, and dynamic instability (translation greater than 2–3 mm in the anteroposterior [AP] direction). Alignment of the cervical spine must also be considered in the context of the entire spine, because pathology below can exacerbate or create poor alignment in the cervical region, and long cassette or 3-ft standing radiographs allow assessment of complete spinal alignment. With respect to DCM, kyphosis is increasingly recognized as an important factor, causing anterior compression and tension on the spinal cord as it is draped over the vertebral bodies (and bulging disks/osteophytes) and imparting a worse prognosis.[18] Flexion/extension radiographs of the cervical spine can determine if kyphosis is reducible or fixed, and the latter case should warrant strong consideration for anterior surgery to allow correction. Flexion/extension views can also detect instability related to ligamentous laxity, which is more common in individuals with inflammatory arthritis (eg, rheumatoid arthritis), and this finding indicates a need for instrumented fixation. Preoperative x-rays are also useful as a baseline examination to compare postoperative films against, particularly to assess issues of alignment and instability. The presence of OPLL spanning several segments should also be taken into consideration, because anterior decompression in these cases requires multilevel corpectomies that increase the surgical risk, warranting stronger consideration for posterior treatment.

CT provides 3-D information that is useful to completely understand the bony anatomy and plan surgical treatment. OPLL is best characterized by CT because it can distinguish between subtypes and clearly define the extent and geometry of pathology. For cases of DCM in which instrumentation is needed, screw trajectories can be measured and planned based on CT data.

Most spinal navigation systems are based on a preoperative CT scan that defines the bony anatomy, and the intraoperative space is registered to the CT to allow real-time tracking and navigation of screws. The quality of bone can also be assessed by CT, which may influence the type of instrumentation and number of levels, although a bone mineral density scan is needed to formally diagnose osteoporosis or osteopenia. Finally, CT and/or CT angiography may be useful to identify anomalous vertebral artery anatomy. This most commonly affects C1 and C2 levels, in which cases CT angiography or MR angiography should be performed, but occasionally subaxial cervical levels have a vertebral artery and foramen transversarium with an abnormally medial position that poses a serious risk of injury (**Fig. 1**).

Although radiographs and CT provide useful information, surgical planning for DCM requires visualization of the spinal cord and the soft tissues of the spinal canal, which is best achieved using MRI. The information provided by MRI includes the degree of spinal cord compression, the cause of compression, the number of compressed levels, and the degree of degeneration of other levels (eg, adjacent disks). When MRI shows that compression is primarily anterior (eg, related to a bulging disc/osteophyte) or posterior (eg, ligamentum flavum hypertrophy), decompression from that direction is preferable to address the source of pathology. The surgeon must always ask the question: If I perform only anterior or posterior surgery, will an adequate decompression be achieved? This question can often be answered based on the preoperative MRI by careful inspection or measurement of the canal diameter at the compressed level and above/below. The number of levels with spinal cord compression is also an important factor, because a greater number may disproportionately increase the risk of anterior surgery due to the complex anatomy, and many surgeons are unfamiliar with anterior cervical procedures that span more than 2 or 3 disk levels. Surgeons should also carefully examine the preoperative MRI for the status of adjacent levels; when there is evidence of advanced degeneration that has not yet caused spinal cord compression, consideration should be given to extending the procedure to include that level, particularly in instrumented cases where the risk of adjacent segment cord compression is elevated. Finally, it is important that the MRI used for surgical planning is up to date, because it is inadvisable to use an MRI that was performed more than 6 months prior to surgical treatment so that new levels of spinal cord compression are not missed.

Monitoring for Progression

Some patients who are diagnosed with DCM are managed nonoperatively due to patient preference or because the patient and/or surgeon do not feel that the risk of surgery is justified by its potential benefits. Often, surgeons or primary care physicians repeat an MRI for these patients to assess if spinal cord compression has progressed, either at a previously compressed level or new level. This concept is akin to monitoring a patient with a benign tumor for growth over time, which typically prompts surgical treatment. Few studies have investigated this population longitudinally, however, and the role of MRI or other types of imaging to monitor for worsening of disease has not been defined. It might be imagined that neurologic

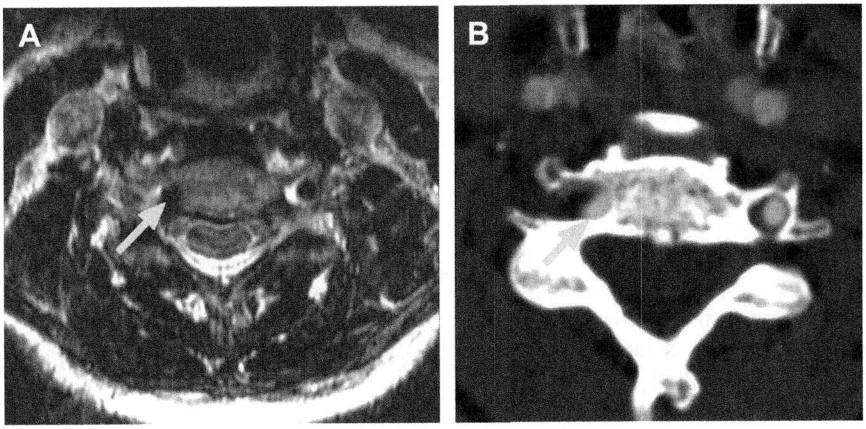

Fig. 1. Imaging showing anomalous vertebral artery. T2-weighted MRI (*A*) and CT (*B*) images show the right vertebral artery (*arrows*) takes an anomalous course medially into the C5 vertebral body. This is important to identify because the medial position of the artery increases the risk of injury during discectomy, corpectomy, or screw placement.

worsening would usually correspond with increased spinal cord compression in DCM, but the authors' data in a cohort of 26 patients revealed that cord compression remained stable in approximately 80% of patients who showed neurologic decline.[19] It is also conceivable that progressive kyphosis on radiographs might be indicative of disease progression, but this has also not been studied. Thus, further investigation the role of imaging for longitudinal monitoring of nonoperative DCM patients is needed.

Postoperative Assessment

After surgical treatment, radiographs, CT, and MRI again provide useful and complementary information. Radiographs are useful to determine the placement and integrity of instrumentation, in addition to the postoperative alignment, which is an issue of potential concern in both instrumented and noninstrumented cases. Flexion/extension views can demonstrate both instability and pseudoarthrosis, which are both reasons to consider a possible reoperation. CT is useful in the immediate postoperative period for determining the exact placement of screws, including the grading of breaches, into the spinal canal, disk space, spinal foramen, or foramen transversarium. CT is also useful for assessment of pseudoarthrosis and bony fusion, although it may take more than 1 year for fusion to occur. MRI is useful to evaluate the degree of compression of the neural elements and ideally should be performed routinely at 3 months to 6 months. In cases of perioperative or postoperative neurologic worsening, MRI is particularly important to determine if a new source of spinal cord compression is present, such as an epidural hematoma. Immediate postoperative MRI images must be interpreted cautiously, however, because there is often a small amount of venous blood in the epidural space.

Prognostication

A large body of literature has investigated imaging features and their associations with postoperative outcomes in DCM, but less research has focused on predicting neurologic deterioration in patients managed nonoperatively. Numerous imaging factors have been identified that correlate with outcomes after surgery, but a large number of clinical prognostic factors that have also been identified, such as preoperative neurologic status, duration of symptoms, age, smoking, and obesity.[20–26] The most important predictor of postoperative outcome in DCM is preoperative neurologic status; therefore, imaging factors that aim to predict outcomes must be measured in terms of what they add to this and other established clinical predictors.[23]

Numerous imaging studies have investigated MRI features for their prognostic value, such as the presence of T2-weighted hyperintensity, T1-weighted hypointensity, degree of spinal cord compression, and number of compressed levels.[8,17,18,25,27–30] The strongest MRI predictors of postoperative neurologic outcome seem to be T1-weighted hypointensity, which reflects cavitation and cell loss in the spinal cord gray and white matter, and the degree of cord compression, which can be measured using numerous techniques, such as maximal spinal cord compression, maximal canal compromise, compression ratio, or cross-sectional area (CSA) (**Fig. 2**).[2,17,27,31] Furthermore, a combined T1/T2 signal change, a higher signal intensity ratio (compressed vs noncompressed segments C7-T1; T2/T1-weighted images) and a greater number of signal intensity segments on T2-weighted images are also significantly predictive of surgical outcome; these 3 imaging characteristics reflect more severe, irreversible histologic damage that may not be reversible after decompression. Finally, the presence of kyphosis on radiographs has been reported as a negative predictor of neurologic outcome in DCM.[18] Only a few studies have evaluated predictors of neurologic deterioration in nonoperative DCM. In a study by Shimomura and colleagues,[32] the presence of circumferential cord compression on axial MRI was an important predictor of functional deterioration and conversion to surgery in mild DCM patients managed nonoperatively. Other studies have failed to identify an association between disease progression and spinal cord diameter (measured by the ratio at the narrowest part of the canal to the C1 level), number of intervertebral disks compressing the spinal cord, presence of high signal intensity on T2-weighted images, AP diameter, canal size, posterior osteophytosis, lordosis in extension, or kyphosis.[33–35] Overall, imaging prognostic factors have not demonstrated substantially better results than clinical data alone, prompting a trend toward the investigation of more advanced imaging modalities for these purposes.[8,17,23]

FUTURE DIRECTIONS OF SPINAL CORD IMAGING

Quantitative Spinal Cord MRI

A vast array of quantitative MRI (qMRI) techniques have become available that can measure specific physical properties of neural tissue,

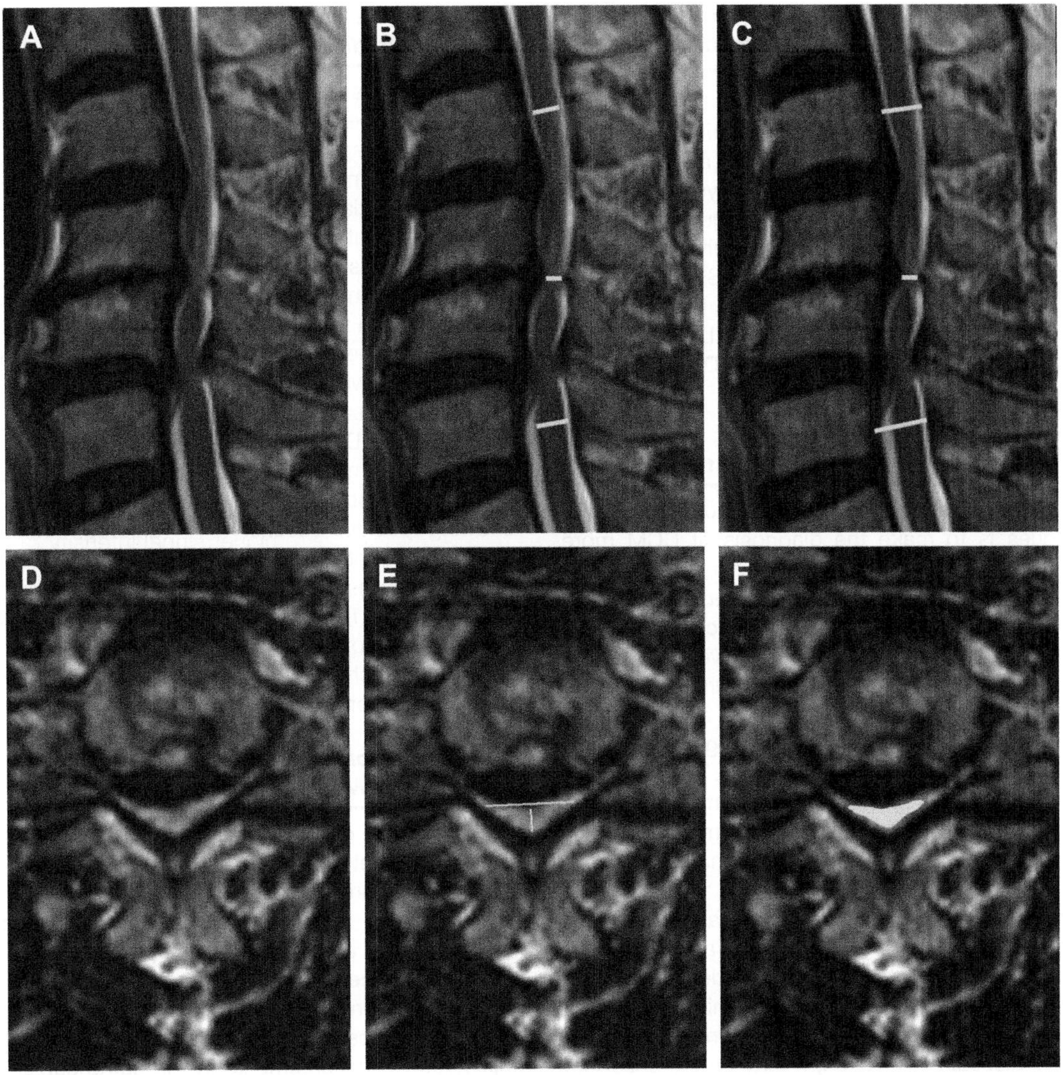

Fig. 2. Methods of measuring the degree of spinal cord compression. (*A*) Sagittal image of a patient with severe DCM. (*B*) Maximum spinal cord compression is measured on the midsagittal slice as the AP diameter at the most compressed level divided by an average of diameters of the uncompressed cord from above and below. (*C*) Maximum canal compromise is similarly the AP canal diameter at the most compressed level divided by the average of uncompressed canal diameters above and below. (*D*) Axial image of a patient with severe DCM. (*E*) Compression ratio is measured on axial images as the AP diameter divided by the transverse diameter. (*F*) CSA is the 2-D area of the spinal cord on axial imaging (if the slice is not perpendicular to the spinal cord, CSA should be corrected by multiplying by sine [θ]).

allowing characterization of microstructure and tissue injury with great implications for the management of DCM.[36–39] The most popular of these techniques is diffusion tensor imaging (DTI), which can measure the directionality and magnitude of water diffusion. This allows the detection of injury to the axons and myelin in white matter, which tends to have highly directional (anisotropic) diffusivity. Demyelination is a general phenomenon of white matter injury that is also present in DCM, and more specific myelin imaging techniques are also available, such as magnetization transfer (MT) and myelin water fraction.[37,40] T2*-weighted imaging also shows promise for characterizing spinal cord pathology, because it shows strong gray-white contrast that allows atrophy measurement of specific spinal cord compartments[41]; furthermore, the degree of contrast is a biomarker of white matter injury that reflects demyelination, iron, and possibly perfusion changes.[40] Magnetic resonance spectroscopy (MRS) is a technique that can characterize molecular and metabolic changes in the spinal cord, reflecting neuronal loss, gliosis, and demyelination.[42,43] Finally, functional MRI (fMRI) provides information about the neural activity and connectivity in the spinal cord and associated brain structures.[37] It is also important to note that the central nervous system (CNS) is intricately connected, and thus injury to the spinal cord causes changes throughout the neuraxis, known as a diaschisis. Several efforts have investigated advanced brain imaging techniques, such as MRS and fMRI, to measure rostral changes in patients with DCM or spinal cord injury (SCI).[44–48]

Improving Diagnosis with Quantitative MRI

One potential use of these advanced MRI techniques is to make the diagnosis of DCM more objective by directly detecting tissue injury within the cervical spinal cord.[38] Few studies, however, have investigated the diagnostic accuracy of these techniques in DCM, and most have shown poor performance.[49–52] One study found that mean diffusivity had a sensitivity of 100% and specificity of 75% for diagnosis,[50] exceeding that of fractional anisotropy in the same study. The remaining studies showed much worse performance of mean diffusivity and only modest performance of fractional anisotropy. Several issues may explain the poor performance of DTI metrics for diagnosis, including their wide range of normal values in the spinal cord (even when the metrics are specifically extracted from white matter), modest test-retest reliability of measurement, and limited sensitivity to pathology (eg, axonal loss may only occur in severe disease).[53] As such, it may be the case that multiple measures of tissue injury are needed to overcome the limitations of individual imaging techniques, which is a growing trend in spinal cord qMRI studies.[53–57] The authors recently reported a multiparametric diagnostic model using CSA, DTI, MT, and T2*-weighted imaging data that showed much higher diagnostic accuracy than was possible using any individual imaging metric.[58] Two studies have also attempted to identify a single symptomatic level in multilevel DCM using DTI, showing good diagnostic accuracy in comparison with detailed clinical examination of deficits in each cervical dermatome and myotome.[59,60] The clinical utility of this approach is unclear, however, because most surgeons elect to decompress all compressed spinal cord levels in cases of multilevel compression. Furthermore, there was no indication from these studies that DTI improved diagnosis over clinical examination.

Using Quantitative MRI to Improve Outcome Prediction

Another proposed use of quantitative imaging has been to improve outcome prediction, as discussed previously. Imaging techniques that can characterize specific microstructural changes may have greater potential to predict outcomes because they can potentially differentiate between reversible (eg, perfusion deficits) and irreversible (eg, axonal loss) changes in neural tissue. To date, DTI has shown the strongest results in characterizing the degree of tissue injury in cross-sectional DCM studies, with moderate to strong correlations with global disability and focal neurologic deficits.[40,50,61–66] DTI metrics, however, have only demonstrated modest performance in predicting postsurgical outcome,[61,62,64–66] with 3 studies showing positive results,[61,65,66] although these did not account for clinical predictors with multivariate analyses, which likely require much larger sample sizes. The same issues that limit qMRI's utility for diagnosis also affect outcome prediction, and further technical improvements and/or multiparametric approaches need to be explored.

Monitoring for Disease Progression with Quantitative MRI

A potential use of qMRI that circumvents the wide range of normal values of these measures is longitudinal monitoring for progressive tissue injury. This is highly relevant in mild DCM, in which many patients are managed nonoperatively, and clinical practice guidelines recommend surgical treatment when deterioration occurs.[5] Assuming that no changes have occurred in terms of tissue injury, qMRI measurements in the same subject separated by a period of time should only be affected by the standard error of measurement and the effect of normal aging. If these parameters have been accurately characterized, then statistical tests can be performed to determine if a subject has experienced progressive tissue injury. The authors implemented this approach using a multiparametric qMRI protocol in a small cohort of DCM subjects and found that qMRI results were highly congruent with patients' subjective impression of neurologic worsening.[19] Furthermore, qMRI seemed more sensitive at identifying deterioration than any clinical or subjective measure, possibly because compensatory mechanisms, such as neuroplasticity and behavioral adaptation, act to mask progressive tissue injury and give the false impression of neurologic stability. A similar approach may also show promise in monitoring for tissue regeneration, as demonstrated in traumatic SCI, once stem cells and other therapies become available over the coming decades.[67] Larger efforts are needed to confirm these findings and establish qMRI as an effective method of identifying progressive tissue injury in DCM, but this approach shows great promise for clinical translation.

Double Diffusion Encoding Technique for the Evaluation of Spinal Cord Axonal Injury

Techniques, such as DTI, which allow measures of axial and radial diffusivity in the spinal cord, have revealed new insights into SCI. For instance, axial diffusivity is decreased with axonal damage and has been correlated with histologically measured axonal injury,[68,69] which in turn has been strongly correlated to functional outcomes in SCI.[70,71] Axial diffusivity has also been correlated with injury severity[72,73] in experimental models of SCI.[64,68] DTI-measured diffusivity, however, is confounded by the presence of cord edema, hemorrhage, demyelination, and inflammation, which greatly limit its sensitivity in the evaluation of SCI.[73]

The double diffusion encoding (DDE) technique applies 2 diffusion gradient weightings within a single measurement. The first diffusion gradient pulse is applied perpendicular to the cord as a filter to suppress the signal from noncord tissues and a second gradient pulse is applied parallel to the cord. Coupling of the filtered signal with a point-resolved spectroscopic (PRESS) readout can then be used for whole-cord measurements without contributions of non-neuronal tissues, which can reduce both the acquisition and post-processing times that are typically required with other diffusion-weighted imaging models.

A recent study by Skinner and colleagues[73] applied the DDE sequence to an in vivo rat model of SCI and compared it to standard DTI. Their results demonstrated that DDE-PRESS was highly sensitive to injury severity, had shorter scan durations, and reduced the need for extensive image postprocessing compared with DTI. Their findings suggest this technique may be used as a sensitive biomarker of SCI severity although further work is needed to better define its limitations.

Resting State Functional MRI for the Evaluation of Spinal Cord Function

Disruption of the afferent and efferent conduits of the spinal cord, such as may be seen after SCI or compressive myelopathy, is associated with dysfunction of efferent response and afferent feedback throughout the neuraxis and subsequently structural and functional alterations.[46,74]

Several task-dependent fMRI studies have demonstrated rearrangement of cortical activation patterns with spatial shifts toward secondary brain areas in SCI patients.[74,75] These shifts are thought to occur due to expansion of the adjoining innervated parts into deafferented regions of the cortex.[46] Unfortunately, task-based fMRI studies lack standardized protocols for application of motor tasks across various SCI grades.[46,76]

In contrast, resting state fMRI (rs-fMRI) is a method for evaluating spontaneous, low-frequency fluctuations in the blood oxygenation level–dependent signal in the absence of a task or voluntary activity. In other words, with rs-fMRI intrinsic neural activity can be evaluated while a patient is at rest and, therefore, may be used for the evaluation of patients with various grades of sensorimotor dysfunction.[46,48,76,77] A prospective rs-fMRI study on 11 complete cervical SCI patients (>2 years postinjury) revealed decreased functional connectivity in motor and sensory cortical regions and increased connectivity between the left postcentral regions of interest and the thalamus compared with controls.[46] The presence of this dynamic reorganization in SCI patients is suggestive of the inherent neural plasticity within the CNS and highlights the potential of rs-fMRI for studying disease progression and treatment effects on neuroplasticity.[46]

More recently, rs-fMRI has been used to evaluate functional connectivity within the spinal cord. Barry and colleagues[78,79] demonstrated robust and reproducible resting state functional connectivity in the human spinal cord using ultra–high-field imaging at 7T. These results were later replicated by Eippert and colleagues[80] using the more widely available field strength of 3T. rs-fMRI has also been used to study the neural development of CSM through amplitude of low-frequency fluctuation measurements. This study of 18 CSM patients revealed a higher amplitude of low-frequency fluctuation values at all cervical segments compared with healthy controls.[47] These studies highlight the potential of this technique as a noninvasive metric of disease progression and treatment response in states of spinal cord compression and SCI.

Spinal Cord Imaging in Degenerative Cervical Myelopathy

There are numerous additional spinal cord imaging techniques currently under development that hold promise to transform clinical management of DCM. The emergence of open and upright MRI scanners can allow flexion/extension MRI to be performed under load-bearing conditions, which seems to increase the degree of cord compression that occurs, particularly in neck extension.[81] These studies tend to be more affected, however, by motion artifact, and further development is needed to improve image quality. Spinal cord perfusion imaging holds great promise to characterize the degree of ischemia in patients with DCM, which may reflect reversible impairment in comparison to microstructural changes that are detected with other techniques. The only reports of successful spinal cord perfusion measurements, however, have used CT with intravenous contrast, and further efforts are needed to develop noncontrast perfusion measures with MRI, such as arterial spin labeling methods that have successfully been used in brain imaging. Diffusion imaging techniques, such as DTI, are capable of showing far greater sensitivity to pathology as MRI hardware with stronger gradients and higher slew rates become available, based on the impressive results achieved using the human connectome scanner.[82] Other diffusion-based techniques, such as diffusion kurtosis imaging, neurite density and dispersion index, and DDE, also show potential to outperform DTI.[73,83–85] In addition, clinical MRI scanners with 7T field strength are now available, offering increased signal-to-noise ratio and opening the door to a host of new imaging approaches. Specifically, T2*-weighted imaging, MRS, and fMRI of the spinal cord are likely to benefit greatly from 7T due to increased signal-to-noise ratio, provided that issues of magnetic field inhomogeneity and specific absorption rate can be sufficiently mitigated. Specifically, rs-fMRI has shown promise as a technique for understanding whole-brain connectivity,[45] and it has recently been applied to the spinal cord including 1 study in DCM.[47] In addition to these advances in MRI, other imaging approaches, such as PET and near-infrared spectroscopy, hold promise for metabolic and functional imaging of the spinal cord, but specific applications to DCM have yet to be investigated. Overall, there are many exciting directions that are being pursued in the field of spinal cord imaging, and it is inevitable that future discoveries will once again transform clinical management of DCM.

SUMMARY

Imaging currently plays several critical roles in the care of patients with DCM, including diagnosis, surgical planning, and postoperative assessment. For most patients, MRI is sufficient for diagnosis, whereas radiographs, CT, and MRI are useful prior to and after surgery, although CT should be used sparingly in younger patients. In the near future, it can be expected that imaging (specifically MRI) will take on an even greater role in the management of DCM patients, including monitoring for progressive tissue injury, improved diagnosis, and outcome prediction.

REFERENCES

1. Nouri A, Tetreault L, Singh A, et al. Degenerative cervical myelopathy: epidemiology, genetics, and pathogenesis. Spine (Phila Pa 1976) 2015;40: E675–93.
2. Nouri A, Martin A, Tetreault L, et al. MRI analysis of the combined prospectively collected AOSpine North America and International Data: the prevalence and spectrum of pathologies in a global cohort of patients with degenerative cervical myelopathy. Spine (Phila Pa 1976) 2017;42(14): 1058–67.
3. New PW, Cripps RA, Bonne Lee B. Global maps of non-traumatic spinal cord injury epidemiology: towards a living data repository. Spinal Cord 2014; 52:97–109.
4. Farry A, Baxter D. The incidence and prevalence of spinal cord injury in Canada: overview and estimates based on current evidence. Vancouver, BC, Canada: Rick Hansen Institute and Urban Futures; 2010.
5. Fehlings MG, Tetreault L, Aarabi B, et al. A clinical practice guideline for the management of patients with degenerative cervical myelopathy: recommendations for patients with mild, moderate and severe disease and non-myelopathic patients with evidence of cord compression. Global Spine J 2017; 7(3_suppl):70S–83S.
6. Karadimas SK, Erwin WM, Ely CG, et al. Pathophysiology and natural history of cervical spondylotic myelopathy. Spine 2013;38:S21–36.
7. Fehlings MG, Wilson JR, Kopjar B, et al. Efficacy and safety of surgical decompression in patients with cervical spondylotic myelopathy: results of the AOSpine North America prospective multi-center study. J Bone Joint Surg Am 2013;95:1651–8.
8. Nouri A, Tetreault L, Cote P, et al. Does magnetic resonance imaging improve the predictive performance of a validated clinical prediction rule developed to evaluate surgical outcome in patients with degenerative cervical myelopathy? Spine 2015;40: 1092–100.
9. Boden SD, McCowin PR, Davis DO, et al. Abnormal magnetic-resonance scans of the cervical spine in asymptomatic subjects. A prospective investigation. J Bone Joint Surg Am 1990;72:1178–84.
10. Teresi LM, Lufkin RB, Reicher MA, et al. Asymptomatic degenerative disk disease and spondylosis of the cervical spine: MR imaging. Radiology 1987; 164:83–8.
11. Kato F, Yukawa Y, Suda K, et al. Normal morphology, age-related changes and abnormal findings of the

cervical spine. Part II: magnetic resonance imaging of over 1,200 asymptomatic subjects. Eur Spine J 2012;21:1499–507.
12. Kovalova I, Kerkovsky M, Kadanka Z, et al. Prevalence and imaging characteristics of nonmyelopathic and myelopathic spondylotic cervical cord compression. Spine (Phila Pa 1976) 2016;41: 1908–16.
13. Lee MJ, Cassinelli EH, Riew KD. Prevalence of cervical spine stenosis. Anatomic study in cadavers. J Bone Joint Surg Am 2007;89:376–80.
14. Martin AR, De Leener B, Cohen-Adad J, et al. Multiparametric spinal cord MRI detects subclinical tissue injury in asymptomatic cervical spinal cord compression. International Society for Magnetic Resonance in Medicine (ISMRM). Honolulu, Hawaii, USA, April 22–27, 2017.
15. Bartlett RJ, Hill CA, Rigby AS, et al. MRI of the cervical spine with neck extension: is it useful? Br J Radiol 2012;85:1044–51.
16. Al-Mefty O, Harkey LH, Middleton TH, et al. Myelopathic cervical spondylotic lesions demonstrated by magnetic resonance imaging. J Neurosurg 1988;68:217–22.
17. Nouri A, Martin AR, Tetreault L, et al. The relationship between MRI signal intensity changes, clinical presentation, and surgical outcome in degenerative cervical myelopathy: analysis of a global cohort. Spine (Phila Pa 1976) 2017. [Epub ahead of print].
18. Shamji MF, Mohanty C, Massicotte EM, et al. The association of cervical spine alignment with neurologic recovery in a prospective cohort of patients with surgical myelopathy: analysis of a series of 124 cases. World Neurosurg 2016;86:112–9.
19. Martin AR, De Leener B, Cohen-Adad J, et al. Toward clinical translation of quantitative spinal cord MRI: serial monitoring to identify disease progression in patients with degenerative cervical myelopathy. International Society for Magnetic Resonance in Medicine. Honolulu, Hawaii, USA, 2017.
20. Tetreault LA, Karpova A, Fehlings MG. Predictors of outcome in patients with degenerative cervical spondylotic myelopathy undergoing surgical treatment: results of a systematic review. Eur Spine J 2015;24(Suppl 2):236–51.
21. Tetreault LA, Dettori JR, Wilson JR, et al. Systematic review of magnetic resonance imaging characteristics that affect treatment decision making and predict clinical outcome in patients with cervical spondylotic myelopathy. Spine (Phila Pa 1976) 2013;38:S89–110.
22. Tetreault L, Nouri A, Singh A, et al. An assessment of the key predictors of perioperative complications in patients with cervical spondylotic myelopathy undergoing surgical treatment: results from a survey of 916 AOSpine international members. World Neurosurg 2015;83:679–90.
23. Tetreault L, Kopjar B, Cote P, et al. A clinical prediction rule for functional outcomes in patients undergoing surgery for degenerative cervical myelopathy: analysis of an international prospective multicenter data set of 757 subjects. J Bone Joint Surg Am 2015;97:2038–46.
24. Nakashima H, Tetreault LA, Nagoshi N, et al. Does age affect surgical outcomes in patients with degenerative cervical myelopathy? Results from the prospective multicenter AOSpine International study on 479 patients. J Neurol Neurosurg Psychiatry 2016;87:734–40.
25. Nakashima H, Tetreault L, Kato S, et al. Prediction of outcome following surgical treatment of cervical myelopathy based on features of ossification of the posterior longitudinal ligament: a systematic review. JBJS Rev 2017;5 [pii:01874474-201702000-00003].
26. Wilson JR, Tetreault LA, Schroeder G, et al. Impact of elevated body mass index and obesity on long-term surgical outcomes for patients with degenerative cervical myelopathy: analysis of a combined prospective dataset. Spine (Phila Pa 1976) 2017; 42:195–201.
27. Nouri A, Tetreault L, Zamorano JJ, et al. Role of magnetic resonance imaging in predicting surgical outcome in patients with cervical spondylotic myelopathy. Spine 2015;40:171–8.
28. Wada E, Ohmura M, Yonenobu K. Intramedullary changes of the spinal cord in cervical spondylotic myelopathy. Spine (Phila Pa 1976) 1995;20: 2226–32.
29. Matsumoto M, Toyama Y, Ishikawa M, et al. Increased signal intensity of the spinal cord on magnetic resonance images in cervical compressive myelopathy. Does it predict the outcome of conservative treatment? Spine (Phila Pa 1976) 2000;25: 677–82.
30. Matsuda Y, Shibata T, Oki S, et al. Outcomes of surgical treatment for cervical myelopathy in patients more than 75 years of age. Spine (Phila Pa 1976) 1999;24:529–34.
31. Yamazaki T, Yanaka K, Sato H, et al. Cervical spondylotic myelopathy: surgical results and factors affecting outcome with special reference to age differences. Neurosurgery 2003;52:122–6 [discussion: 6].
32. Shimomura T, Sumi M, Nishida K, et al. Prognostic factors for deterioration of patients with cervical spondylotic myelopathy after nonsurgical treatment. Spine (Phila Pa 1976) 2007;32:2474–9.
33. Yoshimatsu H, Nagata K, Goto H, et al. Conservative treatment for cervical spondylotic myelopathy. prediction of treatment effects by multivariate analysis. Spine J 2001;1:269–73.
34. Barnes MP, Saunders M. The effect of cervical mobility on the natural history of cervical spondylotic

myelopathy. J Neurol Neurosurg Psychiatry 1984;47: 17–20.
35. Oshima Y, Seichi A, Takeshita K, et al. Natural course and prognostic factors in patients with mild cervical spondylotic myelopathy with increased signal intensity on T2-weighted magnetic resonance imaging. Spine (Phila Pa 1976) 2012;37:1909–13.
36. Wheeler-Kingshott CA, Stroman PW, Schwab JM, et al. The current state-of-the-art of spinal cord imaging: applications. Neuroimage 2014;84:1082–93.
37. Stroman PW, Wheeler-Kingshott C, Bacon M, et al. The current state-of-the-art of spinal cord imaging: methods. Neuroimage 2014;84:1070–81.
38. Martin AR, Aleksanderek I, Cohen-Adad J, et al. Translating state-of-the-art spinal cord MRI techniques to clinical use: a systematic review of clinical studies utilizing DTI, MT, MWF, MRS, and fMRI. Neuroimage Clin 2016;10:192–238.
39. Vedantam A, Jirjis MB, Schmit BD, et al. Diffusion tensor imaging of the spinal cord: insights from animal and human studies. Neurosurgery 2014;74:1–8 [discussion: 8]; [quiz: 8].
40. Martin AR, De Leener B, Cohen-Adad J, et al. A novel MRI biomarker of spinal cord white matter injury: T2*-weighted white matter to gray matter signal intensity ratio. AJNR Am J Neuroradiol 2017; 38(6):1266–73.
41. Grabher P, Mohammadi S, Trachsler A, et al. Voxel-based analysis of grey and white matter degeneration in cervical spondylotic myelopathy. Sci Rep 2016;6:24636.
42. Holly LT, Freitas B, McArthur DL, et al. Proton magnetic resonance spectroscopy to evaluate spinal cord axonal injury in cervical spondylotic myelopathy. J Neurosurg Spine 2009;10:194–200.
43. Holly LT, Ellingson BM, Salamon N. Metabolic imaging using proton magnetic spectroscopy as a predictor of outcome after surgery for cervical spondylotic myelopathy. Clin Spine Surg 2017; 30(5):E615–9.
44. Kowalczyk I, Duggal N, Bartha R. Proton magnetic resonance spectroscopy of the motor cortex in cervical myelopathy. Brain 2012;135:461–8.
45. Zhou F, Gong H, Liu X, et al. Increased low-frequency oscillation amplitude of sensorimotor cortex associated with the severity of structural impairment in cervical myelopathy. PLoS One 2014;9: e104442.
46. Oni-Orisan A, Kaushal M, Li W, et al. Alterations in cortical sensorimotor connectivity following complete cervical spinal cord injury: a prospective resting-state fMRI study. PLoS One 2016;11: e0150351.
47. Liu X, Qian W, Jin R, et al. Amplitude of low frequency fluctuation (ALFF) in the cervical spinal cord with stenosis: a resting state fMRI study. PLoS One 2016;11:e0167279.
48. Kaushal M, Oni-Orisan A, Chen G, et al. Evaluation of whole-brain resting-state functional connectivity in spinal cord injury: a large-scale network analysis using network-based statistic. J Neurotrauma 2017;34(6):1278–82.
49. Ellingson BM, Salamon N, Grinstead JW, et al. Diffusion tensor imaging predicts functional impairment in mild-to-moderate cervical spondylotic myelopathy. Spine J 2014;14:2589–97.
50. Uda T, Takami T, Tsuyuguchi N, et al. Assessment of cervical spondylotic myelopathy using diffusion tensor magnetic resonance imaging parameter at 3.0 tesla. Spine (Phila Pa 1976) 2013;38:407–14.
51. Demir A, Ries M, Moonen CT, et al. Diffusion-weighted MR imaging with apparent diffusion coefficient and apparent diffusion tensor maps in cervical spondylotic myelopathy. Radiology 2003;229:37–43.
52. Facon D, Ozanne A, Fillard P, et al. MR diffusion tensor imaging and fiber tracking in spinal cord compression. AJNR Am J Neuroradiol 2005;26: 1587–94.
53. Martin AR, De Leener B, Cohen-Adad J, et al. Clinically feasible microstructural MRI to quantify cervical spinal cord tissue injury using DTI, MT, and T2*-weighted imaging: assessment of normative data and reliability. AJNR Am J Neuroradiol 2017; 38(6):1257–65.
54. Samson RS, Ciccarelli O, Kachramanoglou C, et al. Tissue- and column-specific measurements from multi-parameter mapping of the human cervical spinal cord at 3 T. NMR Biomed 2013;26:1823–30.
55. Oh J, Zackowski K, Chen M, et al. Multiparametric MRI correlates of sensorimotor function in the spinal cord in multiple sclerosis. Mult Scler 2013;19: 427–35.
56. Cohen-Adad J, El Mendili MM, Lehericy S, et al. Demyelination and degeneration in the injured human spinal cord detected with diffusion and magnetization transfer MRI. Neuroimage 2011;55:1024–33.
57. Ellingson BM, Salamon N, Hardy AJ, et al. Prediction of neurological impairment in cervical spondylotic myelopathy using a combination of diffusion MRI and proton MR Spectroscopy. PLoS One 2015;10: e0139451.
58. Martin AR, De Leener B, Cohen-Adad J, et al. Multiparametric cervical spinal cord MRI provides an accurate diagnostic tool for detecting clinical myelopathy. International Society for Magnetic Resonance in Medicine (ISMRM). Honolulu, Hawaii, USA, 2017.
59. Li X, Cui JL, Mak KC, et al. Potential use of diffusion tensor imaging in level diagnosis of multilevel cervical spondylotic myelopathy. Spine (Phila Pa 1976) 2014;39:E615–22.
60. Wang SQ, Li X, Cui JL, et al. Prediction of myelopathic level in cervical spondylotic myelopathy using diffusion tensor imaging. J Magn Reson Imaging 2015;41:1682–8.

61. Vedantam A, Rao A, Kurpad SN, et al. Diffusion tensor imaging correlates with short-term myelopathy outcome in patients with cervical spondylotic myelopathy. World Neurosurg 2017;97:489–94.
62. Jones JG, Cen SY, Lebel RM, et al. Diffusion tensor imaging correlates with the clinical assessment of disease severity in cervical spondylotic myelopathy and predicts outcome following surgery. AJNR Am J Neuroradiol 2013;34:471–8.
63. Mamata H, Jolesz FA, Maier SE. Apparent diffusion coefficient and fractional anisotropy in spinal cord: age and cervical spondylosis-related changes. J Magn Reson Imaging 2005;22:38–43.
64. Rajasekaran S, Kanna RM, Chittode VS, et al. Efficacy of diffusion tensor imaging indices in assessing postoperative neural recovery in cervical spondylotic myelopathy. Spine (Phila Pa 1976) 2017;42:8–13.
65. Lee JW, Kim JH, Park JB, et al. Diffusion tensor imaging and fiber tractography in cervical compressive myelopathy: preliminary results. Skeletal Radiol 2011;40:1543–51.
66. Wen CY, Cui JL, Liu HS, et al. Is diffusion anisotropy a biomarker for disease severity and surgical prognosis of cervical spondylotic myelopathy? Radiology 2014;270:197–204.
67. Jirjis MB, Valdez C, Vedantam A, et al. Diffusion tensor imaging as a biomarker for assessing neuronal stem cell treatments affecting areas distal to the site of spinal cord injury. J Neurosurg Spine 2017;26:243–51.
68. Kim JH, Loy DN, Wang Q, et al. Diffusion tensor imaging at 3 hours after traumatic spinal cord injury predicts long-term locomotor recovery. J Neurotrauma 2010;27:587–98.
69. Zhang J, Jones M, DeBoy CA, et al. Diffusion tensor magnetic resonance imaging of Wallerian degeneration in rat spinal cord after dorsal root axotomy. J Neurosci 2009;29:3160–71.
70. Ferguson AR, Irvine KA, Gensel JC, et al. Derivation of multivariate syndromic outcome metrics for consistent testing across multiple models of cervical spinal cord injury in rats. PLoS One 2013;8:e59712.
71. Medana IM, Esiri MM. Axonal damage: a key predictor of outcome in human CNS diseases. Brain 2003;126:515–30.
72. Kim JH, Loy DN, Liang HF, et al. Noninvasive diffusion tensor imaging of evolving white matter pathology in a mouse model of acute spinal cord injury. Magn Reson Med 2007;58:253–60.
73. Skinner NP, Kurpad SN, Schmit BD, et al. Rapid in vivo detection of rat spinal cord injury with double-diffusion-encoded magnetic resonance spectroscopy. Magn Reson Med 2017;77:1639–49.
74. Oudega M, Perez MA. Corticospinal reorganization after spinal cord injury. J Physiol 2012;590:3647–63.
75. Freund P, Weiskopf N, Ward NS, et al. Disability, atrophy and cortical reorganization following spinal cord injury. Brain 2011;134:1610–22.
76. Kokotilo KJ, Eng JJ, Curt A. Reorganization and preservation of motor control of the brain in spinal cord injury: a systematic review. J Neurotrauma 2009;26:2113–26.
77. Biswal B, Yetkin FZ, Haughton VM, et al. Functional connectivity in the motor cortex of resting human brain using echo-planar MRI. Magn Reson Med 1995;34:537–41.
78. Barry RL, Smith SA, Dula AN, et al. Resting state functional connectivity in the human spinal cord. Elife 2014;3:e02812.
79. Barry RL, Rogers BP, Conrad BN, et al. Reproducibility of resting state spinal cord networks in healthy volunteers at 7 Tesla. Neuroimage 2016;133:31–40.
80. Eippert F, Kong Y, Winkler AM, et al. Investigating resting-state functional connectivity in the cervical spinal cord at 3T. Neuroimage 2017;147:589–601.
81. Jinkins JR, Dworkin J. Proceedings of the State-of-the-Art Symposium on Diagnostic and Interventional Radiology of the Spine, Antwerp, September 7, 2002 (Part two). Upright, weight-bearing, dynamic-kinetic MRI of the spine: pMRI/kMRI. JBR-BTR 2003;86:286–93.
82. Duval T, McNab JA, Setsompop K, et al. In vivo mapping of human spinal cord microstructure at 300 mT/m. Neuroimage 2015;118:494–507.
83. Raz E, Bester M, Sigmund EE, et al. A better characterization of spinal cord damage in multiple sclerosis: a diffusional kurtosis imaging study. AJNR Am J Neuroradiol 2013;34:1846–52.
84. Hori M, Fukunaga I, Masutani Y, et al. New diffusion metrics for spondylotic myelopathy at an early clinical stage. Eur Radiol 2012;22:1797–802.
85. Grussu F, Schneider T, Zhang H, et al. Neurite orientation dispersion and density imaging of the healthy cervical spinal cord in vivo. Neuroimage 2015;111:590–601.

Pathophysiology of Calcification and Ossification of the Ligamentum Flavum in the Cervical Spine

Toshiyuki Takahashi, MD*, Junya Hanakita, MD, Manabu Minami, MD

KEYWORDS

• Calcification • Ossification • Ligamentum flavum • Cervical spine • Myelopathy
• Calcium pyrophosphate dehydrate

KEY POINTS

- Symptomatic calcification of the ligamentum flavum and ossification of the ligamentum flavum in the cervical spine are relatively rare compared with other degenerative cervical diseases.
- These diseases are associated with degenerative hypertrophy and a metaplastic mechanism of the ligamentum flavum related to the aging process; but mechanical, metabolic, and genetic factors are also involved.
- Clinical features are nonspecific compared with other degenerative cervical diseases; however, radiological and histopathologic studies can provide a precise diagnosis.
- Surgical decompression with adequate timing is required in most patients who present with relevant or progressive radiculomyelopathy.

INTRODUCTION

Degenerative change of the ligamentum flavum is a common finding associated with the intervertebral aging process. The main categories of ligamentous degeneration are hypertrophy, calcification, and ossification.[1] Symptomatic calcification of the ligamentum flavum (CLF) and ossification of the ligamentum flavum (OLF) in the cervical spine are relatively rare compared with other degenerative cervical diseases, although the performance of clinical and histopathologic investigations is increasing. This article summarizes the epidemiology, clinical appearances, radiological characteristics, and histopathologic findings of CLF and OLF in the cervical spine.

Calcification of the Ligamentum Flavum

Epidemiology and pathogenesis

CLF is a crystal deposition disease that mainly affects the central portion of the ligamentum flavum. Many previous articles have differentiated calcium pyrophosphate dihydrate (CPPD) crystal deposition disease from CLF. However, many patients develop compressive radiculomyelopathy without the painful arthropathy typically seen in CPPD deposition disease, also known

Conflicts of Interest Disclosure: The authors report no conflict of interest concerning the materials or methods used in this study or the findings specified in this article.
Spinal Disorders Center, Fujieda Heisei Memorial Hospital, Fujieda, Shizuoka, Japan
* Corresponding author. Spinal Disorders Center, Fujieda Heisei Memorial Hospital, 123-1 Mizukami, Fujieda city 426-8662, Japan.
E-mail address: heisei.t-taka@ny.tokai.or.jp

Neurosurg Clin N Am 29 (2018) 47–54
https://doi.org/10.1016/j.nec.2017.09.016
1042-3680/18/© 2017 Elsevier Inc. All rights reserved.

as articular chondrocalcinosis or pseudogout.[2] Crystallographic analysis of patients with CLF frequently demonstrates not only CPPD but also other mineralized deposits, such as hydroxyapatite, calcium orthophosphate, and combinations of these.[3–5] Therefore, discrimination among these disorders is still difficult in many cases. The pathogenesis of CLF has been described in relation to the degenerated and thickened ligaments. Calcium deposits mainly occur in the central part of the ligamentum flavum, which is surrounded by degenerated elastic fibers. CLF ordinarily has no continuity with the lamina, and the superficial and deep layers of the ligamentum flavum are preserved.[1,6] Various factors reportedly play relevant roles in the development of CLF, including the aging process, endocrine imbalance, mechanical stress of the cervical spine, metabolic diseases, and chondrocytic metaplasia.[7,8] According to their histologic investigation, Kawano and colleagues[9] speculated that CPPD was first deposited in the ligamentum flavum and then transformation from CPPD to the stable final form of the hydroxyapatite crystal was induced particularly in the central area of the calcification.

Although the prevalence of CLF in the general population is unclear, Watanabe and colleagues[10] found that radiographic evaluation revealed positive findings of CLF in the cervical spine in only 15 of 1619 (0.9%) patients who complained of neck problems. Symptomatic CLF in the cervical spine was first reported by Nanko and colleagues[11] in 1976. The investigators described a 70-year-old woman with radiculomyelopathy at the C5-6 and C6-7 levels. Baba and colleagues[12] experienced 8 cases and reviewed 91 reported cases involving patients who underwent surgical treatment of cervical myeloradiculopathy caused by CLF. The investigators found that 85% of all patients were female and had an average age of 64.8 years (range, 39–80 years). Additionally, 81% of the lesions were between the C4-5 and C6-7 levels.[12] Previous reports have identified the following characteristics of patients with symptomatic CLF: most patients are female; most are aged greater than 60 years; the lower cervical spine is frequently affected; 1- or 2-level lesions are common; it is mostly reported in Asian populations; it is sometimes associated with cervical disc disease; acute neck pain accompanied by crystal-induced arthritis is uncommon; and concomitant calcium deposits are often observed in other articular or periarticular sites (commonly the knee joint, intervertebral disc, hip joint, pubic symphysis, and shoulder).[3,5,13,14] Almost all clinical reports of CLF describe involvement in the cervical spine; it is extremely rare in the thoracic spine.[15–17] Several cases of symptomatic CLF in the cervical spine have been reported from non-Asian countries.[18–21]

Clinical features and radiographic appearance

There are no characteristic neurologic symptoms or signs that distinguish CLF from cervical spondylosis and ossification of the posterior longitudinal ligament (OPLL). According to data compiled by clinical reviews, the most common initial symptom is a sensory disturbance, such as numbness, dysesthesia, or pain, with an incidence of greater than 80%.[22] A common symptom in patients on hospital visits is gait disturbance coexisting with an abnormal deep tendon reflex or objective sensory disturbance. Hand clumsiness is also frequently observed.[12,22] Mwaka and colleagues[23] described 26 patients with clinical, radiological, and histologic evidence of cervical cord compression by CPPD crystal deposition among 465 Japanese patients who underwent posterior decompression surgery. All patients complained of numbness in the upper and lower extremities except 4 who did not have numbness in the lower extremities. Gait disturbance, bladder dysfunction, and a radicular sign in the arm were observed in 85%, 42%, and 38% of patients, respectively. Abnormal reflexes were also apparent in 85%.

Many affected patients do not present with abnormal laboratory data related to inflammatory, calcium metabolism, and hormonal imbalances.[12] However, Imai and Hukuda[24] reported that the preoperative erythrocyte sedimentation rate and serum C-reactive protein concentration were abnormally high in 4 of 8 patients and the white blood cell count was transiently but abnormally high in one. After surgery, these data were normalized in all patients except one. Histologic analysis of the resected specimens showed that the 4 patients with a high preoperative erythrocyte sedimentation rate and C-reactive protein concentration had inflammatory granulation tissue adjacent to the ligamentum flavum. Although the calcification itself does not usually induce acute neck pain, Kobayashi and colleagues[25] reported an atypical case of severe acute neck pain caused by CLF in the cervical spine with an inflammatory blood examination. In that case, conservative treatment was not effective and surgical removal of the CLF provided complete resolution of the patient's symptom. The investigators speculated that a relationship was present between CPPD crystal deposition in the ligamentum flavum, which was histologically proven, and acute neck pain similar to a pseudogout attack.

Plain lateral radiographs often demonstrate a nodular calcified mass that bulges from the interlaminar space to the intraspinal canal. However, this finding is rarely detected in patients with severe degeneration in the cervical spine. CLF lesions can sometimes be easily identified by oblique or lateral radiographs in the flexion position (**Fig. 1**A, **Fig. 2**A). Plain computed tomography (CT) is the most useful technique with which to diagnose CLF and typically reveals round or oval masses of high density located in the interlaminar part of the ligament flavum (**Figs. 2**C–E).[26] A less common form of symptomatic CLF is mainly localized in the capsular part around the facet joints.[27] Advanced and detailed CT neuroimaging has increased the reported prevalence of CLF, including that characterized by the depositions of small crystal particles, especially in the lumbar levels.[28] CT myelography clearly shows not only hypertrophic and calcified ligaments but also severe spinal cord compression from the posterolateral aspect (**Fig. 1**B).[13] MRI ordinarily shows a hypointense nodular mass on both T1- and T2-weighted imaging (**Figs. 1**C–E, **Fig. 2**B). Round lesions that compress the cervical cord are distinctive, although absolute differentiation from hypertrophy of the ligamentum flavum is impossible compared with a CT scan. Peripheral enhancement by gadolinium–diethylenetriamine pentaacetic was also found in a case report.[29]

Histopathologic findings

The estimated incidence of histologic calcium deposition is 22.0% to 24.5% among specimens resected during decompression lumbar surgery for the treatment of degenerative disease.[30,31] Yayama and colleagues[32] histologically analyzed

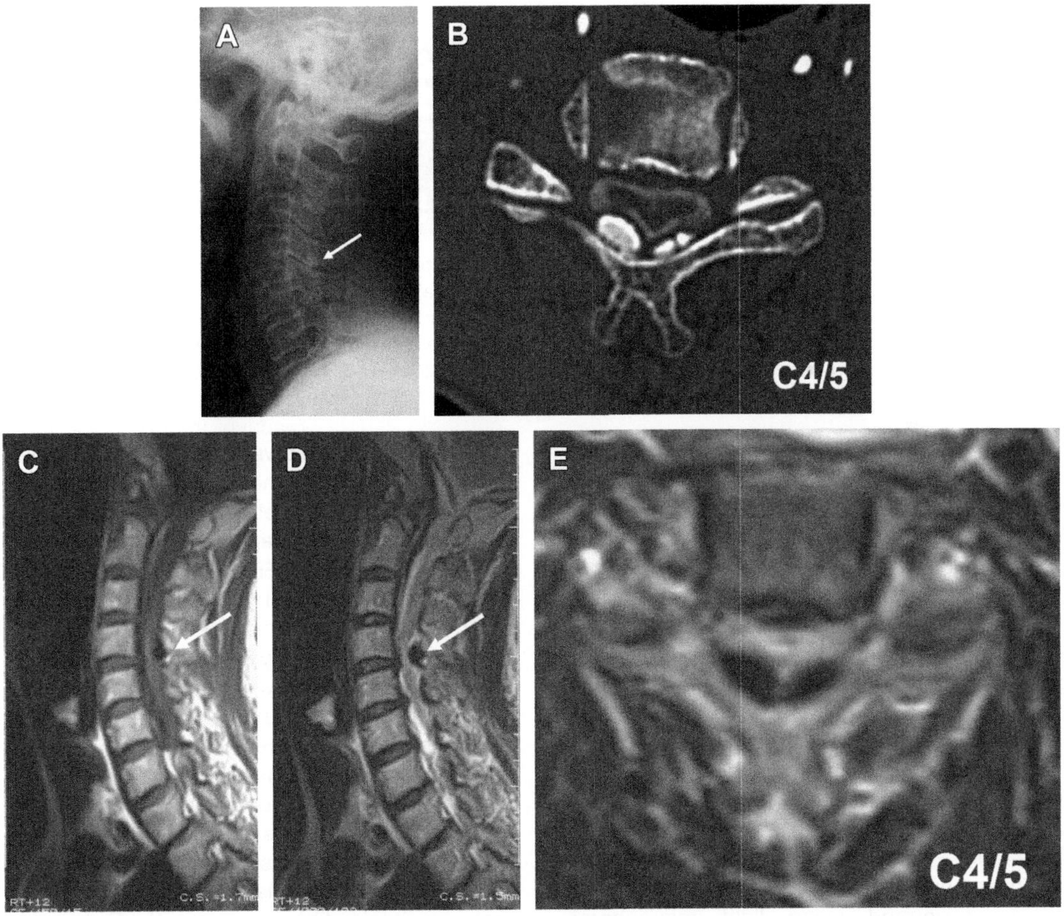

Fig. 1. Radiologic imaging of CLF in a 78-year-old woman who presented with a 5-month history of myelopathy. (*A*) Lateral radiography of the cervical spine shows a round mass (*arrow*) at the C4-5 level. (*B*) Computed tomography myelography reveals hyperdense masses in the bilateral medial parts of the ligamentum flavum. The cervical cord is remarkably compressed from the dorsal sites. MRI of the cervical spine demonstrates round hypointense masses (*arrow*) on (*C*) T1- and (*D, E*) T2-weighted imaging at the C4-5 level with compression of the cervical cord.

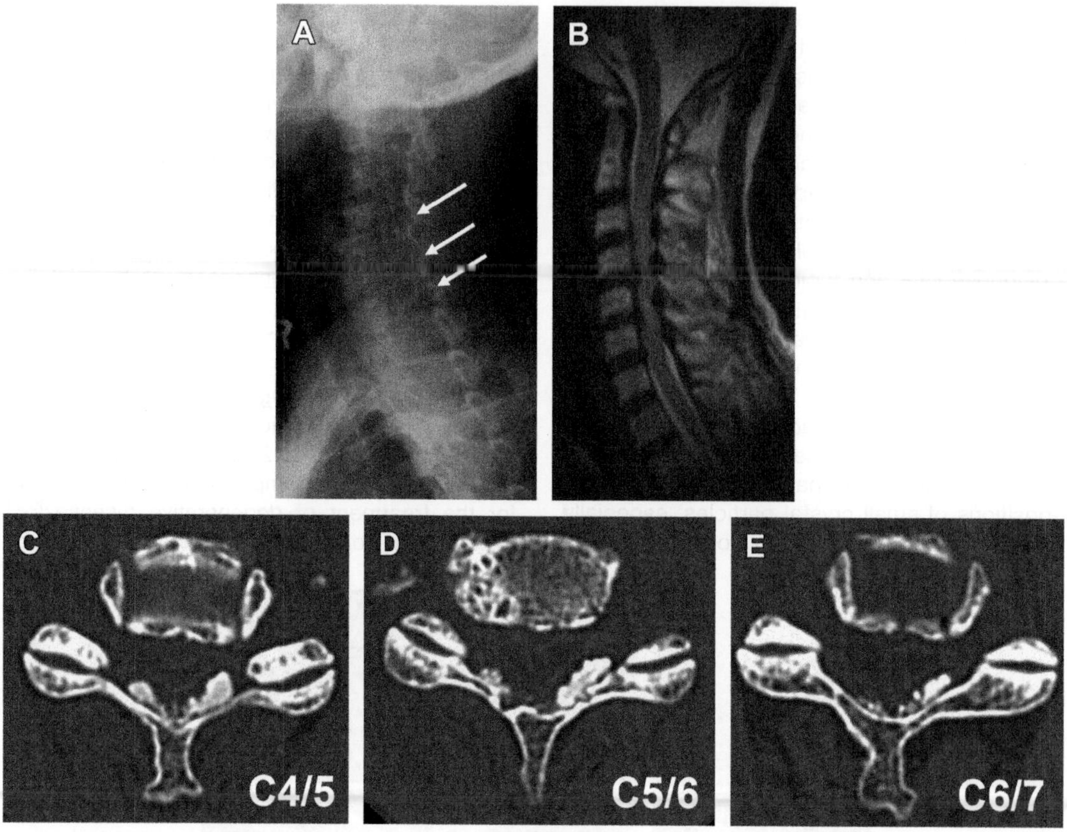

Fig. 2. A 74-year-old woman who presented with an 18-month history of myelopathy caused by multilevel cervical CLF. (*A*) Cervical radiograph (oblique view) shows a nodular calcified mass (*arrows*) through the foraminal space. (*B*) T2-weighted MR imaging also reveals a thickened hypointense mass corresponding to the site of the ligamentum flavum from the C3-4 to C6-7 levels. Cervical disc disease is also present. (*C–E*) Computed tomography demonstrates a nodular mass in the ligamentum flavum in multiple levels of the cervical spine.

180 specimens of the lumbar ligamentum flavum from 119 patients with lumbar degenerative disease. Calcium deposits were seen in 56 of 148 (38%) specimens from patients with degenerative spondylosis and in 17 of 32 (53%) specimens from patients with degenerative spondylolisthesis. Mwaka and colleagues[23] found histologic evidence of CPPD crystal deposition in 5.6% of 465 Japanese patients who underwent posterior cervical decompression surgery.

Macroscopically, CLF is observed as a white, chalky, rough, granular substance surrounded by degenerated ligamentum (**Figs. 3**A–D). Calcified lesions do not extend to the surface of the ligamentum flavum and adhere neither to the lamina nor dura matter. Histopathologic analysis is performed using light microscopy, including immunohistochemical staining, scanning electron microscopy, and transmission electron microscopy. Energy-dispersive x-ray microanalysis and x-ray diffraction studies are applied to define the crystal compositions.[9,29]

Light microscopy shows that calcified granules are deposited within the degenerated ligamentum, in which depleted elastic fibers are confirmed with an irregular arrangement and fragmented changes (**Figs. 4**A, B). These findings are accompanied by an increasing number of collagen fibers sometimes coexisting with chondrocytes.[31–33] Yayama and colleagues[32] performed a histologic evaluation and found that elastic fiber rupture is the initial change that produces crystal deposition in the ligamentum flavum of the lumbar spine. Collagen fibers increase as a reaction to rupture of the elastic fibers, and chondrocytes are induced from fibroblasts. In an immunohistochemical study of the cervical ligamentum flavum, some cytokines, such as basic fibroblast growth factor and transforming growth factor-β, were found in hypertrophic chondrocytes and fibroblastlike mesenchymal calls that infiltrated the area surrounding the calcified deposits.[23] Scanning electron microscopy shows various formations of

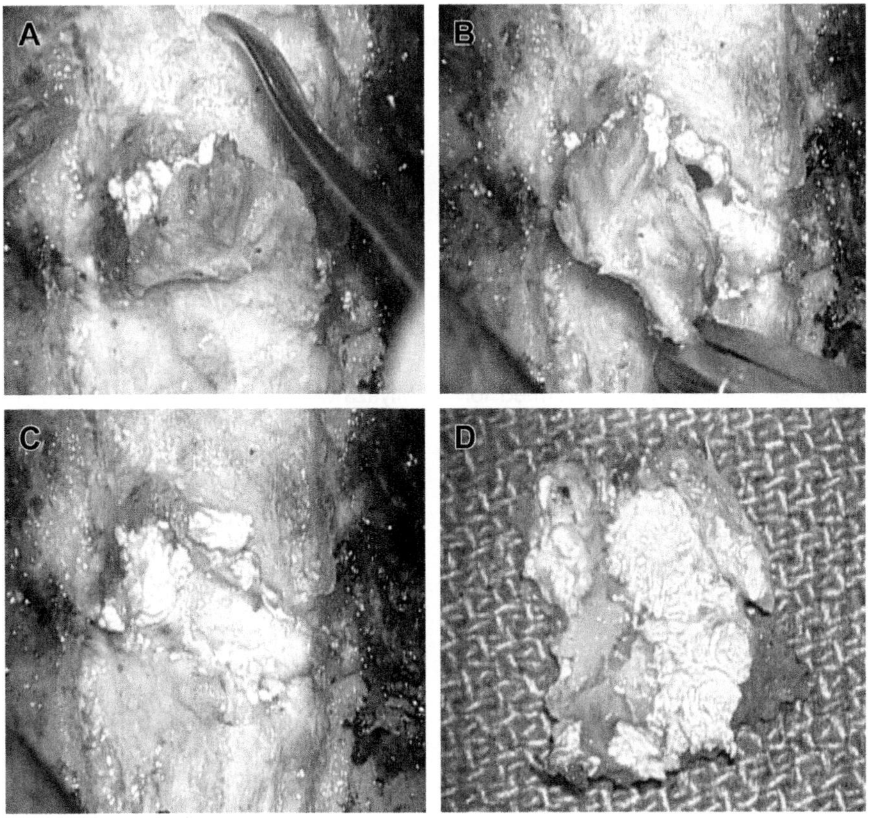

Fig. 3. Intraoperative findings of removal of cervical CLF. (*A*) after cervical laminectomy, calcified lesion in the ligamentum flavum was seen. Superficial layer of the ligamentum flavum was removed (*B*); CLFs are observed as a white, chalky, and rough granular substance surrounded by degenerated ligamentum (*C*, *D*).

the deposited calcium crystals, which appear as pinlike, rodlike, spherelike, or rectangular crystals.[32] Kawano and colleagues[9] reported that many plate-shaped crystals were distributed between the elastic fibers and that some of them were phagocytosed by macrophages on transmission electron microscopy.

Treatment options

Many cases of CLF are subclinical because histologic changes involving calcium deposition in the ligamentum flavum, including minor histologic changes, frequently occur in the aged spine. Some medications can reportedly induce neurologic and radiologic improvement. And, in a few

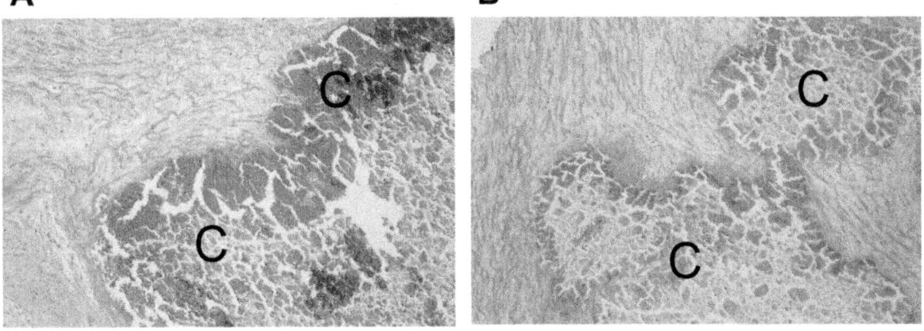

Fig. 4. (*A*, *B*) Light microscopy shows calcium deposits within the degenerated ligamentum, in which depleted elastic fibers exhibit an irregular arrangement and fragmented changes (hematoxylin and eosin [H-E] stain, original magnification ×40). C, calcified lesion.

cases, spontaneous regression has been reported.[8,10] Takehana and colleagues[34] reported that the administration of ethane-1-hydroxy-1 diphosphate to a patient resulted in significant diminution of the calcium deposits. However, immediate surgical decompression is recommended when patients present with apparent or progressive neurologic deficits. Few adverse events have been reported after surgery. Both laminectomy and expansive laminoplasty are expected to achieve adequate neural decompression. Mwaka and colleagues[23] described 26 patients with CPPD crystal deposition who underwent cervical posterior decompression. Laminoplasty was performed for almost all patients, and 77% achieved an excellent or good postoperative prognosis. Four of 6 patients with unsatisfactory surgical results were greater than 79 years old at the time of the operation. Yabuki and Kikuchi[35] described the clinical application of endoscopic partial laminectomy and removal of calcified ligaments in patients with CLF-induced cervical myelopathy.

Ossification of the Ligamentum Flavum

Epidemiology and pathogenesis

OLF was first reported by Polgár[36] in 1920; since then, it has been reported predominantly in Asian countries. OLF tends to arise from the lateral capsular portion of the ligamentum flavum and exhibits continuity with the bony laminae, in contrast to CLF. Details of the transitional process from a normal ligament to an ossified ligament remain unclear. However, degenerative hypertrophy and a metaplastic mechanism are suspected to play a role in the process. Additionally, pathologic change in the ligamentous enthesis will induce and increase local ossification, and endochondral ossification leads to laminar bone formation.[1,37,38] Systematic factors, including hormones and growth factors, have also been thought to contribute the pathogenesis of OLF. Moreover, genetic factors are suspected based on the selectively high prevalence of the condition in certain geographic areas and racial groups.[39,40]

In a whole-spine radiograph study of 232 elderly patients (mostly >60 years of age) in Japan, OLF at any level was detected in 34.5% of all patients and was significantly dominant in men. OLF in the cervical spine was present in only 2.6% of patients, whereas it was present in the thoracic and lumbar spine in 32.8% and 16.4% of patients, respectively.[41] In a study of 1736 volunteers of southern Chinese origin, radiological OLF in the cervical spine was present in only 0.23% of individuals, whereas OLF at any level was found in a total 3.8% of individuals.[42] In a recent whole-spine CT study from Japan, thoracic OLF was detected in 12.0% (male 15.0%, female 7.7%) of 1500 healthy persons who underwent PET-CT examinations for screening of cancer.[43]

The lower thoracic spine is a common site of symptomatic OLF, whereas involvement of the cervical spine is extremely rare.[44] An absent or decreased capsular portion of the ligamentum flavum above the midcervical level supports the fact that OLF in the cervical spine is infrequent compared with OLF at the thoracic level.[38]

Clinical features and radiographic appearance

Miyazawa and Akiyama[45] reviewed 50 cases of OLF in the cervical spine reported from 1962 to 2005, including Japanese articles, and established an extensive review of 23 detailed reports. The mean age of the patients was 56.3 years (range, 27–75 years), and the male/female ratio was 1.44:1. Among the 22 cases in which the spinal levels were described, 82% involved a single intervertebral level and the other cases involved 2 intervertebral levels. The involved spinal level varied from C1-2 to C7-T1 and had no common location. However, high rates of local kyphosis were involved in the formation of OLF of the upper cervical spine at C2-4. Almost all patients presented with sensorimotor deficits, whereas muscle atrophy and sphincter dysfunction were rare. The initial symptom is commonly a sensory disturbance of the extremities, as in other cervical degenerative diseases.[46] CT is the most useful technique with which to clarify the type of OLF and distinguish OLF from CLF. MRI can detect hypertrophy of the ligamentum flavum and the condition of cord compression in the cervical spine despite the fact that a definitive diagnosis of ossification is impossible. In the review by Miyazawa and Akiyama,[45] OLF of the cervical spine was either the lateral type or the continuous type. The incidence of coexisting OPLL and diffuse idiopathic skeletal hyperostosis was 35% and 33%, respectively. Concurrent OLF in other spinal regions was also observed in 33% of patients. Kotani and colleagues[47] reviewed 6 cases of OLF, including their own cases, of symptomatic cervical OLF with cervical OPLL. The investigators found that cervical OLF arose adjacent to the cervical OPLL margin, suggesting that increased mechanical stress at the OPLL junction may be a causative factor.

Histopathologic findings

The histopathologic characteristics of cervical OLF are presumed to be similar to those of thoracic OLF. In OLF of the thoracic spine, hypertrophic and degenerative changes of elastic fiber are accompanied by ossified lesions predominantly at the surface of the capsular portion. Cartilaginous cell proliferation and matrix hyperplasia with endochondral ossification are seen in these areas.[37] Yayama and colleagues[40] suggested that mechanical stimuli and certain metabolic disorders promote the appearance and development of ossification with the involvement of specific osteogenetic cytokines, such as bone morphogenetic protein 2 and transforming growth factor-β. However, the histopathologic details of OLF in the cervical spine are still unclear; there are some conflicting points in comparison with thoracic OLF.

Treatment options

Sufficient information regarding the natural course and optimal treatment of cervical OLF is lacking because clinical reports are extremely rare. Surgical removal is the first choice if patients have apparent or progressive neurologic deficits similar to those associated with other degenerative cervical lesions. Dural adhesion is possible, and attention should be paid to prevent dural injury during removal of OLF in contrast to CLF.

SUMMARY

CLF and OLF in the cervical spine are differential diagnoses in patients with posterior extradural compressive lesions related to cervical degenerative disease. Preoperative CT can facilitate the detection of characteristic findings and help distinguish between CLF and OLF. Although these are rare entities in the cervical spine, adequately timed surgical decompression is required in most patients who present with radiculomyelopathy.

REFERENCES

1. Nouri A, Tetreault L, Singh A, et al. Degenerative cervical myelopathy: epidemiology, genetics, and pathogenesis. Spine (Phila Pa 1976) 2015;40:E675–93.
2. McCarty DJ Jr, Kohn NN, Faires JS. The significance of calcium phosphate crystals in the synovial fluid of arthritic patients: the "pseudogout syndrome". I. Clinical aspects. Ann Intern Med 1962;56:711–32.
3. Haraguchi K, Yamaki K, Kurokawa Y, et al. A case of calcification of the cervical ligamentum flavum. No Shinkei Geka 1996;24:69–73 [in Japanese].
4. Hijioka A, Suzuki K, Nakamura T, et al. Light and electron microscopy of hydroxyapatite depositions in the ligamentum flavum. Spine (Phila Pa 1976) 1994;19:2626–31.
5. Koyama Y, Nishimura T, Kubokura T, et al. A case with myelopathy caused by calcified nodules of cervical ligamentum flavum. No Sinkei Geka 1988;16: 1179–85 [in Japanese].
6. Nagashima C, Takahama M, Shibata T, et al. Calcium pyrophosphate dihydrate deposits in the cervical ligamenta flava causing myeloradiculopathy. J Neurosurg 1984;60:69–80.
7. Pascal-Moussellard H, Cabre P, Smadja D, et al. Myelopathy due to calcification of the cervical ligamenta flava: a report of two cases in West Indian patients. Eur Spine J 1999;8:238–40.
8. Yamanuro K, Kikkawa I, Nakama S, et al. Calcification of ligamentum flavum. Spine Spinal Cord 2007;20:125–30 [in Japanese].
9. Kawano N, Matsuno T, Miyazawa S, et al. Calcium pyrophosphate dihydrate crystal deposition disease in the cervical ligamentum flavum. J Neurosurg 1988;68:613–20.
10. Watababe W, Arai M, Sakou K, et al. Radiological study on calcification of the yellow ligament of the cervical spine. Rinsho Seikei Geka (Clin Orthop Surg 1990;25:1006–11 [in Japanese].
11. Nanko S, Takagi A, Mannen T, et al. A case of cervical radiculo-myelopathy due to calcification of the ligamentum flavum. Neurol Med 1976;4:205–10 [in Japanese].
12. Baba H, Maezawa Y, Kawahara N, et al. Calcium crystal deposition in the ligamentum flavum of the cervical spine. Spine (Phila Pa 1976) 1993;18:2174–81.
13. Iwasaki Y, Akino M, Abe H, et al. Calcification of the ligamentum flavum of the cervical spine. Report of four cases. J Neurosurg 1983;59:531–4.
14. Iwasaki Y, Isu T, Abe H, et al. Two cases of calcification of cervical ligamentum flavum. The figure of early stage on CT scan. Rinsho Hoshasen 1985;30: 821–3 [in Japanese].
15. Giulioni M, Zucchelli M, Damiani S. Thoracic myelopathy caused by calcified ligamentum flavum. Joint Bone Spine 2007;74:504–5.
16. Muthukumar N, Karuppaswamy U, Sankarasubbu B. Calcium pyrophosphate dihydrate deposition disease causing thoracic cord compression: case report. Neurosurgery 2000;46:222–5.
17. Paolini S, Ciappetta P, Guiducci A, et al. Foraminal deposition of calcium pyrophosphate dihydrate crystals in the thoracic spine: possible relationship with disc herniation and implications for surgical planning. Report of two cases. J Neurosurg Spine 2005;2:75–8.
18. Cabre P, Pascal-Moussellard H, Kaidomar S, et al. Six cases of cervical ligamentum flavum calcification in blacks in the French West Indies. Joint Bone Spine 2001;68:158–65.
19. Khan MH, Smith PN, Donaldson WF 3rd. Acute quadriparesis caused by calcification of the entire cervical ligamentum flavum in a white female–report of an unusual case and a brief review of the literature: case report. Spine (Phila Pa 1976) 2005;30:E687–91.
20. Roet M, Spoor JK, de Waal M, et al. Extensive calcification of the ligamentum flavum causing cervical

myelopathy in a Caucasian woman. Springerplus 2016;5:1927. eCollection.
21. Ugarriza LF, Cabezudo JM, Porras LF, et al. Cord compression secondary to cervical disc herniation associated with calcification of the ligamentum flavum: case report. Neurosurgery 2001;48:673–6.
22. Takahashi K, Murakami Y, Ohta K. Cervical myelopathy due to the calcification of the yellow ligament. Spine and Spinal Cord 1991;4:421–7 [in Japanese].
23. Mwaka ES, Yayama T, Uchida K, et al. Calcium pyrophosphate dehydrate crystal deposition in the ligamentum flavum of the cervical spine: histopathological and immunohistochemical findings. Clin Exp Rheumatol 2009;27:430–8.
24. Imai S, Hukuda S. Cervical radiculomyelopathy due to deposition of calcium pyrophosphate dihydrate crystals in the ligamentum flavum: historical and histological evaluation of attendant inflammation. J Spinal Disord 1994;7:513–7.
25. Kobayashi T, Miyakoshi N, Abe T, et al. Acute neck pain caused by pseudogout attack of calcified cervical yellow ligament: a case report. J Med Case Rep 2016;10:133.
26. Miyasaka K, Kaneda K, Sato S, et al. Myelopathy due to ossification or calcification of the ligamentum flavum: radiologic and histologic evaluations. AJNR Am J Neuroradiol 1983;4:629–32.
27. Omura K, Hukuda S, Matsumoto K, et al. Cervical myelopathy caused by calcium pyrophosphate dihydrate crystal deposition in facet joints. A case report. Spine (Phila Pa 1976) 1996;21:2372–5.
28. Avrahami E, Wigler I, Stern D, et al. Computed tomographic (CT) demonstration of calcification of the ligamenta flava of the lumbosacral spine associated with protrusion of the intervertebral disc. Spine (Phila Pa 1976) 1990;15:21–3.
29. Yamagami T, Kawano N, Nakano H. Calcification of the cervical ligamentum flavum–case report. Neurol Med Chir (tokyo) 2000;40:234–8.
30. Markiewitz AD, Boumphrey FR, Bauer TW, et al. Calcium pyrophosphate dihydrate crystal deposition disease as a cause of lumbar canal stenosis. Spine (Phila Pa 1976) 1996;21:506–11.
31. Okuda T, Baba I, Fujimoto Y, et al. The pathology of ligamentum flavum in degenerative lumbar disease. Spine (Phila Pa 1976) 2004;29:1689–97.
32. Yayama T, Baba H, Furusawa N, et al. Pathogenesis of calcium crystal deposition in the ligamentum flavum correlates with lumbar spinal canal stenosis. Clin Exp Rheumatol 2005;23:637–43.
33. Kubota T, Kawano H, Yamashima T, et al. Ultrastructural study of calcification process in the ligamentum flavum of the cervical spine. Spine (Phila Pa 1976) 1987;12:317–23.
34. Takehana T, Shingu H, Shiotani A, et al. Treatment of calcification of the cervical ligamentum flavum with EHDP. Seikei Geka (Orthop Surg 1989;10:1543–5 [in Japanese].
35. Yabuki S, Kikuchi S. Endoscopic surgery for cervical myelopathy due to calcification of the ligamentum flavum. J Spinal Disord Tech 2008;21:518–23.
36. Polgár F. Über interarkuelle Wirbelverkalkung. Fortschr Geb Röntogenstr 1929;40:292.
37. Ono K, Yonenobu K, Miyamoto S, et al. Pathology of ossification of the posterior longitudinal ligament and ligamentum flavum. Clin Orthop Relat Res 1999;359:18–26.
38. Tanaka H, Tsuzuki N, Seichi A, et al. Anatomical study of ossification and calcification of the yellow ligament of spine with reference to the distribution of the yellow ligament. Rinsho Seikei Geka (clin Orthop Surg 1988;23:411–7 [in Japanese].
39. Inoue H, Seichi A, Kimura A, et al. Multiple-level ossification of the ligamentum flavum in the cervical spine combined with calcification of the cervical ligamentum flavum and posterior atlanto-axial membrane. Eur Spine J 2013;22:S416–20.
40. Yayama T, Uchida K, Kobayashi S, et al. Thoracic ossification of the human ligamentum flavum: histopathological and immunohistochemical findings around the ossified lesion. J Neurosurg Spine 2007;7:184–93.
41. Hasue M, Kikuchi S, Fujiwara M, et al. Roentgenographic analysis of ossification of the spinal ligament; with special reference to the findings of the whole spine. (Jpn) Seikei Geka (Orthop Surg) 1980;31:1179–86.
42. Guo JJ, Luk KD, Karppinen J, et al. Prevalence, distribution, and morphology of ossification of the ligamentum flavum: a population study of one thousand seven hundred thirty-six magnetic resonance imaging scans. Spine (Phila Pa 1976) 2010;35:51–6.
43. Fujimori T, Watabe T, Iwamoto Y, et al. Prevalence, concomitance, and distribution of ossification of the spinal ligaments: results of whole spine CT scans in 1500 Japanese patients. Spine (Phila Pa 1976) 2016;41:1668–76.
44. Kruse JJ, Awasthi D, Harris M, et al. Ossification of the ligamentum flavum as a cause of myelopathy in North America: report of three cases. J Spinal Disord 2000;13:22–5.
45. Miyazawa N, Akiyama I. Ossification of the ligamentum flavum of the cervical spine. J Neurosurg Sci 2007;51:139–44.
46. Kobayashi S, Okada K, Onoda K, et al. Ossification of the cervical ligamentum flavum. Surg Neurol 1991;35:234–8.
47. Kotani Y, Takahata M, Abumi K, et al. Cervical myelopathy resulting from combined ossification of the ligamentum flavum and posterior longitudinal ligament: report of two cases and literature review. Spine J 2013;13:e1–6.

Radiologic Evaluation of Ossification of the Posterior Longitudinal Ligament with Dural Ossification

Junichi Mizuno, MD, PhD

KEYWORDS

• Ossification • Posterior longitudinal ligament • Cervical spine • Dural ossification • CT

KEY POINTS

- The shape of dural ossification (DO) is classified into 3 types: isolated type, double-layer type, and masse type, based on relationship with OPLL.
- Bone window CT is most useful for identification of DO as well as ossification of the posterior longitudinal ligament (OPLL), whereas MRI is ineffective in recognizing DO.
- Nonsegmental OPLL is prone to accompaniment by DO, although segmental OPLL appears without dural involvement.
- Preoperative recognition of DO in conjunction with OPLL is beneficial in planning the surgical tactics to reduce complications as well as to yield good outcome.

INTRODUCTION

When an epidural mass, such as an intervertebral herniated disk, a posterior spur, or ossification of the posterior longitudinal ligament (OPLL), begins to grow and occupy the spinal column, the dura mater and the spinal cord are compressed, and the space between the dura mater and the spinal cord becomes narrow. Once the dura mater becomes ossified or calcified in conjunction with OPLL in the long-term process, operative manipulation for removal of the ossified mass via an anterior approach may increase unexpected complications. Cerebrospinal fluid (CSF) leakage through the resected portion of the dura mater is one of the major complications in the anterior approach for direct removal of cervical OPLL.[1–4] Increasing opportunity for spinal cord or nerve roots damage may cause a disastrous irreversible neurologic deterioration in this condition. Although anterior procedures of a cervical OPLL can achieve more satisfactory results than posterior procedures, surgical tactics are of importance to avoid unnecessary complications, including CSF leakage and spinal cord damage.[5–7]

Radiological recognition of dural ossification (DO) associated with OPLL provides significant information in considering the surgical approach preoperatively.[2,8] DO is sometimes ignored because of lack of awareness or knowledge of this condition. DO coexists in approximately 10% of OPLL cases. Although many radiological modalities are performed preoperatively, CT is the most detectable tool for identifying DO.[9]

Disclosure Statement: J. Mizuno is a Consultant for Ammtec, Inc, Tokyo, Japan.
Center for Minimally Invasive Spinal Surgery, Shin-Yurigaoka General Hospital, 255 Furusawa, Asao-ku, Kawasaki, Kanagawa 215-0026, Japan
E-mail address: mizuno@shibire.com

Neurosurg Clin N Am 29 (2018) 55–61
https://doi.org/10.1016/j.nec.2017.09.007
1042-3680/18/© 2017 Elsevier Inc. All rights reserved.

HISTORICAL REVIEW OF OSSIFICATION OF THE POSTERIOR LONGITUDINAL LIGAMENT

Key[10] reported the OPLL in 1838, and this is considered the first article to introduce the ectopic OPLL. Since the concept of infection or spondylitis was not well understood in this era, this report did not fully explain the clinical entity of OPLL. This report, however, discussed cases of spinal stenosis due to OPLL causing paraplegia, and autopsy of these 2 cases demonstrated the spinal cord compression due to thickening of the posterior longitudinal ligament. Case 1 showed that OPLL at L2-3 occupied the spinal canal in 30%, and the cauda equina was seriously compressed. Case 2 showed hypertrophy and ossification of the posterior longitudinal ligament causing paraplegia in a 44-year-old man. Oppenheimer[11] later reported 18 cases of calcification or ossification of the anterior and posterior longitudinal ligaments. In Japan, Tsukimoto[12] reported the first autopsy case of cervical OPLL in 1969. He described a 47-year-old man developing quadriparesis due to OPLL at C3-4. The ossified mass was completely separated from the posterior surface of the vertebral body, and the height of the mass became 3 mm. After this autopsy case was reported, the Japanese Ministry of Public Health and Welfare organized the Investigation Committee of OPLL for understanding these unique clinical and radiological manifestations in the aspects of etiology, epidemiology, pathogenesis, diagnosis, and treatment in 1975. Numerous reports of OPLL have been published in Japan, and as a result OPLL is called a "Japanese disease." It is clear that OPLL has a genetic background, and this is supported by family studies, twin studies, and HLA haplotype analysis.[13,14] Although OPLL is rare among whites, it is a significant cause of myelopathy in middle-aged and older Asian adults.

OPLL sometimes appears long with multiple lesions and sometimes as ossification of the dura mater. Surgical treatment of OPLL always demands correct preoperative diagnosis and optimal surgical treatment.[15]

RADIOLOGICAL EVALUATION OF OSSIFICATION OF THE POSTERIOR LONGITUDINAL LIGAMENT

OPLL is usually diagnosed on lateral plain radiographs as an abnormal radiopacity along the posterior aspects of the vertebral bodies. According to the Investigation Committee on OPLL of the Japanese Ministry of Public Health and Welfare, OPLL is classified into 3 basic types based on the sagittal plane appearance (**Fig. 1**). There are segmental, continuous, and mixed-type OPLLs, and segmental type is the most common. Segmental OPLL is defined as OPLL behind the vertebral bodies. Continuous OPLL is defined as 1 longitudinally large ossified mass, and mixed-type OPLL is a mixture of segmental and continuous OPLLs. CT is more sensitive than plain radiography. CT is helpful to understand the shape and size of the ossified mass as well as the extent of narrowing of the spinal canal. MRI is less useful

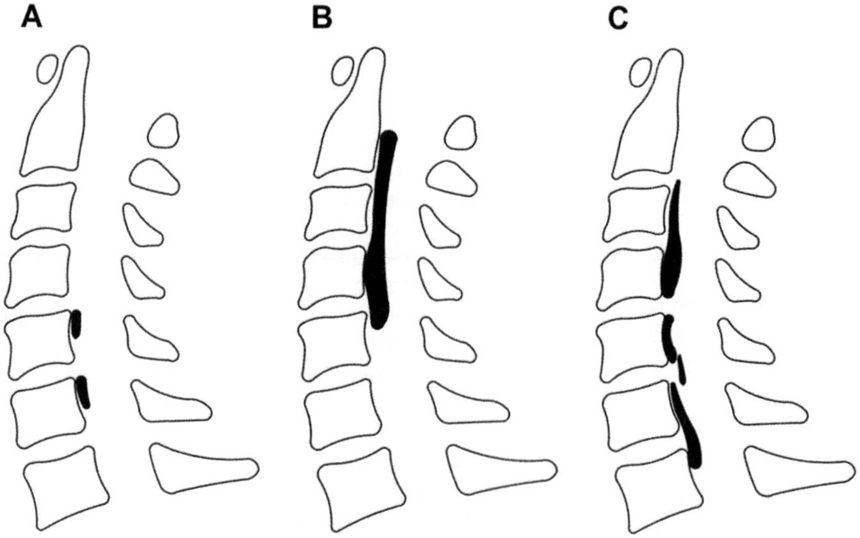

Fig. 1. Schematic drawings of 3 basic figures of OPLL. (*A*) Segmental OPLL is defined as OPLL behind the vertebral bodies. (*B*) Continuous OPLL is defined as 1 longitudinally large ossified mass. (*C*) Mixed-type OPLL is a mixture of segmental and continuous OPLLs.

than CT for diagnosis of OPLL. The basic role of MR imaging is the assessment of severity of the spinal cord deformity as well as the intramedullary cord lesions, such as cavity formation and edematous conditions.[16]

MECHANISM OF SPINAL CORD DAMAGE BY OSSIFICATION OF THE POSTERIOR LONGITUDINAL LIGAMENT

Not only direct compression that is mechanically induced by ossification but also the secondary circulatory disturbance should be taken into consideration as important factors in the damage to the spinal cord. Mair and Druckman[17] considered, from pathologic examination of cervical spondylosis, that the lesions had resulted from compression of the anterior spinal artery and its branches by the protruded disk. Yamazaki and colleagues[18] reported an autopsy case of OPLL showing occlusion of the anterior spinal artery. Kameyama and colleagues[19] showed that the location of cysts on a transverse plane commonly extended from the intermediate zone and the posterior horn to the lateral aspects of the posterior column bilaterally in the cervical cord of OPLL. There were prominent thick-walled vessels, predominantly venules, within and around the cysts accompanied by dilated perivascular spaces. Thus, venous congestion and subsequent necrosis play a significant role in the pathogenesis of spinal cord cysts secondary to chronic compression by OPLL growth. Karadimas and colleagues[20] proposed that elucidation of the role of ischemia as well as the complex cascade of biomolecular events as a result of the unique pathophysiology in cervical spondylotic myelopathy will pave the way for further neuroprotective strategies to be developed to attenuate the physiologic consequences of surgical decompression and augment its benefits. Moreover, Yu and colleagues[21] showed Fas-mediated apoptosis and inflammation may play an important role in the pathobiology of human cervical spondylotic myelopathy in their animal models.

Box 1
Basic 3 radiological patterns of dural ossification

- Isolated DO
  - DO apart from OPLL
  - Small and localized DO
- Double-layer DO
  - Positive surgical plane between OPLL and DO
  - Most common DO
- Masse-type DO
  - En bloc DO with OPLL
  - Usually large OPLL
  - Recommendation of posterior approach

DURAL OSSIFICATION

Type of Dural Ossification

DO is categorized into 3 different patterns (**Box 1**). The posterior longitudinal ligament is a connective band running along the posterior aspect of the vertebral body. Longitudinal evaluation in addition to axial examination should be studied in cases of OPLL. Therefore, sagittal reformation of CT or sagittal polytomography combined with axial bone window CT is essential for elucidating the type of DO. Among the 3 basic patterns of DO, double-layer DO was most common. Double-layer DO is characterized by concomitant DO and OPLL at the same level (**Fig. 2**). The ossified

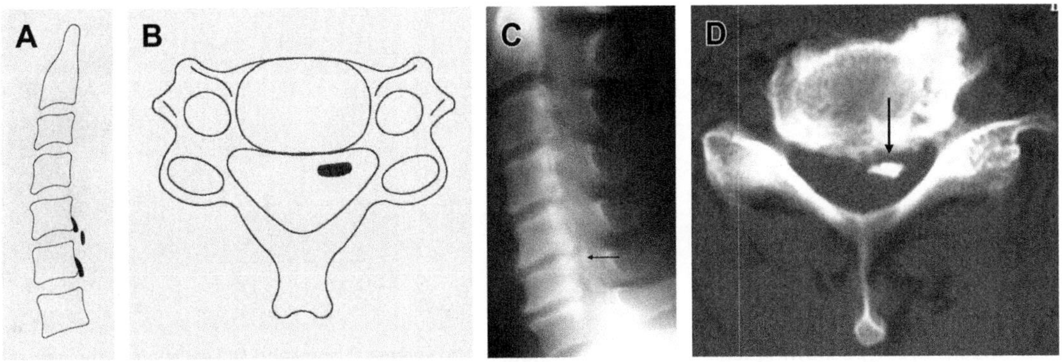

Fig. 2. Isolated type showing small ossification (*arrows*) apart from the posterior aspect of vertebral body at C5–6. (*A, B*) Schematic drawing of isolated DO and (*C, D*) illustrative CT images.

portion of the dura mater can be separated from the OPLL as a low-density space between high-density OPLL and high-density DO. Isolated DO features ossification of the dura mater without a correlation to OPLL; therefore, this type of DO might not be identified by examination of only the OPLL level. Precise examination of sagittal CT reformation and multislice axial CT are essential for identifying isolated DO (**Fig. 3**). Masse DO is characterized by a single hyperdense mass on CT, which cannot be differentiated between DO and OPLL. Sagittal reformation of CT or polytomography revealing OPLL with a hyperdense meningeal tail sign can make a diagnosis of this type of DO (**Fig. 4**). Although double-layer DO is more common in this radiological categorization of DO, it is clinically useful to know that DO develops in 3 patterns, not only the double-layer pattern but also the single and masse patterns to avoid unnecessary dural injury.

Relationship Between Type of Ossification of the Posterior Longitudinal Ligament Associated with Dural Ossification and Type of Dural Ossification

There is no significant difference between segmental and nonsegmental (continuous and mixed types) OPLLs and type of DO or between type of OPLL associated with DO and type of OPLL.

Relationship Between Type of Ossification of the Posterior Longitudinal Ligament and Frequency of Dural Ossification

There is a significant difference between segmental type and nonsegmental type regarding type of OPLL and frequency of DO. Comparison among segmental, continuous, and mixed-type OPLLs shows that nonsegmental OPLL, which is larger than segmental OPLL, is prone to accompaniment by DO. Therefore, DO might firmly attach to nonsegmental large OPLL, and the separation of DO from OPLL during surgical manipulation might be difficult, resulting in CSF leakage. Thus, that nonsegmental OPLL associated with DO should be treated by posterior procedures to obtain a better outcome must be considered.[22,23]

RELATIONSHIP AMONG PLAIN LATERAL RADIOGRAPHY, COMPUTED TOMOGRAPHY, AND MRI AND CAPABILITY OF IDENTIFICATION OF OSSIFICATION OF THE POSTERIOR LONGITUDINAL LIGAMENT AND DURAL OSSIFICATION

Lateral plain radiography, axial view and sagittal reformation on CT, and sagittal and axial T2-weighted views on MRI are regularly used for the preoperative radiological evaluation for degenerative cervical myelopathy. Bone window CT can always detect DO as well as OPLL. Lateral plain radiography can reveal a majority of OPLL cases, unless the ossified mass is minimal. Unlike bone window CT, plain lateral radiography cannot visualize DO well. Although MRI is useful in revealing the degree of cord compression due to ossified mass, OPLL and DO are not identified well. Because the existence of OPLL is defined as a signal intensity with a partial isointensity mass behind the posterior aspect of the vertebral body beyond the intervertebral disk level, OPLL cannot be differentiated from the posterior spur or the degenerated hypertrophied ligament on MRI.

Regarding capability of identifying OPLL and radiological modalities, there is no significant correlation between CT and plain radiography; however, there is a significant correlation between CT and MRI.

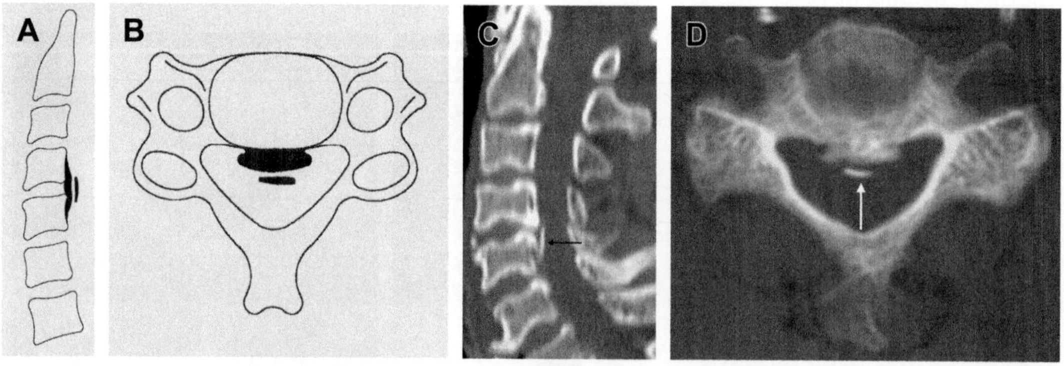

Fig. 3. Double-layer type showing segmental OPLL attaching to the vertebral body and DO locating at the ventral portion of the spinal cord (*arrows*) at C4–5. (*A, B*) Schematic drawings of double-layer DO and (*C, D*) illustrative CT images.

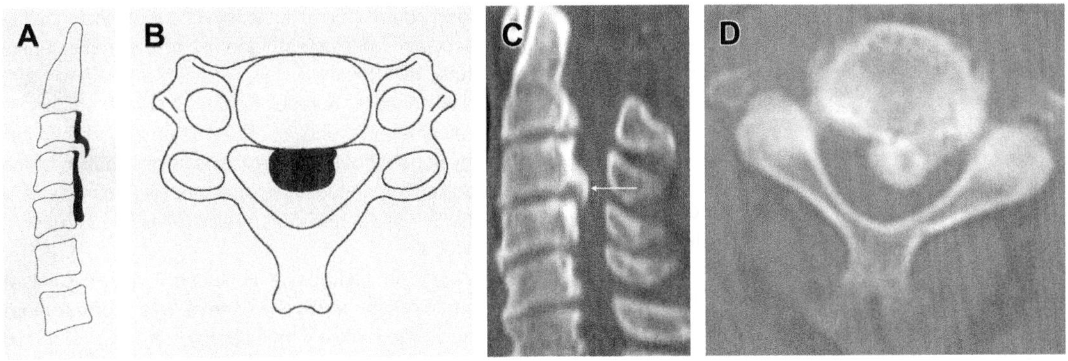

Fig. 4. Masse type showing OPLL containing DO (*arrow*). (*A,B*) Schematic drawings of masse-type DO and (*C,D*) illustrative CT images.

DURAL OSSIFICATION AND SURGICAL TACTICS

Preoperative recognition of DO associated with OPLL of the cervical spine would facilitate the surgical tactics for decompression, in particular those in anterior procedures. Several investigators have reported CSF leakage during anterior decompression and fusion for OPLL.[1–4] Anticipation of dural involvement in OPLL is important for avoiding CSF leakage and accidental damage of the spinal cord or nerve roots in planning anterior procedures for OPLL.[1,2] Thus, preoperative radiological identification of DO becomes essential. According to Hida and colleagues,[2] the single-layer sign, consisting of the demonstration of a single homogeneous ossified OPLL mass, appears somewhat less specific for focal dural penetration. On the contrary, the double-layer sign, characterized by anterior and posterior ossified rims separated by a centrally hypertrophied posterior longitudinal ligament, is more pathognomonic for multilevel absent dura. Hida and colleagues[2] speculated that ossification of the superficial layer as well as the deep layer of the posterior longitudinal ligament separated by a hypertrophied portion of the ligament might form a double-layer sign and cause a dural penetration.

The dura mater is the thick connective membrane covering the spinal cord and the nerve roots. One of the important functions of the dura mater is protection of the nerve tissues from epidural masses, such as OPLL. Once the dura mater is ossified in OPLL, however, surgical manipulation may cause serious injury of the nerve tissues as well as the dura mater without knowledge of the relationship between the OPLL, the dura mater, and the nerve tissues.[24–27] Thus, preoperative identification of DO in OPLL plays an important role in planning an anterior procedure with direct removal of OPLL.[28,29] Lateral plain radiography, CT, and MRI should be evaluated, because these radiological modalities are performed for diagnosis of OPLL preoperatively.

CAPABILITY OF IDENTIFYING DURAL OSSIFICATION ASSOCIATED WITH OSSIFICATION OF THE POSTERIOR LONGITUDINAL LIGAMENT

There is no significant difference in identifying OPLL between plain radiography and CT, but there is a significant difference in identifying DO between plain radiography and CT. Thus, plain radiography should be performed as a screening radiological examination regardless of whether the patient has OPLL. It is almost inherently obvious that CT is most accurate for this type of problem.

MRI was not sufficient to visualize OPLL or DO. The ossified mass in the posterior longitudinal ligament is visualized as asignal intensity both in T1-weighted and T2-weighted images with partial isointensity to high signal intensity.[30,31] Therefore, only asignal OPLL behind the vertebral body cannot be differentiated from posterior spur or associated DO. Although MRI is useful in revealing the degree of cord compression due to the ossified mass, OPLL and DO were not identified well.

SUMMARY

There are 3 basic radiological patterns of DO. Although double-layer DO is most common, examiners of the neuroimaging of OPLL should keep isolated DO or masse DO in mind. Bone window CT is most sufficient in identifying any type of DO associated with OPLL. MRI is not optimal for identification of DO and OPLL.

REFERENCES

1. Epstein NE, Hollingsworth R. Anterior cervical microdural repair of cerebrospinal fluid fistula after surgery for ossification of the posterior longitudinal ligament. Technical note. Surg Neurol 1999;52:511–4.
2. Hida K, Iwasaki Y, Koyanagi I, et al. Bone window computed tomography for detection of dural defect associated with cervical ossified posterior longitudinal ligament. Neurol Med Chir (Tokyo) 1997;37:173–6.
3. Macdonald RL, Fehling MG, Tator CH, et al. Multilevel anterior cervical corpectomy and fibular allograft fusion for cervical myelopathy. J Neurosurg 1997;86:990–7.
4. Smith MD, Bolesta MJ, Leventhal M, et al. Postoperative cerebrospinal fluid fistula associated with erosion of the dura. Findings after anterior resection of ossification of the posterior longitudinal ligament in the cervical spine. J Bone Joint Surg Am 1992;74:270–7.
5. Abe H, Tsuru M, Iwasaki Y, et al. Anterior decompression for ossification of the posterior longitudinal ligament of the cervical spine. J Neurosurg 1981;55:108–16.
6. Harsh GR, Sypert GW, Weinstein PR, et al. Cervical spine stenosis secondary to ossification of the posterior longitudinal ligament. J Neurosurg 1987;67:349–57.
7. Kojima T, Waga S, Kubo Y, et al. Anterior cervical vertebrectomy and interbody fusion for multi-level spondylosis and ossification of the posterior longitudinal ligament. Neurosurgery 1989;24:864–72.
8. Epstein NE. Identification of ossification of the posterior longitudinal ligament extending through the dura on preoperative computed tomographic examinations of the cervical spine. Spine 2000;26:182–6.
9. Mizuno J, Nakagawa H, Matsuo N, et al. Dural ossification associated with cervical ossification of the posterior longitudinal ligament: frequency of dural ossification and comparison of neuroimaging modalities in ability to identify the disease. J Neurosurg Spine 2005;2:425–30.
10. Key CA. On paraplegia, depending on disease of the logaments of the spine. Guys Hosp Rep 1838;3:17–34.
11. Oppenheimer A. Calcification and ossification of vertebral ligaments (spondylitis ossificans ligamentosa): Roentogen study of pathogenesis and clinical significance. Radiology 1942;38:160–73.
12. Tsukimoto H. A case report: autopsy of syndrome of compression of spinal cord owing to ossification within spinal canal of cervical spines. Nippon Geka Hokan (Arch Jpn Chir) 1960;17:1003–7 (in Japanese).
13. Sakou T, Takemoto E, Matsunaga S, et al. Genetic study of ossification of the posterior longitudinal ligament in the cervical spine with human leukocyte antigen halotype. Spine 1991;6:1249–52.
14. Terayama K. Genetic study on ossification of the posterior longitudinal ligament of the spine. Spine 1989;14:1184–91.
15. Nakashima H, Tetreault L, Kato S, et al. Prediction of outcome following surgical treatment of cervical myelopathy based on features of ossification of the posterior longitudinal ligament: a systematic review. JBJS Rev 2017;5(2) [pii:01874474-201702000-00003].
16. Mizuno J, Nakagawa H, Inoue T, et al. Clinicopathological study of "snake eye appearance" in compressive myelopathy of the cervical spinal cord. J Neurosurg 2003;99(2 Suppl):162–8.
17. Mair WGP, Druckman R. The pathology of spinal cord lesions and their relation to the clinical features in protrusions of cervical intervertebral discs. Brain 1953;76:70–91.
18. Yamazaki Y, Toda N, Nubotani T, et al. Anterior spinal artery syndrome by the ossification of the posterior longitudinal ligament in the cervical spine. An autopsy case. Chubuseisaishi 1972;15:849–58 (in Japanese).
19. Kameyama T, Hashizume Y, Ando T, et al. Spinal cord morphology and pathology in ossification of the posterior longitudinal ligament. Brain 1995;118:263–78.
20. Karadimas SK, Gatzounis G, Fehlings MG. Pathobiology of cervical spondylotic myelopathy. Eur Spine J 2015;24(Suppl 2):132–8.
21. Yu WR, Liu T, Kiehl TR, et al. Human neuropathological and animal model eveidence supporting a role for Fas-mediated apoptosis and inflammation in cervical spondylotic myelopathy. Brain 2011;134:1277–92.
22. Ohmori K, Ishida Y, Suzuki K. Suspension laminotomy: a new surgical technique for compression myelopathy. Neurosurgery 1987;21:950–7.
23. Hashizume Y, Iijima S, Kishimoto H, et al. Pathology of spinal cord lesions caused by ossification of the posterior longitudinal ligament. Acta Neuropathol 1984;63:123–30.
24. Hashizume Y, Kameyama T, Mizuno J, et al. Pathology of spinal cord lesions caused by ossification of the posterior longitudinal ligament. In: Yonenobu K, Sakou T, Ono K, editors. OPLL: ossification of the posterior longitudinal ligament. Tokyo: Springer-Verlag; 1997. p. 59–64.
25. Inoue K, Mannen T, Nakanishi T, et al. An autopsy case of ossification of the posterior longitudinal ligament of the cervical spine. Shinkei Kenkyu No Shimpo 1976;20:425–33 [in Japanese].
26. Mizuno J, Nakagawa H, Hashizume Y, et al. Pathological study of ossification of the posterior longitudinal ligament, with special reference to mechanism of ossification and spinal cord damage. Spinal Surg 1988;2:81–7 [in Japanese].

27. Epstein NE. The surgical management of ossification of the posterior longitudinal ligament in 51 patients. J Spinal Disord 1993;6:432–55.
28. Epstein NE. Evaluation and treatment of clinical instability associated pseudoarthrosis after anterior cervical surgery for ossification of the posterior longitudinal ligament. Surg Neurol 1998;49:246–52.
29. Mizuno J, Nakagawa H. Outcome analysis of anterior decompressive surgery and fusion for cervical ossification of the posterior longitudinal ligament: report of 107 cases and review of the literature. Neurosurg Focus 2001;10:E6.
30. Yone K, Sakou T, Yanase M, et al. Preoperative and postoperative magnetic resonance image evaluations of spinjal cord in cervical myelopathy. Spine 1992;17:388–92.
31. Yone K, Komiya S. Ossification of the posterior longitudinal ligament. Spine and Spinal Cord 2001;14:542–4 [in Japanese].

Ossification of the Ligaments in the Cervical Spine, Including Ossification of the Anterior Longitudinal Ligament, Ossification of the Posterior Longitudinal Ligament, and Ossification of the Ligamentum Flavum

Yukoh Ohara, MD

KEYWORDS

• OPLL • OALL • OLF • Prevalence

KEY POINTS

- Ossification of spinal ligaments includes ossification of the posterior longitudinal ligament (OPLL), ossification of the anterior longitudinal ligament (OALL), ossification of the ligamentum flavum (OLF) or ossification of yellow ligament, and ossification of supra/interspinous ligament.
- These conditions sometimes coexist in the same patients.
- Ossification of the spinal ligaments has common pathologic features, while at the same time exhibiting unique features specific to each entity.

INTRODUCTION

Ossification of spinal ligaments includes ossification of the posterior longitudinal ligament (OPLL), ossification of the anterior longitudinal ligament (OALL), ossification of the ligamentum flavum (OLF) or ossification of yellow ligament, and ossification of supra/interspinous ligament. These conditions sometimes coexist in the same patients. Ossification of the spinal ligaments has common pathologic features, while at the same time exhibiting unique features specific to each entity. In this article the relationship between these ossifications of spinal ligament and points to remember in clinical situations are discussed.

OSSIFICATION OF POSTERIOR LONGITUDINAL LIGAMENT

OPLL was first described in the English literature by Onji and colleagues.[1] They reported 18 Japanese patients, one-third of whom showed cervical myelopathy. OPLL mainly affects the cervical spine and is the most common cause of myelopathy in the ossification of spinal ligaments.[2] The most frequent level of OPLL is C5 vertebral level.[3,4] C5 is the site that is most vulnerable to degeneration[5] and OPLL is more common in older patients. Degenerative factors might be related to progress of OPLL. A genetic factor is thought to be related to the onset of OPLL.[6,7] Some studies have found

Disclosures: The author has no potential conflicts of interest to declare.
Center for Minimally Invasive Spinal Surgery, ShinYurigaoka General Hospital, 255 Furusawa Asao-ku, Kawasaki, Kanagawa 215-0026, Japan
E-mail address: yukoh@juntendo.ac.jp

Neurosurg Clin N Am 29 (2018) 63–68
https://doi.org/10.1016/j.nec.2017.09.018
1042-3680/18/© 2017 Elsevier Inc. All rights reserved.

neurosurgery.theclinics.com

that genetic background is strongly related to OPLL but few significant candidate genes were found for other disorders associated with ossification of spinal ligaments.[8–11] The incidence of cervical OPLL is estimated to be 1.9% to 4.3% in the Japanese general population. The difference between races is well known.[10,12] Previous studies using computed tomography (CT) scans reported the prevalence of cervical OPLL to be 6.3% in the Japanese healthy population,[13] 5.7% in Korean,[14] and 4.8% in an Asian American population.[15]

OSSIFICATION OF ANTERIOR LONGITUDINAL LIGAMENT

OALL was first reported by Forestier and Lagier[16] and Forestier and Rostes-Querol.[17] They named this pathology ankylosing hyperostosis (Forestier disease) to distinguish cervical spondylosis and ankylosing spondylitis. Resnick and coworkers[18,19] established specific radiologic criteria for its diagnosis as diffuse idiopathic skeletal hyperostosis (DISH) or Forestier disease. They defined DISH as showing calcification or ossification along the anterior to anterolateral aspect of four contiguous vertebral bodies with relative preservation of the height of the intervertebral disk in the affected areas, distinguishing it from degenerative diskogenic disease.[18,19] The spinal form of DISH is characterized by OALL with involvement of the cervical spine in approximately 76% of the patients.[20,21] Segmental OALL and anterior osteophyte may be confused because each of them shows radiologic similarity. OALL does not show decrease in disk height at the affected level.

The cause of OALL and DISH is unknown but the associations with obesity, type 2 diabetes mellitus, and advanced age have been reported.[22,23] The rate of progression of OALL may be related to increased cervical motion.[24,25] The prevalence of DISH is different between races ranging from 2.9% to 25%.[26,27]

OALL is frequently located at thoracic spine and the most frequent spinal level of OALL was T8/9.[13,28] In the cervical portion the most involved levels of OALL are C4-C5 and C5-C6.[29] Although cervical OALL is usually asymptomatic,[30] patients with OALL may show some characteristic clinical symptoms. The main causes of these symptoms are compression of the esophagus and trachea.[19,31,32] Some authors commented that not only compression but also inflammation and fibrosis might introduce the symptoms.[33] Dysphagia is one the most frequent symptom. Song and colleagues[33] described that the thickness and shape on axial CT scans in patients with OALL were important contributing factors to dysphagia and hoarseness. Some authors reported challenges with orotracheal intubation in patients with OALL undergoing general anesthesia.[34,35]

When the patient with symptomatic OALL exhibits severe dysphagia, with/without aspiration of food, surgical decompression of these structures may be required.[36,37] However, this type of surgery is required in fewer than 10% of patients.

OALL is not directly associated with development of myelopathy. However, the patient with DISH can have the possibility of severe cervical spinal cord injury because of extension-distraction injuries of the spinal column after minor trauma.[38] Spinal fractures and following spinal cord injuries are easily caused by low-energy trauma in patients with DISH because of the rigidity of the spinal column.[39,40] Most fractures are localized in cervical spine.[40] The fracture spreads transversely resulting in posterior element injuries and spinal column dislocation. DISH fractures tend to occur at the level of the vertebral body end plate.[41] Patients with unrecognized fractures commonly complain of only low back pain until abrupt neurologic deterioration occurs.[38] Initially neurologically intact patients may develop secondary neurologic deterioration after unprotected transfer.[39,42] Patients with DISH should be handled with great care when they complain of neck pain after even minor injury. Oppenlander and coworkers[34] emphasized catastrophic neurologic deterioration after emergency intubation caused by cervical fracture-dislocation.

OSSIFICATION OF LIGAMENTUM FLAVUM OR OSSIFICATION OF YELLOW LIGAMENT

Thoracic myelopathy caused by OLF was first described in 1920 by Polgar. The prevalence of OLF has been described to be 3.8% to 26%.[43–45] Fujimori and colleagues[13] reported CT data of 1500 healthy Japanese subjects. They found 12% in thoracic OLF and 0.3% in lumbar OLF. OLF is predominantly observed at the upper or lower third of the thoracic spine.[46,47] A few case reports were available in patients with cervical OLF.[4,48,49] The affected sites ranged from the middle to lower cervical spine.[50] The reasons for the high frequency of OLFs at upper and lower thoracic levels include increased mechanical stress where the thoracic vertebrae form the junction between the rigid rib cage and elastic cervical or lumbar spine.[51] Symptomatic OLF is usually located at the lower thoracic spine (38.5%) and the lumbar spine (26.5%), and the cervical spine (0.9%).[52]

RELATION BETWEEN OSSIFICATION OF THE POSTERIOR LONGITUDINAL LIGAMENT AND OSSIFICATION OF THE ANTERIOR LONGITUDINAL LIGAMENT

OPLL is frequently associated with OALL.[33,53–55] In a Japanese healthy population 36% of cervical OPLL occurred with DISH.[13] The same mechanism may enhance ossification of these two spinal ligaments.[56,57] An increase in cervical motion is positively correlated with more rapid progression of OALL and OPLL.[24,25] Some authors think that OPLL is one subtype of DISH, which involves OALL.[58–61] In patients with DISH OPLL and OALL frequently coexist in cervical spine. But the most frequent level of OPLL is the cervical portion and that of OALL is thoracic spine levels. The posterior longitudinal ligament runs along the vertebral body from clivus to sacrum. The posterior longitudinal ligament is thickest and widest in the transition portion of the head-neck junction and becomes thin and narrow in the lumbar spine.[62] However, the anterior longitudinal ligament is thin in the cervical spine and becomes thick and wide in the caudal direction. These anatomic features are associated with the frequent levels of OALL and OPLL.

RELATIONSHIP BETWEEN OSSIFICATION OF THE POSTERIOR LONGITUDINAL LIGAMENT AND OSSIFICATION OF THE LIGAMENTUM FLAVUM

OPLL and OLF may coexist in the same patients, but the frequency is lesser than OPLL and OALL.[13,63] Ligamentum flavum differs anatomically from anterior and posterior longitudinal ligaments. Both the anterior and posterior longitudinal ligaments spread across multiple intervertebral levels but ligamentum flavum spans a single intervertebral level. This anatomic feature causes the wide spread of OPLL and OALL but limited spread of OLF. The incidence of coexisting OPLL and OLF has been reported as 30% to 50% at the thoracic spine.[64] Kawaguchi and colleagues[3] investigated whole-spine CT of 117 patients with cervical OPLL. They found 9.6% of all patients had OPLL and OLF at the same spinal level. All the levels with coexisting OPLL and OLF were thoracic spine. A total of 64.6% of all patients with cervical OPLL had OLF at any levels of the whole spine. They emphasized the differences in affected lesions, genetics, and acquired factors and concluded that OPLL and OLF are not directly affected by each other. Fujimori and colleagues[13] reported high concomitance rate of each spinal ligament ossification. They found 34% of cervical OPLL ossification occurred with thoracic OLF. However, the combination of cervical OLF and OPLL is extremely rare.[4,50,65–67]

RELATIONSHIP BETWEEN OSSIFICATION OF THE LIGAMENTUM FLAVUM AND OSSIFICATION OF THE ANTERIOR LONGITUDINAL LIGAMENT

OALL is seen in patients with an OLF.[68] The rate of progression of an OALL also may be related to increased motion as with OLF.[24,25] Ando and colleagues[68] reported that OALLs present around vertebral levels were affected OLFs. This correlation may be caused by the mechanical stress arising from the OALL and the OLFs.

DISCUSSION

In many reports, authors have discussed the relationship between symptomatic OPLL and other spinal ossifications. It is difficult to investigate ossification of spinal ligaments in healthy general populations, and there is the problem about the diagnostic tool. Diagnosis of spinal ligament ossification has been performed using plain radiograph.[69] Some ossifications, especially at thoracic spine, are difficult to diagnose by using plain radiographs. CT has been shown have higher diagnostic accuracy for identifying ossification of the spinal ligaments at any level.[70–72] The prevalence of spinal ligament ossification in recent reports was higher than that of previous ones because of high-sensitivity CT.[13]

Biomechanical stability and inherent anatomic stability contributes to the growth of ossification of the spinal ligament.[43] There are several reports that support the relationship between the growing factors of the ossification of the spinal ligaments and static or dynamic factors.[73,74] However, the anatomic characters of each ligament are different. The ossification of the spinal ligaments might be included in the same category of disease but all of the factors might enhance the frequent lesions.

SUMMARY

Ossification of the spinal ligaments includes OPLL, OALL, and OLF. Dynamic stress induces the growth of ossified lesion. Anatomic differences might enhance the frequent levels and prevalence of each ossification. There are no data about common genetic factors of all ossification of the spinal ligaments, but these diseases might be included in same category. Many reports describe the coexisting ossification in patients with symptomatic OPLL because OPLL is the most frequent type of ossification of the spinal ligaments. There are limitations in the availability of suitable screening diagnostic tools for the healthy population. More studies are needed about these pathologies especially in asymptomatic patients with special consideration for relevant racial and genetic factors.

REFERENCES

1. Onji Y, Akiyama H, Shimomura Y, et al. Paravertebral ossification causing cervical myelopathy. A report of 18 cases. J Bone Joint Surg Am 1967; 49:1314–28.
2. Matsunaga S, Sakou T. 78 ossification of the posterior longitudinal ligaments. Prevalence, presentation and natural history. In: Clark CR, editor. The cervical spine. 4th edition. Philadelphia: Lippincott Williams & Wilkins; 2005. p. P1091–8.
3. Kawaguchi Y, Nakano M, Yasuda T, et al. Characteristics of ossification of the spinal ligament; incidence of ossification of the ligamentum flavum in patients with cervical ossification of the posterior longitudinal ligament: analysis of the whole spine using multidetector CT. J Ortho Sci 2016;21:439–45.
4. Kim K, Isu T. Cervical ligamentum flavum ossification: two case report. Neurol Med Chir (Tokyo) 2008;48(4):183–7.
5. Freedenberg ZEBU, Ezekiel J, Spencer HEN, et al. Degenerative changes in the cervical spine. J Bone Joint Surg Am 1959;41:61–70.
6. Liu Y, Zhao Y, Chen Y, et al. RUN polymorphisms associated with OPLL and OLF in the Han population. Clin Orthop Relat Res 2010;468:3333–41.
7. Nakamura I, Ikebana S, Odawa A, et al. Association of the human NAPS gene with ossification of the posterior longitudinal ligament of the spine (OPLL). Hum Genet 1999;104:492–7.
8. Iwasaki M, Piao J, Kimura A, et al. Runx2 haploinsufficiency ameliorates the development of ossification of the posterior longitudinal ligament. PLoS One 2012;7(8):e43372.
9. Karasugi T, Nakajima M, Ikari K, et al. A genome-wide sib-pair linkage analysis of ossification of the posterior longitudinal ligament of the spine. J Bone Miner Metab 2013;31:136–43.
10. Matsunaga S, Sakou T. Overview of epidemiology and genetics. In: Yanenobu K, Nakamura K, Toyone Y, editors. Ossification of the posterior longitudinal ligament. Tokyo: Springer; 2006. p. 7–9.
11. Nakajima M, Takahashi A, Tsuji T, et al, Genetic study group of investigation committee on ossification of the spinal ligaments. A genome-wide association study identifies susceptibility loci for ossification of the posterior longitudinal ligament of the spine. Nat Genet 2014;46(9):1012–6.
12. Matusnaga S, Sakou T. Ossification of the posterior longitudinal ligament of the cervical spine: etiology and natural history. Spine 2012;37:E309–14.
13. Fujimori T, Watabe T, Iwamoto Y, et al. Prevalence, concomitance, and distribution of ossification of the spinal ligaments. Result of whole spine CT scan in 1500 Japanese patients. Spine 2016;41: 1668–76.
14. Sohn S, Chung CK, Yun TJ, et al. Epidemiological survey of ossification of the posterior longitudinal ligament in an adult Korean population: three-dimensional computed tomographic observation of 3240 cases. Calcif Tissue Int 2014;94:613–20.
15. Fujimori T, Le H, Hu SS, et al. Ossification of the posterior longitudinal ligament of the cervical spine in 3161 patients: a CT-based study. Spine 2015;40: E394–403.
16. Forestier J, Lagier R. Ankylosing hyperostosis of the spine. Clin Orthop 1971;74:65–83.
17. Forestier J, Rostes-Querol J. Senile ankylosing hyperostosis of the spine. Ann Rheum Dis 1950;9: 321–30.
18. Resnick D, Shaul SR, Robins JM. Diffuse idiopathic skeletal hyperostosis (DISH): Forestier's disease with extraspinal manifestations. Radiology 1975; 115:513–24.
19. Resnick D, Shapiro RF, Wiesner KB, et al. Diffuse idiopathic skeletal hyperostosis (DISH) (ankylosing hyperostosis of Forester and Rotes-Querol). Semin Arthritis Rheum 1978;7:153–87.
20. Mader R. Clinical manifestations of diffuse idiopathic skeletal hyperostosis of the cervical spine. Semin Arthritis Rheum 2002;32:130–5.
21. Meyer PR Jr. Diffuse idiopathic skeletal hyperostosis in the cervical spine. Clin Orthop Relat Res 1999; 359:49–57.
22. Denko CW, Malemud CJ. Body mass index and blood glucose: correlations with serum insulin, growth hormone, and insulin-like growth factor-1 levels in patients with diffuse idiopathic skeletal hyperostosis (DISH). Rheumatol Int 2006;26:292–7.
23. Kiss SK, Szilagyi M, Paksy A, et al. Risk factors for diffuse idiopathic skeletal hyperostosis; a case-control study. Rheumatology(Oxford) 2002; 41:27–30.
24. Oga M, Mashima T, Iwakuma T, et al. Dysphasia complications in ankylosing spinal hyperostosis and ossification of the posterior longitudinal ligament. Roentgenographic findings of the developmental process of cervical osteophytes causing by dysphasia. Spine 1993;18:391–4.
25. Suzuki K, Ishida Y, Ohmori K. Long term follow-up of diffuse idiopathic skeletal hyperostosis in the cervical spine. Analysis of progression of ossification. Neuroradiology 1991;33:427–31.

26. Kim SK, Choi BR, Kim CG, et al. The prevalence of diffuse idiopathic skeletal hyperostosis in Korea. J Rheumatol 2004;31:2032–5.
27. Weinfeld RM, Olson PN, Maki DD, et al. The prevalence of diffuse idiopathic skeletal hyperostosis (DISH) in two large American Midwest metropolitan populations. Skeletal Radiol 1997;26:222–5.
28. Kagotani R, Yoshida M, Muraki S, et al. Prevalence of diffuse idiopathic skeletal hyperostosis (DISH) of the whole spine and its association with lumber spondylosis and knee osteoarthritis: the ROAD study. J Bone Miner Metab 2015;33:221–9.
29. Gamache FW Jr, Voorhies RM. Hypertrophic cervical osteophytes causing dysphasia. A review. J Neurosurg 1980;16:338–44.
30. Mizuno J, Nakagawa H, Song J. Symptomatic ossification of the anterior longitudinal ligament with stenosis of the cervical spine. A report of seven cases. J Bone Joint Surg 2005;87:1375–9.
31. Stuart D. Dysphasia due to cervical osteophytes: a description of five patients and a review of the literature. Int Orthop 1989;13:95–9.
32. Underberg-Devis S, Levine MS. Giant thoracic osteophyte causing oesophageal food impaction. Am J Roentgenol 1991;157:319–20.
33. Song J, Mizuno J, Nakagawa H. Clinical and radiological analysis of ossification of the anterior longitudinal ligament causing dysphasia and hoarseness. Neurosurgery 2006;58:913–9.
34. Oppenlander ME, Hsu FD, Bolton P, et al. Catastrophic neurological complications of emergent endotracheal intubation: report of 2 cases. J Neurosurg Spine 2015;22:454–8.
35. Yamada N, Katou Y, Kimura O, et al. Difficult airway management of a patient with the ossification of anterior longitudinal ligament. Masui 2015;64:392–5.
36. McCaffery RR, Harrison MJ, Tamas LB, et al. Ossification of the anterior longitudinal ligament and Forestier's disease: an analysis of seven cases. J Neurosurg 1995;83:13–7.
37. Warwick C, Sherman MS, Lesser RW. Aspiration pneumonia due to diffuse cervical hyperostosis. Chest 1990;98:763–4.
38. Yamamoto T, Kabayashi Y, Ogura Y, et al. Delayed leg paraplegia associated with hyperextension injury in patients with diffuse idiopathic skeletal hyperostosis (DISH): case report and review of the literature. J Surg Case Rep 2017;3:1–4.
39. Westerveld LA, Verlaan JJ, Oner FC. Spinal fractures in patient with ankylosing spinal disorders: a systemic review of the literature on treatment, neurological status and complications. Eur Spine J 2009;18:145–56.
40. Westerveld LA, van Bemmel JC, Dhert WJ, et al. Clinical outcome after traumatic spinal fractures in patients with ankylosing spinal disorders compared with control patients. Spine J 2014;14:279–740.
41. Graham B, Van Peteghem PK. Fractures of the spine in ankylosing spondylitis. Diagnosis, treatment and complications. Spine 1989;14:803–7.
42. Einsiedel T, Kleimann M, Nothofer W, et al. Special problems and management in lesions of cervical spine affected by Bechterew's disease. Unfallchirung 2001;104:1129–33.
43. Guo JJ, Luk KD, Karppinen J, et al. Prevalence, distribution, and morphology of ossification of the ligamentum flavum: a population study of one thousand seven hundred thirty-six magnetic resonance imaging scans. Spine 2010;35:52–6.
44. Kudo S, Ono M, Russell WJ. Ossification of thoracic ligamenta flava. AJR Am J Roentgenol 1983;141:117–21.
45. Williams DM, Gabrielsen TO, Latack JT, et al. Ossification in cephalic attachment of the ligamentum flavum. An anatomical and CT study. Radiology 1984;150:423–6.
46. Aizawa T, Sato T, Sasaki H, et al. Thoracic myelopathy caused by ossification of the ligamentum flavum: clinical features and surgical results in the Japanese population. J Neurosurg Spine 2006;5:514–9.
47. Kawaguchi Y, Yasuda T, Seki S, et al. Variables affecting postsurgical prognosis of thoracic myelopathy caused by ossification of the ligamentum flavum. Spine J 2013;13:1095–107.
48. Fotakopoulos GI, Alexiou GA, Mihos E, et al. Ossification of the ligamentum flavum in cervical and thoracic spine. Report of three cases. Acta Neurol Belg 2010;110:186–9.
49. Inoue H, Seichi A, Kimura A, et al. Multiple-level ossification of the ligamentum flavum in the cervical spine combined with calcification of the cervical ligamentum flavum and posterior atlanto-axial membrane. Eur Spine J 2013;22:S416–20.
50. Kotani Y, Takahata M, Abumi K, et al. Cervical myelopathy resulting from combined ossification of the ligamentum flavum and posterior longitudinal ligament: report of two cases and literature review. Spine J 2013;13:e1–6.
51. Okada K, Oka S, Tohge K, et al. Thoracic myelopathy caused by ossification of the ligamentum flavum. Clinicopathologic study and surgical treatment. Spine 1991;16:280–7.
52. Hasue M, Kikuchi S, Fijiwara M, et al. Roentgenographic analysis of ossification of the spinal ligament; with special reference to the findings of the whole spine. Seikei Geka 1980;31:1179–86 [in Japanese].
53. Chacko AG, Daniel RT. Multilevel cervical oblique corpectomy in the treatment of ossified posterior longitudinal ligament in the presence of ossified anterior longitudinal ligament. Spine 2007;32:E575–80.
54. Ehara S, Shimamura T, Nakamura R, et al. Paravertebral ligamentous ossification: DISH, OPLL and OLF. Eur J Radiol 1998;27:196–205.

55. Epstein NE. Simultaneous cercal diffuse idiopathic skeletal hyperostosis and ossification of the posterior longitudinal ligament resulting in dysphasia or myelopathy in two geriatric North Americans. Surg Neurol 2000;53:427–31.
56. Resnick D, Niwayama G. Radiographic and pathologic features of spinal involvement in diffuse idiopathic skeletal hyperostosis (DISH). Radiology 1976;119:559–68.
57. Yamada T, Mizuno J, Isobe M, et al. Analysis of ossification of the anterior longitudinal ligament: report five cases. J Jpn Med Soc Paraplegia 2000;13:70–1 [in Japanese].
58. Griffiths ID, Fitzjohn TP. Cervical myelopathy, ossification of the posterior longitudinal ligament, and diffuse idiopathic skeletal hyperostosis: problems in investigation. Ann Rheum Dis 1987;46:166–8.
59. McAfee PC, Regan JJ, Bohlmann HH. Cervical cord compression from ossification of the posterior longitudinal ligament in nonorientals. J Bone Joint Surg Br 1987;69:569–75.
60. Resnick D, Guerra J Jr, Robinson CA, et al. Association of diffuse idiopathic skeletal hyperostosis (DISH) and calcification and ossification of the posterior longitudinal ligament. AJR Am J Roentgenol 1978;131:1049–53.
61. Tsukahara S, Miyazawa N, Akagawa H, et al. COL6A1, the candidate gene for ossification of the posterior longitudinal ligament, is associated with diffuse idiopathic skeletal hyperostosis in Japanese. Spine 2005;30:2321–4.
62. Schuenke M, Schulte E, Schumacher U. Thieme atlas of anatomy general anatomy and musculoskeletal system. 1st edition. Stuttgart (Germany): Thieme; 2010. p. 76–117.
63. Ohtsuka K, Yanagihara M. The epidemiology of the hyperostosis of the spine. Seikeigeka MOOK 1987; 50:E394–403.
64. Inamasu J, Guiot BH. A review of factors predictive of surgical outcome for ossification of the ligamentum flavum of the thoracic spine. J Neurosurg Spine 2006;5:133–9.
65. Kobayashi S, Okada K, Onoda K, et al. Ossification of the cervical ligamentum flavum. Surg Neurol 1991;35:234–8.
66. Kubota M, Baba I, Sumida T. Myelopathy due to ossification of the ligamentum flavum of the cervical spine. A report of two cases. Spine 1981;6: 553–9.
67. Mizuno J, Nakagawa H. Unilateral ossification of the ligamentum flavum in the cervical spine with atypical radiological appearance. J Clin Neurosci 2002;9: 452–64.
68. Ando K, Imagama S, Wakao M, et al. Examination of the influence of ossification of the anterior longitudinal ligament on symptom progression and surgical outcome of ossification of the thoracic ligamentum flavum: a multicenter study. J Neurosurg Spine 2012;16:147–53.
69. Tsuyama N. Ossification of the posterior longitudinal ligament of the pine. Clin Orthop Relat Res 1984;(184):71–84.
70. Chang H, Kong CG, Won HY, et al. Inter- and intraobserver variability of a cervical OPLL classification using reconstructed CT images. Clin Orthop Surg 2010;2:8–12.
71. Fujimori T, Iwasaki M, Nagamoto Y, et al. Three-dimensional measurement of growth of the posterior longitudinal ligament. J Neurosurg Spine 2012;16: 289–95.
72. Kawaguchi Y, Matsumoto M, Iwasaki M, et al. New classification system for ossification of the posterior longitudinal ligament using CT images. J Orthop Sci 2014;19:530–6.
73. Azuma Y, Kato Y, Taguchi T. Etiology of cervical myelopathy induced by ossification of the posterior longitude ligament: determining the response level of OPLL myelopathy by correlating static compression and dynamic factors. J Spinal Disord Tech 2010;23:166–9.
74. Fukuyama S, Nakamura T, Ikeda T, et al. The effect of mechanical stress on hypertrophy of the lumbar ligamentum flavum. J Spinal Disord 1995;8:126–30.

Importance of Sagittal Alignment of the Cervical Spine in the Management of Degenerative Cervical Myelopathy

Thomas J. Buell, MD*, Avery L. Buchholz, MD, MPH,
John C. Quinn, MD, Christopher I. Shaffrey, MD,
Justin S. Smith, MD, PhD

KEYWORDS

• Cervical myelopathy • Sagittal alignment • Kyphosis • Scoliosis • Deformity

KEY POINTS

- Cervical spine sagittal malalignment may be associated with worse clinical symptoms and poor outcomes in patients with degenerative cervical myelopathy (DCM).
- DCM may cause progressive neurologic deficits; therefore, there is little evidence to support nonsurgical management, especially in the setting of moderate or severe myelopathy.
- Clinical improvement following surgical management of DCM has been demonstrated using both anterior-only and posterior-only approaches, with cervical sagittal alignment (lordosis vs kyphosis) often cited as a primary factor in surgical approach planning.
- Surgical approach may not significantly impact outcomes in patients with preoperative lordotic alignment, and these patients generally have greater clinical improvement compared with those with preoperative kyphotic alignment.
- Although there is no clear consensus, most studies suggest that patients with DCM with kyphotic cervical deformity have improved outcomes when adequate correction of local sagittal alignment is obtained through an anterior or a combined anterior-posterior approach.

INTRODUCTION

Cervical spondylotic myelopathy, or degenerative cervical myelopathy (DCM), is often a progressive disease and is the most common cause of spinal cord dysfunction in patients older than 55 years.[1–3] The etiology of DCM has been primarily attributed to multilevel spondylosis involving disc degeneration and osteophyte formation.[2,3] However, DCM may also be associated with and potentially exacerbated by loss of normal

Disclosures: C.I. Shaffrey is a consultant for Medtronic, Nuvasive, Zimmer Biomet, and K2M. He has received royalties from Medtronic, Nuvasive, and Zimmer Biomet. He is also a stockholder of Nuvasive. He has received grant funding from NIH (grant no. GO10989), Department of Defense, and NACTN (grant no. GF12318). J.S. Smith is a consultant for Zimmer Biomet, Nuvasive, K2M, and Cerapedics. In addition to receiving royalties from Zimmer Biomet, he has received honoraria for teaching from Zimmer Biomet, Nuvasive, and K2M. He has received research grant support from DePuy Synthes/ISSG (grant no. GI12651), NIH ASLS (grant no. 1R01AR055176-01A2), NACTN (grant no. W81XWH-16-C-0031), and fellowship support from NREF and AOSpine. All other authors have no disclosures.
Department of Neurological Surgery, University of Virginia Health System, Box 800212, Charlottesville, VA 22908, USA
* Corresponding author. Department of Neurological Surgery, University of Virginia Health System, Box 800212, Charlottesville, VA 22908.
E-mail address: tjb4p@virginia.edu

Neurosurg Clin N Am 29 (2018) 69–82
https://doi.org/10.1016/j.nec.2017.09.004
1042-3680/18/© 2017 Elsevier Inc. All rights reserved.

sagittal alignment of the cervical spine as a result of primary cervical disease or related to changes in subjacent spinal regions.[3] As a result of the growing recognition of the importance of sagittal alignment as a contributor to DCM, there has been increasing emphasis on the importance of cervical sagittal malalignment in the management of DCM.[3]

Kyphotic alignment of the cervical spine may contribute to myelopathy development by forced draping of the spinal cord against the vertebral bodies and disc-osteophyte complexes, inducing anterior cord pathology and increasing the longitudinal cord tension from tethering by the dentate ligaments and cervical nerve roots (**Fig. 1**).[3,4] As

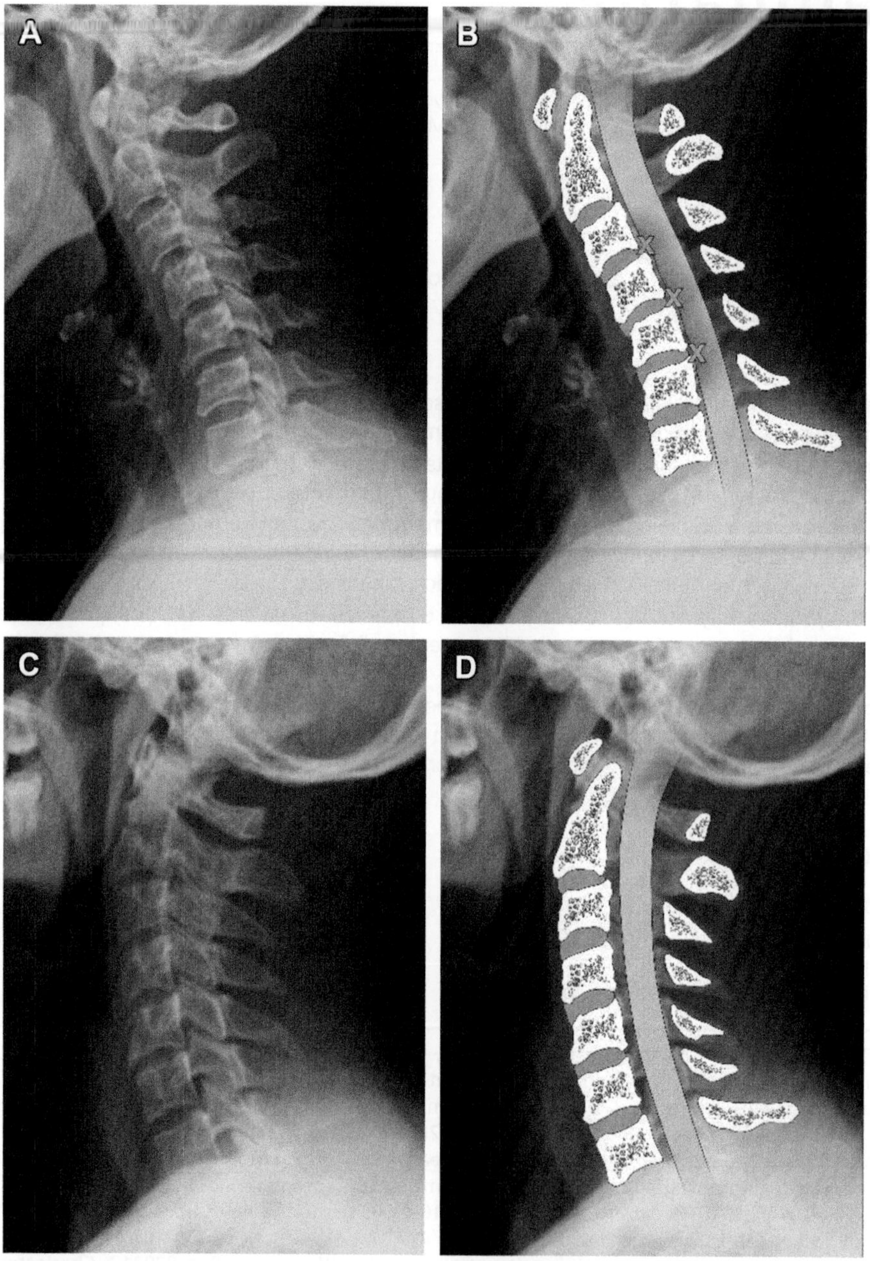

Fig. 1. In kyphotic alignment of the cervical spine, the spinal cord may be "draped" over the anterior vertebral bodies and disc-osteophyte complexes (x) (*A, B*). A mechanism for myelopathy development results from this kyphosis draping the spinal cord against the vertebral bodies inducing anterior cord pathology and increasing the longitudinal cord tension. The objective of surgery, in addition to direct decompression, is stabilization in lordosis of the operated segment to allow the posterior shifting and relaxation of the spinal cord (*C, D*). (*Courtesy of* Emma C. Vought, MS, CMI, Department of Neurosurgery, Medical University of South Carolina, Charleston.)

the kyphotic deformity worsens, the anterior and posterior cord margins compress and the lateral margins expand.[3] Shimizu and colleagues[5] supported this observation by inducing cervical kyphosis in small game fowls and analyzing histologic sections of their spinal cords. The investigators found a significant correlation between kyphosis progression and the degree of cord flattening. As kyphosis progresses, tethering of the spinal cord may increase intramedullary pressure and result in neuronal loss and demyelination.[3,5] The pattern of demyelination tends to begin with the anterior fasciculus, with subsequent progression to the lateral and posterior fasciculi.[3,5] Along with these pathologic changes, the smaller arterial feeders to the cord may become compressed and flattened, resulting in further cord injury due to compromised blood supply.[3,5] These results suggest that sagittal alignment of the cervical spine may significantly influence the development of cervical myelopathy.[3]

DYNAMIC SAGITTAL PLANE MOTION ANALYSIS IN DEGENERATIVE CERVICAL MYELOPATHY

In addition to the static forces from mechanical compression caused by cervical stenosis and kyphosis, DCM may be exacerbated by the repetitive insult of dynamic factors during neck flexion and extension.[6] Static factors that contribute to stenosis include protruding discs, ligamentous hypertrophy, and age-related changes of the vertebrae and facets that represent the osseous degenerative cascade known as spondylosis. However, cervical spondylosis is not invariably pathognomonic for clinical myelopathy. A consecutive autopsy series in 200 adults demonstrated spondylosis in 53.5% of specimens, with only 7.5% of these having documented clinical evidence of myelopathy.[7]

Whereas degenerative changes associated with spondylosis typically reduce the spinal canal diameter, there may be more to DCM than is evident from a static MRI study.[6] Dynamic factors associated with neck flexion and extension may exacerbate static compressive elements.[6] With flexion, the spinal cord is draped over the posterior aspect of the vertebral bodies and can be further compressed against osteophytic spurs and protruding discs.[3,8–10] With hyperextension, a hypertrophied ligamentum flavum or lamina may also compress the cord.[10] Chronic, repetitive cervical movements may result in irreversible spinal cord changes from neuronal loss or demyelination, which may help to explain why some patients do not improve after decompression alone, but rather experience a plateau of previously deteriorating symptoms.[11,12]

DYNAMIC CERVICAL MOTION ANALYSIS WITH THE CONE OF KINESIS

Dynamic motion analysis may play an important role in understanding cervical myelopathy. Dubousset[13] visualized a cone of balance for the standing position, in which the feet are located within a zone called the "polygon of sustentation" and the body, under the influence of muscle function and ligamentous support, can move in a conical fashion without moving the feet.[6] Dubousset further described the concept of a "conus of economy," where the body can stay balanced with minimal muscle action.[13] With Dubousset's conus of economy in mind, Liu and colleagues[6] proposed to model the dynamic cervical spine in DCM patients as a "cone of kinesis" to examine the pathology in a kinetic fashion (**Fig. 2**). Liu and colleagues[6] studied patients, who at baseline, had mean health-related quality of life (HRQOL) measures and radiographic parameters that demonstrated disability and sagittal malalignment, respectively. The investigators found that reduced flexion/extension motion cones, a more posterior center of rotation, and smaller range of motion correlated with worse myelopathy grades. Furthermore, the investigators postulated that loss of cone size may be at least initially more a consequence of neurologic compression and not necessarily the inability to move, culminating in a cycle of intentional hypomobility and stiffness. Therefore,

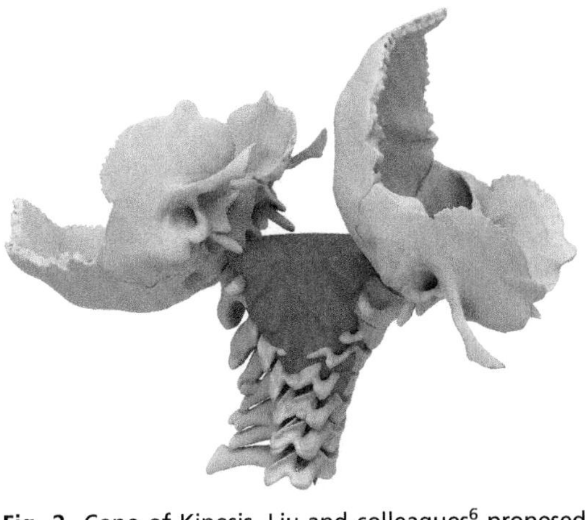

Fig. 2. Cone of Kinesis. Liu and colleagues[6] proposed the "cone of kinesis" as a model for dynamic motion analysis of the cervical spine in patients with degenerative cervical myelopathy. This concept is an application of Dubousset's cone of economy. (*Courtesy of* Emma C. Vought, MS, CMI, Department of Neurosurgery, Medical University of South Carolina, Charleston.)

when surgery is performed, the goal may be to achieve what patients are already doing in the course of their disease: stabilizing sagittal movement of the cervical spine.[9]

CERVICAL ALIGNMENT PARAMETERS

Over the past decade, there have been several reports that identify important radiographic parameters in the thoracolumbar spine that have direct effects on HRQOL.[3,14–16] Normative global and regional parameters have been defined and critical thresholds for sagittal realignment planning have been established.[3,16] However, in comparison, there are relatively fewer reports that identify these normative values for cervical spine alignment.[3,17] The major parameters used to assess cervical spine alignment include Cobb angles, Jackson stress lines, and Harrison posterior tangent lines for sagittal curvature; center of gravity of the head (COG) line or C2 plumb line for sagittal vertical axis (cSVA); and the chin-brow vertical angle (CBVA) for horizontal gaze.[3] There are also multiple other radiographic measures that can be used to assess the cervical spine.[3] **Table 1** presents important radiographic sagittal plane parameters for cervical alignment. **Fig. 3** provides an illustration of several of these parameters on a lateral cervical radiograph.

CORRELATIONS BETWEEN RADIOGRAPHIC PARAMETERS AND MYELOPATHY SCORES

Smith and colleagues[18] performed a post hoc analysis of the prospective, multicenter AOSpine North America cervical spondylotic myelopathy study. The investigators found that modified Japanese Orthopedic Association (mJOA) scores correlated negatively with C2-C7 SVA, C1-C7 SVA, C2 tilt, and C2 slope.[18] The mJOA score correlated weakly with T1 slope minus C2-C7 Cobb angle. The mJOA score was not found to correlate significantly with COG-C7 SVA, C2-C7 Cobb angle, or the posterior or anterior length of the spinal column.[18]

CORRELATIONS AMONG RADIOGRAPHIC PARAMETERS

In the same post hoc analysis, Smith and colleagues[18] found significant correlations among

Table 1
Radiographic cervical sagittal parameters

Radiographic Cervical Sagittal Parameter	Definition
Cervical sagittal vertical axis (cSVA)	Horizontal offset between a chosen plumbline and the posterosuperior corner of the C7 vertebral body. Measured using plumblines from the barycenter of C1 (C1-C7 SVA), the barycenter of C2 (C2-C7 SVA), or the center of gravity of the head (COG), taken as the midpoint of the line between the 2 external auditory canals (COG-C7 SVA).
C2 tilt	Angle between the posterior aspect of the C2 vertebral body and the vertical. (−) for posterior inclination and (+) for anterior inclination.
C2 slope	Angle between the C2 inferior endplate and horizontal reference line.
C7 slope	Angle between the C7 superior endplate and horizontal reference line.
T1 slope	Angle between the T1 superior endplate and horizontal reference line.
C2-C7 Cobb angle	Sagittal cervical curvature from C2 to C7, using the Cobb method. (−) for lordosis and (+) for kyphosis.
C2-C7 Harrison angle	Sagittal cervical curvature from C2 to C7, using Harrison method.[3] (−) for lordosis and (+) for kyphosis.
Posterior length	The summation of the lengths of the posterior aspects of the vertebral bodies and disk heights from the C7 inferior endplate to the C2 inferior endplate.
Anterior length	The summation of the lengths of the anterior aspects of vertebral bodies and disk heights from the C7 inferior endplate to the C2 inferior endplate.
Anterior length/posterior length	Anterior length divided by posterior length.

Data from Smith JS, Lafage V, Ryan DJ, et al. Association of myelopathy scores with cervical sagittal balance and normalized spinal cord volume: analysis of 56 preoperative cases from the AOSpine North America Myelopathy study. Spine (Phila Pa 1976) 2013;38(22 Suppl 1):S161–70.

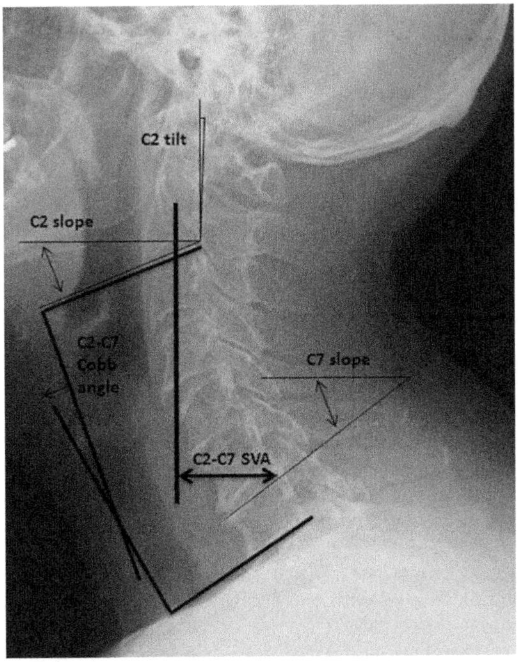

Fig. 3. Lateral cervical spine radiograph illustrating important radiographic measurements (C2-C7 sagittal vertical axis [SVA], C2 tilt, C2 slope, C7 slope, C2-C7 Cobb angle).

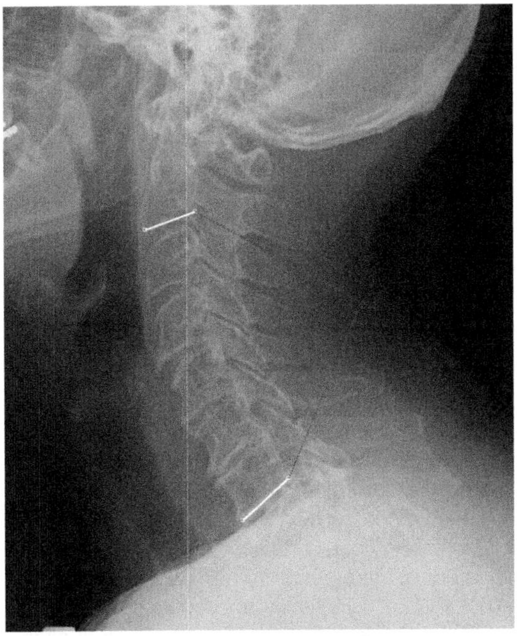

Fig. 4. Traditional cervical sagittal alignment measurement (C2-C7 Cobb angle). Lateral radiographic image showing measurement of the C2-C7 Cobb angle between the C2 and C7 interior endplates.

radiographic parameters. Within the radiographic parameters, C2-C7 SVA correlated with T1 slope minus C2-C7 Cobb angle, as well as with the anterior and posterior lengths of the cervical spine.[18] In addition, the anterior length of the cervical spine correlated with C2-C7 Cobb angle and the posterior length of the cervical spine.[18] The ratio between anterior and posterior lengths of the cervical spine correlated to C2 tilt, C2 slope, C7 slope, T1 slope, C2-C7 Cobb angle, C2-C7 Harrison angle, and the T1 slope minus C2-C7 Cobb angle.[18]

STRAIGHT-LINE METHOD FOR MEASUREMENT OF EFFECTIVE SPINAL CANAL LORDOSIS

Gwinn and colleagues[19] hypothesized that traditional methods for taking angular measurements of sagittal cervical spine alignment, such as the C2-C7 Cobb angle and C2-C7 posterior tangent method (**Figs. 4** and **5**), do not take into account ventral obstructions to the spinal cord. The investigators introduced the "effective lordosis" measurement, which may provide a simple and more reliable means for determining clinically significant lordosis.[19] The effective lordosis of the spinal canal was calculated by drawing a line from the dorsal-caudal aspect of the C2 vertebral body to

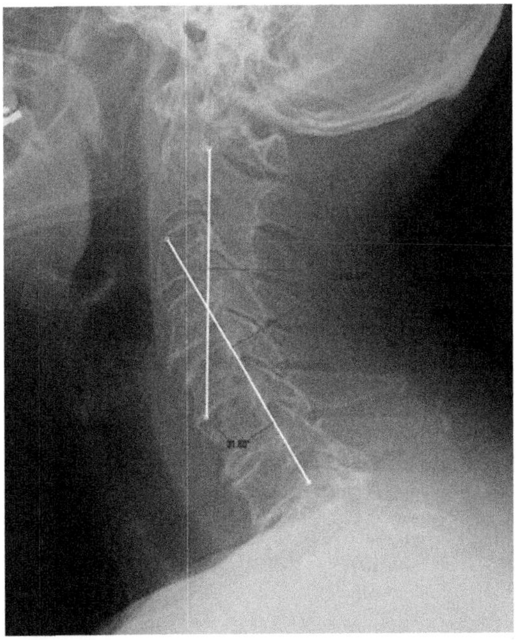

Fig. 5. Traditional cervical sagittal alignment measurement (C2-C7 posterior tangent method). Lateral radiographic image showing measurement of the absolute rotation angle of C2-C7, according to the posterior tangent method, between the tangents drawn from the posterior aspect of the C2 and C7 vertebral bodies.

the dorsal-caudal aspect of the C7 vertebral body.[19] Effective lordosis was considered to be maintained if no ventral bone structures (vertebral body, disc-osteophyte complexes, hypertrophic calcifications) projected dorsally to the line; otherwise, effective lordosis was considered lost (**Figs. 6** and **7**).

SURGICAL APPROACH FOR CERVICAL OSSIFICATION OF THE POSTERIOR LONGITUDINAL LIGAMENT: THE K-LINE

The concept of the effective lordosis line is similar to the K-line (**Fig. 8**) for helping to determine the surgical approach in patients with cervical ossification of the posterior longitudinal ligament (OPLL).[20] Prior studies that aimed to identify factors associated with poor surgical outcomes after laminoplasty for cervical OPLL identified: (1) kyphotic alignment of the cervical spine,[21] and (2) relatively large OPLL.[22,23] Fujiyoshi and colleagues[20] introduced the K-line to better evaluate cervical alignment and the OPLL size in a single parameter. The K-line is a straight line that connects the midpoints of the spinal canal at C2 and C7 on the lateral cervical radiographs. OPLL does not exceed the K-line in the K-line (+) group and does exceed it in the K-line (–) group. The investigators demonstrated that a sufficient posterior shift of the spinal cord and neurologic improvement are unlikely to be obtained after posterior decompression surgery in the K-line (–) group.[20]

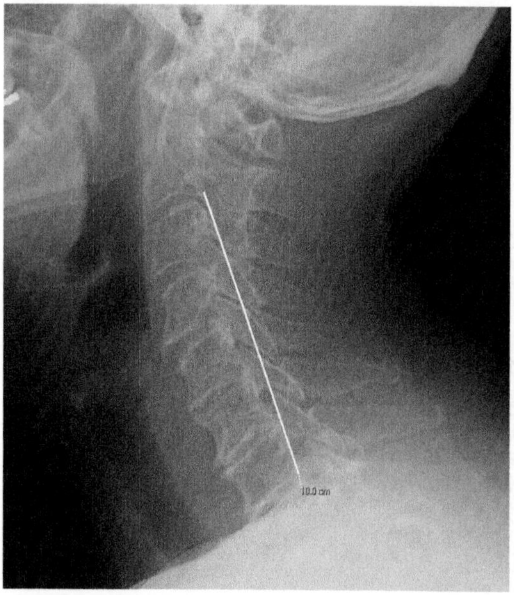

Fig. 6. Effective cervical lordosis line. Lateral radiographic image, with the line drawn from the dorsal-caudal aspect of C2 to the dorsal-caudal aspect of C7. This line can be used as a reference to measure effective cervical lordosis. In this image, effective canal lordosis is maintained, because no osteophytes or bone project posterior to the line.

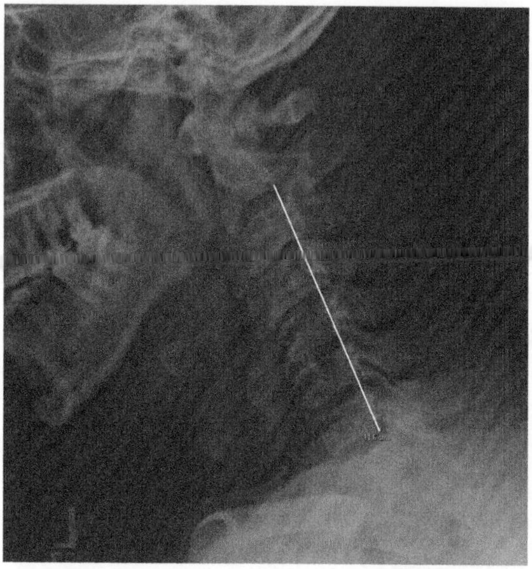

Fig. 7. Effective cervical lordosis line. Lateral radiographic image, with the line drawn from the dorsal-caudal aspect of C2 to the dorsal-caudal aspect of C7. Vertebral endplates and osteophytes protrude dorsal to the effective lordosis line, indicating loss of lordosis within the spinal canal.

MODIFIED K-LINE IN MRI AND CERVICAL SPONDYLOTIC MYELOPATHY

Taniyama and colleagues[24] modified the K-line for MRI to determine whether residual anterior spinal cord compression (after laminoplasty for DCM) is significantly correlated with preoperative anterior spinal cord clearance. The investigators defined the modified K-line (mK-line) as a line connecting midpoints of the spinal cord at C2 and C7 on a T1-weighted sagittal MRI. They then measured the minimum interval distance (INT) between the mK-line and anterior compressive factors (such as disc bulges or osteophytes) on the midsagittal image. They reported that residual anterior spinal cord compression likely occurs in nonlordotic patients when preoperative INT is less than 4 mm.[24] In a subsequent study, Taniyama and colleagues[25] found that INT was also a significant predictive factor for clinical outcomes in patients with preoperative nonlordotic alignment.

CERVICAL SPINE DEFORMITY CLASSIFICATION SYSTEM

In contrast to adult thoracolumbar deformity,[26] until recently, there was no comprehensive cervical

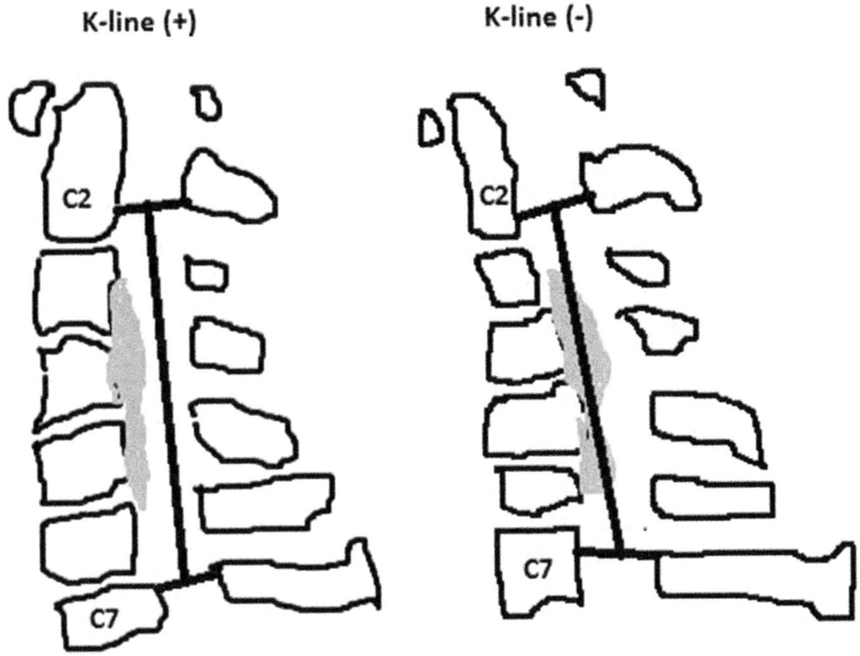

Fig. 8. The K-line is a line connecting the midpoints of the spinal canal from C2 and C7. K-line (+) group have OPLL that does not exceed this line while K-line (–) group does. (*Modified from* Fujiyoshi T, Yamazaki M, Kawabe J, et al. A new concept for making decisions regarding the surgical approach for cervical ossification of the posterior longitudinal ligament: the K-line. Spine (Phila Pa 1976) 2008;33(26):E990–3; with permission.)

spine deformity classification system. To guide patient management and develop a foundation for evidence-based care, Ames and colleagues[27] introduced a novel cervical spine deformity classification system based on clinical and radiographic parameters determined by literature review and a modified Delphi approach with an expert panel (**Fig. 9**).[28]

The classification system included a deformity descriptor and 5 modifiers that incorporate sagittal, regional, and global spinopelvic alignment and neurologic status.[27] The descriptors included: "C," "CT," and "T" for primary cervical kyphotic deformities with an apex in the cervical spine, cervicothoracic junction, or thoracic spine, respectively; "S" for primary coronal deformity with a coronal Cobb angle $\geq$ 15°; and "CVJ" for primary craniovertebral junction deformity.[27] The modifiers included C2-C7 SVA, horizontal gaze (assessed by the CBVA), T1 slope (TS) minus C2-C7 lordosis (TS-CL), myelopathy (mJOA scale score), and the Scoliosis Research Society (SRS)-Schwab classification for thoracolumbar deformity.[26,27] inclusion of the mJOA score in this deformity classification is reflective of the frequent presence of myelopathy in the setting of cervical deformity. The authors readily acknowledge that this classification will likely undergo iterative improvements as we continue to learn more regarding the impact of various clinical and radiographic factors.

NONOPERATIVE MANAGEMENT OF PATIENTS WITH DEGENERATIVE CERVICAL MYELOPATHY

Nonoperative management of patients with DCM may include physical therapy, spinal injections, cervical immobilization with braces or collars, activity restriction, and cervical traction.[29] However, these measures may have limited efficacy, especially in patients with moderate or severe myelopathy and abnormal sagittal alignment.[30] In a systematic review by Ghobrial and colleagues.[31] the investigators concluded that the effectiveness of nonsurgical management may greatly depend on patient-specific factors and the etiology of myelopathy (soft disk herniation, spondylosis, OPLL, circumferential compression). They also found that there was limited evidence to support nonsurgical management for mildly myelopathic patients. On the contrary, in a randomized controlled trial, Kadanka and colleagues[32] demonstrated that surgical management was not superior in mild myelopathic patients; however, to our knowledge, there have been no

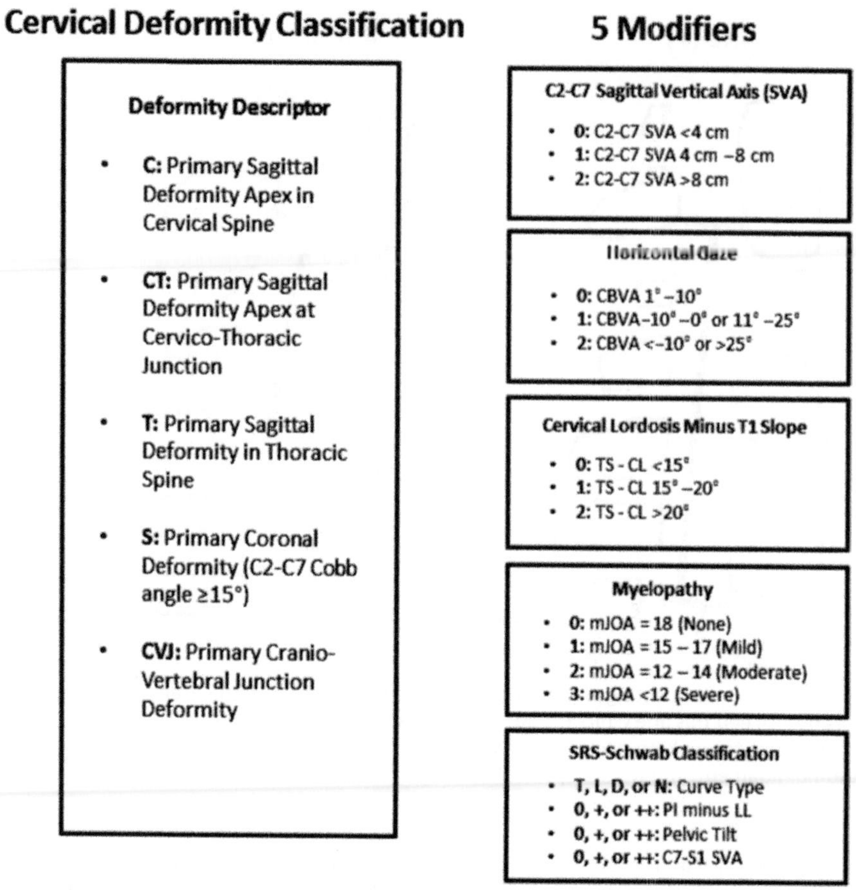

Cervical Deformity Classification
5 Modifiers
Deformity Descriptor
C: Primary Sagittal Deformity Apex in Cervical Spine
CT: Primary Sagittal Deformity Apex at Cervico-Thoracic Junction
T: Primary Sagittal Deformity in Thoracic Spine
S: Primary Coronal Deformity (C2-C7 Cobb angle ≥15°)
CVJ: Primary Cranio-Vertebral Junction Deformity
C2-C7 Sagittal Vertical Axis (SVA)
0: C2-C7 SVA <4 cm
1: C2-C7 SVA 4 cm –8 cm
2: C2-C7 SVA >8 cm
Horizontal Gaze
0: CBVA 1°–10°
1: CBVA-10°–0° or 11°–25°
2: CBVA <-10° or >25°
Cervical Lordosis Minus T1 Slope
0: TS - CL <15°
1: TS - CL 15°–20°
2: TS - CL >20°
Myelopathy
0: mJOA = 18 (None)
1: mJOA = 15 – 17 (Mild)
2: mJOA = 12 – 14 (Moderate)
3: mJOA <12 (Severe)
SRS-Schwab Classification
T, L, D, or N: Curve Type
0, +, or ++: PI minus LL
0, +, or ++: Pelvic Tilt
0, +, or ++: C7-S1 SVA

Fig. 9. The cervical spinal deformity classification system includes a deformity descriptor and 5 modifiers. D, double; L, lordosis; N, none; T, thoracic. (*Modified from* Ames CP, Smith JS, Eastlack R, et al. Reliability assessment of a novel cervical spine deformity classification system. J Neurosurg Spine 2015;23(6):673–83; with permission.)

further studies to support this conclusion. For patients with moderate or severe myelopathy, surgical management may be the best treatment option[33,34]; therefore, early risk stratification is important to identify patients more likely to experience disease progression and thus benefit from early surgery.[29]

SURGICAL MANAGEMENT OF PATIENTS WITH DEGENERATIVE CERVICAL MYELOPATHY

Surgical management of patients with DCM should include both decompression of the spinal cord, along with appropriate restoration of cervical sagittal alignment if indicated.[29,35] This may involve an anterior-only or posterior-only approach or may be achieved through combined anterior and posterior procedures.[29,35–37] Traditionally, the surgical management of cervical myelopathy via posterior-only approaches has been considered primarily in patients with maintained preoperative cervical lordosis, flexible kyphosis that is correctable with traction, or semi-rigid kyphosis that can be corrected with posterior-only osteotomies.[21,29,37,38] A posterior approach for decompression and fusion can enable circumferential decompression.[39] Posterior compressive bone and hypertrophied ligamentum flavum can be directly removed.[40] Furthermore, posterior decompression allows for dorsal migration of the spinal cord for indirect decompression of the anterior spinal cord.[41–45] In other patients with abnormal rigid cervical kyphosis, reconstruction using lordotic interbody spacers through an anterior approach may be necessary to restore the natural lordotic cervical curvature.[46,47] However, symptoms of myelopathy may persist or worsen if posterior decompression alone is performed, and the cervical spine remains kyphotic.[48] Currently, the literature lacks high-level objective evidence regarding which of these surgical approaches, anterior versus posterior, is superior in terms of patient outcomes and complication profiles.[34,36,37,49–53]

SURGICAL MANAGEMENT (POSTERIOR APPROACH)

Posterior surgical techniques for cervical myelopathy and sagittal alignment correction have evolved considerably over the past 40 years.[54] In the past, treatment for DCM often involved decompressive laminectomy alone. This procedure involves removal of compressive bony elements and hypertrophied ligamentum flavum at the desired levels.[55] In general, decompressive laminectomy without fusion should be reserved for patients with preserved lordosis who may be poor candidates for fusion. However, studies have demonstrated significant rates of progressive postoperative kyphosis and segmental instability,[56,57] which may result in additional surgery with instrumentation and fusion.[54,58] As a result, instrumented fusion should be considered, especially in patients with correctable kyphosis and instability. A multitude of instrumentation and screw techniques as well as graft choices exist and can be used at the discretion of the surgeon.[55] In cases of long multilevel laminectomy and fusion, caudal fixation in the C7 lateral masses is suboptimal due to their small size. Pedicle screws at either C7 or the top 2 thoracic vertebrae may decrease the chance of distal fixation failure in these long constructs.[55]

Sielatycki and colleagues[59] studied laminectomy and fusion in DCM for lordotic patients. Although the investigators found that creating more lordosis and decreasing cSVA are associated with improved myelopathy and outcomes in patients with kyphosis, they did not find such associations in patients with lordosis undergoing posterior laminectomy and fusion for cervical spondylotic myelopathy. This suggests that any amount of lordosis may be sufficient.[59]

Although many investigators consider preoperative kyphosis to be a contraindication to a posterior-only surgical approach for DCM,[60,61] Tashjian and colleagues[45] found that preoperative cervical alignment does not statistically correlate with postoperative spinal cord drift in patients undergoing multisegmental decompressive laminectomy and fusion for DCM. The observation of significant posterior shifting of the spinal cord in the context of straight or kyphotic preoperative alignment suggests that posterior decompression and arthrodesis may represent a viable option in the surgical management of some patients with DCM with nonlordotic preoperative alignment.[45]

Another posterior cervical surgical technique for patients with DCM is the expansive laminoplasty.[21,62,63] In comparison with laminectomy and fusion, laminoplasty may be associated with higher rates of postoperative cervical kyphosis and segmental instability.[36] However, laminectomy and fusion changes normal cervical biomechanics, as axial and rotational forces are no longer physiologically distributed to subjacent spinal structures.[54] In contrast, expansive laminoplasty preserves motion with less substantial changes to natural cervical spine biomechanics, but may result in a less extensive cord decompression.[64]

Lee and colleagues[65] performed a meta-analysis comparing posterior cervical laminoplasty versus laminectomy and instrumented fusion for multilevel (at least 3 levels) cervical spondylotic myelopathy. Both treatment groups showed slight cervical lordosis and moderate neck pain in the baseline state. After surgery, expansive laminoplasty and laminectomy plus fusion both led to clinical improvement and loss of lordosis evenly. In the laminectomy plus fusion group, cervical lordosis was preserved in long-term follow-up studies, although the difference compared with the laminoplasty group was not statistically significant. Therefore, the investigators concluded that, in select patients with comorbidities that do not restrict the surgical plan, there may be insufficient evidence to support laminoplasty over laminectomy plus fusion for the treatment of multilevel DCM.[65]

CERVICAL SPINAL CORD POSTERIOR DRIFT AFTER POSTERIOR DECOMPRESSION

Posterior decompression and stabilization in lordosis allows spinal cord to shift posteriorly, leading to indirect decompression of the anterior spinal cord (**Fig. 10**).[44] Denaro and colleagues[44] performed a study to investigate the efficacy of posterior decompression and stabilization in lordosis for multilevel cervical spondylotic myelopathy.[66] The investigators concluded that posterior decompression and stabilization in lordosis is a valuable procedure for patients affected by multilevel cervical spondylotic myelopathy, and may result in significant clinical improvement due to the posterior shift of the spinal cord.[44]

The influence of preoperative cervical sagittal alignment on the outcome of posterior cervical surgical approaches is currently debated in the literature.[45] Many investigators have studied this relationship with the spinal cord posterior shift, but an unequivocal conclusion has not been established. One study showed that posterior cord migration correlated significantly with preoperative and postoperative cervical spine lordosis.[42] However, subsequent studies did not

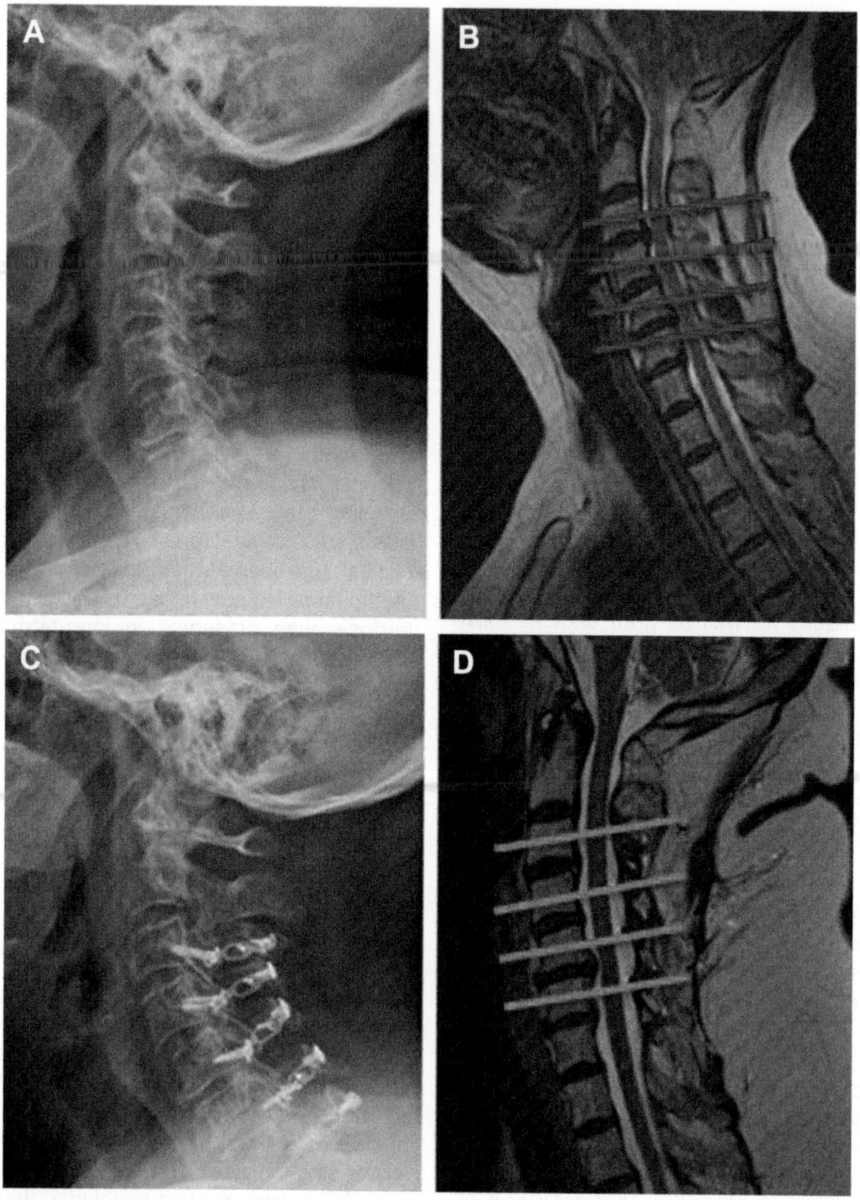

Fig. 10. Posterior shift of the spinal cord after decompression. Lateral cervical radiographs and MR imaging of a patient with degenerative cervical myelopathy and preoperative cervical lordosis (*A, B*). Postoperative imaging demonstrates posterior shift of the cervical spinal cord after C3-C7 laminoplasty in which lordosis was maintained (*C, D*). Decompression with stabilization of the cervical spine in lordosis of the operated segment allows the posterior shift of the spinal cord. The *red horizontal lines* represent a compressed cervical spinal cord. The *green horizontal lines* represent a "decompressed" cervical spinal cord after posterior shift. This allows for indirect decompression of the spinal cord after posterior approaches.

confirm this result.[45] Sodeyama and colleagues[67] found no significant difference in the mean posterior cord shift among neck alignment groups of patients undergoing conventional or extended laminoplasty. Further studies also have not demonstrated a significant correlation between posterior cord migration with preoperative and postoperative cervical spine lordosis.[45,68,69]

SURGICAL MANAGEMENT (ANTERIOR APPROACH)

Significant fixed local or global kyphosis is a relative contraindication to posterior decompression and fusion since the spinal cord may remain "draped" over the anterior compressive elements following decompression.[19] However, as described previously, studies that correlated the magnitude of the posterior cord shifting with neck alignment are discordant, and a certain number of patients with preoperative and postoperative cervical malalignment had acceptable or even satisfactory surgical results.[44,66–69] Denaro and colleagues[44] recommended anterior decompression for patients with preoperative cervical kyphosis exceeding 13°. In patients with a lower degree of cervical kyphosis, the investigators perform posterior decompression, correction of the kyphosis, and fusion in improved alignment.[66] However, posterior surgical techniques alone may not be sufficient to obtain adequate cervical lordotic alignment in the subaxial spine above C7. Therefore, reconstruction using lordotic interbody spacers through an anterior approach may be needed to help restore the natural lordotic curve of the cervical spine.[70]

ANTERIOR VERSUS POSTERIOR APPROACHES

The surgical approach to addressing DCM depends on numerous factors, including patient age, number of involved levels, prior surgical approaches, location of the compressive lesions, and cervical alignment and flexibility. There are multiple studies that compare anterior versus posterior approaches for surgical management of DCM.[48] Sakai and colleagues[48] reported that laminoplasty is inferior to multilevel anterior cervical diskectomy and fusion, especially in patients with sagittal imbalance. Shamji and colleagues[71] studied the association of cervical spine alignment with neurologic recovery in a prospective cohort of patients with surgical myelopathy. Most patients with DCM showed postoperative neurologic improvement, but those with preoperative lordotic alignment exhibited greater improvement compared with patients with preoperative kyphotic alignment. Furthermore, the choice of surgical approach impacted neurologic recovery among kyphotic patients. The investigators found that lordotic patients exhibited similar improvement when approached anteriorly or posteriorly, whereas kyphotic patients exhibited greater improvement when approached by an anterior or combined approach.[71]

In another study by Uchida and colleagues,[47] outcomes after anterior or posterior decompression for DCM associated with kyphosis or sagittal sigmoid alignment were analyzed. The investigators analyzed patients with cervical kyphosis exceeding 10° on preoperative sagittal lateral radiographs obtained in the neutral position. Some patients underwent anterior decompression with interbody fusion whereas others received en bloc open-door C3-7 laminoplasty. mJOA scores at 4 to 6 weeks after surgery were significantly better in the anterior approach group compared with those in the laminoplasty group, but the difference became insignificant on further follow-up. Also, postoperatively the transverse area of the spinal cord was significantly greater in the anterior approach group than in the laminoplasty group. These results may suggest that in a select group of patients with kyphotic deformity ≥10°, improvement of sagittal alignment with an anterior approach may maximize the chances of recovering spinal cord function.[47]

SUMMARY

DCM is often a progressive disease and is the most common cause of spinal cord dysfunction in patients older than 55 years. The etiology of DCM has traditionally been described as multilevel spondylosis involving disc degeneration and osteophyte formation. More recently, attention has been given to the importance of cervical sagittal alignment in the management of DCM. In patients with DCM and cervical sagittal imbalance, myelopathy may worsen due to kyphosis that drapes the cord over the vertebral bodies, increases longitudinal cord tension and intramedullary pressures, and reduces blood supply due to loss of small arterial feeders. Decompressive laminectomy has historically been the surgical treatment for DCM. However, with increasing emphasis on the restoration of cervical lordosis, instrumentation has become more commonly used. However, fixed local or global kyphosis is a relative contraindication to posterior-only techniques, such as laminoplasty or decompression with fusion, because the spinal cord may remain "draped" to the anterior compressive elements without sufficient posterior cord shift. For these reasons, we do not recommend laminoplasty for patients with kyphosis (exceeding 10°) or an S-shaped cervical spine. In such patients, we recommend an anterior approach (with possible combined posterior instrumentation). Use of the K-line or effective cervical lordosis may also help guide the correct surgical approach. Further research, with prospective randomized trials, may help elucidate other factors that further guide proper management of patients with DCM and cervical sagittal malalignment.

ACKNOWLEDGMENTS

Emma C. Vought, MS, CMI, Certified Medical Illustration & Animator, Department of Neurosurgery, Medical University of South Carolina.

REFERENCES

1. Young WF. Cervical spondylotic myelopathy: a common cause of spinal cord dysfunction in older persons. Am Fam Physician 2000;62(5):1064–70, 1073.
2. Karadimas SK, Erwin WM, Ely CG, et al. Pathophysiology and natural history of cervical spondylotic myelopathy. Spine (Phila Pa 1976) 2013;38(22 Suppl 1):S21–36.
3. Scheer JK, Tang JA, Smith JS, et al. Cervical spine alignment, sagittal deformity, and clinical implications: a review. J Neurosurg Spine 2013;19(2):141–59.
4. Albert TJ, Vacarro A. Postlaminectomy kyphosis. Spine (Phila Pa 1976) 1998;23(24):2738–45.
5. Shimizu K, Nakamura M, Nishikawa Y, et al. Spinal kyphosis causes demyelination and neuronal loss in the spinal cord: a new model of kyphotic deformity using juvenile Japanese small game fowls. Spine (Phila Pa 1976) 2005;30(21):2388–92.
6. Liu S, Lafage R, Smith JS, et al. Impact of dynamic alignment, motion, and center of rotation on myelopathy grade and regional disability in cervical spondylotic myelopathy. J Neurosurg Spine 2015;23(6):690–700.
7. Hughes JT, Brownell B. Necropsy observations on the spinal cord in cervical spondylosis. Riv Patol Nerv Ment 1965;86(2):196–204.
8. Ames CP, Blondel B, Scheer JK, et al. Cervical radiographical alignment: comprehensive assessment techniques and potential importance in cervical myelopathy. Spine (Phila Pa 1976) 2013;38(22 Suppl 1):S149–60.
9. Gruninger W, Gruss P. Stenosis and movement of the cervical spine in cervical myelopathy. Paraplegia 1982;20(3):121–30.
10. Toledano M, Bartleson JD. Cervical spondylotic myelopathy. Neurol Clin 2013;31(1):287–305.
11. Breig A, Turnbull I, Hassler O. Effects of mechanical stresses on the spinal cord in cervical spondylosis. A study on fresh cadaver material. J Neurosurg 1966;25(1):45–56.
12. Reid JD. Effects of flexion-extension movements of the head and spine upon the spinal cord and nerve roots. J Neurol Neurosurg Psychiatry 1960;23:214–21.
13. Dubousset J. Three-dimensional analysis of the scoliotic deformity, Vol. 2. New York: Raven Press; 1994.
14. Protopsaltis TS, Scheer JK, Terran JS, et al. How the neck affects the back: changes in regional cervical sagittal alignment correlate to HRQOL improvement in adult thoracolumbar deformity patients at 2-year follow-up. J Neurosurg Spine 2015;23(2):153–8.
15. Smith JS, Shaffrey CI, Glassman SD, et al. Clinical and radiographic parameters that distinguish between the best and worst outcomes of scoliosis surgery for adults. Eur Spine J 2013;22(2):402–10.
16. Schwab F, Patel A, Ungar B, et al. Adult spinal deformity-postoperative standing imbalance: how much can you tolerate? An overview of key parameters in assessing alignment and planning corrective surgery. Spine (Phila Pa 1976) 2010;35(25):2224–31.
17. Villavicencio AT, Babuska JM, Ashton A, et al. Prospective, randomized, double-blind clinical study evaluating the correlation of clinical outcomes and cervical sagittal alignment. Neurosurgery 2011;68(5):1309–16 [discussion: 1316].
18. Smith JS, Lafage V, Ryan DJ, et al. Association of myelopathy scores with cervical sagittal balance and normalized spinal cord volume: analysis of 56 preoperative cases from the AOSpine North America Myelopathy study. Spine (Phila Pa 1976) 2013;38(22 Suppl 1):S161–70.
19. Gwinn DE, Iannotti CA, Benzel EC, et al. Effective lordosis: analysis of sagittal spinal canal alignment in cervical spondylotic myelopathy. J Neurosurg Spine 2009;11(6):667–72.
20. Fujiyoshi T, Yamazaki M, Kawabe J, et al. A new concept for making decisions regarding the surgical approach for cervical ossification of the posterior longitudinal ligament: the K-line. Spine (Phila Pa 1976) 2008;33(26):E990–3.
21. Chiba K, Ogawa Y, Ishii K, et al. Long-term results of expansive open-door laminoplasty for cervical myelopathy–average 14-year follow-up study. Spine (Phila Pa 1976) 2006;31(26):2998–3005.
22. Iwasaki M, Okuda S, Miyauchi A, et al. Surgical strategy for cervical myelopathy due to ossification of the posterior longitudinal ligament: Part 1: clinical results and limitations of laminoplasty. Spine (Phila Pa 1976) 2007;32(6):647–53.
23. Yamazaki A, Homma T, Uchiyama S, et al. Morphologic limitations of posterior decompression by midsagittal splitting method for myelopathy caused by ossification of the posterior longitudinal ligament in the cervical spine. Spine (Phila Pa 1976) 1999;24(1):32–4.
24. Taniyama T, Hirai T, Yamada T, et al. Modified K-line in magnetic resonance imaging predicts insufficient decompression of cervical laminoplasty. Spine (Phila Pa 1976) 2013;38(6):496–501.
25. Taniyama T, Hirai T, Yoshii T, et al. Modified K-line in magnetic resonance imaging predicts clinical outcome in patients with nonlordotic alignment after laminoplasty for cervical spondylotic myelopathy. Spine (Phila Pa 1976) 2014;39(21):E1261–8.
26. Schwab F, Ungar B, Blondel B, et al. Scoliosis Research Society-Schwab adult spinal deformity classification: a validation study. Spine (Phila Pa 1976) 2012;37(12):1077–82.
27. Ames CP, Smith JS, Eastlack R, et al. Reliability assessment of a novel cervical spine deformity

classification system. J Neurosurg Spine 2015; 23(6):673–83.
28. Boulkedid R, Abdoul H, Loustau M, et al. Using and reporting the Delphi method for selecting healthcare quality indicators: a systematic review. PLoS One 2011;6(6):e20476.
29. Kato S, Fehlings M. Degenerative cervical myelopathy. Curr Rev Musculoskelet Med 2016;9(3):263–71.
30. Karpova A, Arun R, Davis AM, et al. Predictors of surgical outcome in cervical spondylotic myelopathy. Spine (Phila Pa 1976) 2013;38(5):392–400.
31. Ghobrial GM, Harrop JS. Surgery vs conservative care for cervical spondylotic myelopathy: nonoperative operative management. Neurosurgery 2015; 62(Suppl 1):62–5.
32. Kadanka Z, Bednarik J, Novotny O, et al. Cervical spondylotic myelopathy: conservative versus surgical treatment after 10 years. Eur Spine J 2011; 20(9):1533–8.
33. Fehlings MG, Wilson JR, Yoon ST, et al. Symptomatic progression of cervical myelopathy and the role of nonsurgical management: a consensus statement. Spine (Phila Pa 1976) 2013;38(22 Suppl 1):S19–20.
34. Fehlings MG, Wilson JR, Kopjar B, et al. Efficacy and safety of surgical decompression in patients with cervical spondylotic myelopathy: results of the AOSpine North America prospective multi-center study. J Bone Joint Surg Am 2013;95(18):1651–8.
35. Lawrence BD, Shamji MF, Traynelis VC, et al. Surgical management of degenerative cervical myelopathy: a consensus statement. Spine (Phila Pa 1976) 2013;38(22 Suppl 1):S171–2.
36. Yoon ST, Hashimoto RE, Raich A, et al. Outcomes after laminoplasty compared with laminectomy and fusion in patients with cervical myelopathy: a systematic review. Spine (Phila Pa 1976) 2013;38(22 Suppl 1):S183–94.
37. Han K, Lu C, Li J, et al. Surgical treatment of cervical kyphosis. Eur Spine J 2011;20(4):523–36.
38. Miyamoto H, Maeno K, Uno K, et al. Outcomes of surgical intervention for cervical spondylotic myelopathy accompanying local kyphosis (comparison between laminoplasty alone and posterior reconstruction surgery using the screw-rod system). Eur Spine J 2014;23(2):341–6.
39. Sekhon LH. Posterior cervical decompression and fusion for circumferential spondylotic cervical stenosis: review of 50 consecutive cases. J Clin Neurosci 2006;13(1):23–30.
40. Epstein NE. Laminectomy for cervical myelopathy. Spinal Cord 2003;41(6):317–27.
41. Choi BW, Song KJ, Chang H. Ossification of the posterior longitudinal ligament: a review of literature. Asian Spine J 2011;5(4):267–76.
42. Baba H, Uchida K, Maezawa Y, et al. Lordotic alignment and posterior migration of the spinal cord following en bloc open-door laminoplasty for cervical myelopathy: a magnetic resonance imaging study. J Neurol 1996;243(9):626–32.
43. Yoshihara H. Indirect decompression in spinal surgery. J Clin Neurosci 2017;44:63–8.
44. Denaro V, Longo UG, Berton A, et al. Favourable outcome of posterior decompression and stabilization in lordosis for cervical spondylotic myelopathy: the spinal cord "back shift" concept. Eur Spine J 2015;24(Suppl 7):826–31.
45. Tashjian VS, Kohan E, McArthur DL, et al. The relationship between preoperative cervical alignment and postoperative spinal cord drift after decompressive laminectomy and arthrodesis for cervical spondylotic myelopathy. Surg Neurol 2009;72(2):112–7.
46. Quinn JC, Kiely PD, Lebl DR, et al. Anterior surgical treatment of cervical spondylotic myelopathy: review article. HSS J 2015;11(1):15–25.
47. Uchida K, Nakajima H, Sato R, et al. Cervical spondylotic myelopathy associated with kyphosis or sagittal sigmoid alignment: outcome after anterior or posterior decompression. J Neurosurg Spine 2009;11(5):521–8.
48. Sakai K, Yoshii T, Hirai T, et al. Impact of the surgical treatment for degenerative cervical myelopathy on the preoperative cervical sagittal balance: a review of prospective comparative cohort between anterior decompression with fusion and laminoplasty. Eur Spine J 2017;26(1):104–12.
49. Fehlings MG, Smith JS, Kopjar B, et al. Perioperative and delayed complications associated with the surgical treatment of cervical spondylotic myelopathy based on 302 patients from the AOSpine North America cervical spondylotic myelopathy study. J Neurosurg Spine 2012;16(5):425–32.
50. Fehlings MG, Barry S, Kopjar B, et al. Anterior versus posterior surgical approaches to treat cervical spondylotic myelopathy: outcomes of the prospective multicenter AOSpine North America CSM study in 264 patients. Spine (Phila Pa 1976) 2013; 38(26):2247–52.
51. Lawrence BD, Jacobs WB, Norvell DC, et al. Anterior versus posterior approach for treatment of cervical spondylotic myelopathy: a systematic review. Spine (Phila Pa 1976) 2013;38(22 Suppl 1):S173–82.
52. Kim B, Yoon DH, Shin HC, et al. Surgical outcome and prognostic factors of anterior decompression and fusion for cervical compressive myelopathy due to ossification of the posterior longitudinal ligament. Spine J 2015;15(5):875–84.
53. Kato S, Nouri A, Wu D, et al. Comparison of anterior and posterior surgery for degenerative cervical myelopathy: an MRI-based propensity-score-matched analysis using data from the prospective multicenter AOSpine CSM North America and international studies. J Bone Joint Surg Am 2017;99(12): 1013–21.

54. Woods BI, Hohl J, Lee J, et al. Laminoplasty versus laminectomy and fusion for multilevel cervical spondylotic myelopathy. Clin Orthop Relat Res 2011; 469(3):688–95.
55. Yalamanchili PK, Vives MJ, Chaudhary SB. Cervical spondylotic myelopathy: factors in choosing the surgical approach. Adv Orthop 2012;2012:783762.
56. Matsunaga S, Sakou T, Nakanisi K. Analysis of the cervical spine alignment following laminoplasty and laminectomy. Spinal Cord 1999;37(1):20–4.
57. Ryken TC, Heary RF, Matz PG, et al. Cervical laminectomy for the treatment of cervical degenerative myelopathy. J Neurosurg Spine 2009;11(2):142–9.
58. Kumar VG, Rea GL, Mervis LJ, et al. Cervical spondylotic myelopathy: functional and radiographic long-term outcome after laminectomy and posterior fusion. Neurosurgery 1999;44(4): 771–7 [discussion: 777–8].
59. Sielatycki JA, Armaghani S, Silverberg A, et al. Is more lordosis associated with improved outcomes in cervical laminectomy and fusion when baseline alignment is lordotic? Spine J 2016;16(8):982–8.
60. Suda K, Abumi K, Ito M, et al. Local kyphosis reduces surgical outcomes of expansive open-door laminoplasty for cervical spondylotic myelopathy. Spine (Phila Pa 1976) 2003;28(12):1258–62.
61. Yonenobu K, Oda T. Posterior approach to the degenerative cervical spine. Eur Spine J 2003; 12(Suppl 2):S195–201.
62. Lee TT, Green BA, Gromelski EB. Safety and stability of open-door cervical expansive laminoplasty. J Spinal Disord 1998;11(1):12–5.
63. Houten JK, Cooper PR. Laminectomy and posterior cervical plating for multilevel cervical spondylotic myelopathy and ossification of the posterior longitudinal ligament: effects on cervical alignment, spinal cord compression, and neurological outcome. Neurosurgery 2003;52(5):1081–7 [discussion: 1087–8].
64. Hyun SJ, Riew KD, Rhim SC. Range of motion loss after cervical laminoplasty: a prospective study with minimum 5-year follow-up data. Spine J 2013; 13(4):384–90.
65. Lee CH, Lee J, Kang JD, et al. Laminoplasty versus laminectomy and fusion for multilevel cervical myelopathy: a meta-analysis of clinical and radiological outcomes. J Neurosurg Spine 2015; 22(6):589–95.
66. Denaro V, Longo UG, Berton A, et al. Cervical spondylotic myelopathy: the relevance of the spinal cord back shift after posterior multilevel decompression. A systematic review. Eur Spine J 2015;24(Suppl 7): 832–41.
67. Sodeyama T, Goto S, Mochizuki M, et al. Effect of decompression enlargement laminoplasty for posterior shifting of the spinal cord. Spine (Phila Pa 1976) 1999;24(15):1527–31 [discussion: 1531–2].
68. Xia G, Tian R, Xu T, et al. Spinal posterior movement after posterior cervical decompression surgery: clinical findings and factors affecting postoperative functional recovery. Orthopedics 2011;34(12): e911–8.
69. Shiozaki T, Otsuka H, Nakata Y, et al. Spinal cord shift on magnetic resonance imaging at 24 hours after cervical laminoplasty. Spine (Phila Pa 1976) 2009;34(3):274–9.
70. Roguski M, Benzel EC, Curran JN, et al. Postoperative cervical sagittal imbalance negatively affects outcomes after surgery for cervical spondylotic myelopathy. Spine (Phila Pa 1976) 2014;39(25): 2070–7.
71. Shamji MF, Mohanty C, Massicotte EM, et al. The association of cervical spine alignment with neurologic recovery in a prospective cohort of patients with surgical myelopathy: analysis of a series of 124 cases. World Neurosurg 2016;86:112–9.

Anterior Cervical Option to Manage Degenerative Cervical Myelopathy

Zoher Ghogawala, MD

KEYWORDS

• Anterior cervical discectomy and fusion • Cervical spondylotic myelopathy • Corpectomy

KEY POINTS

- Anterior decompression and fusion surgery for degenerative cervical myelopathy (DCM) is ideal for patients with 2 to 3 levels of cervical stenosis with spinal cord compression.
- Multilevel anterior cervical decompression and fusion can be used to treat DCM in the context of cervical kyphosis.
- Dysphagia is a common and sometimes significant complication of anterior approaches to treating DCM.
- Anterior surgery for DCM may be less costly than posterior surgery and associated with greater health-related quality of life.

INTRODUCTION

Degenerative cervical myelopathy (DCM) is the most common cause of spinal cord dysfunction in the world.[1] The condition presents insidiously and is defined in terms of its clinical symptoms (gait instability, bladder dysfunction, fine finger motor difficulties) and signs (hyperreflexia, weakness, alteration of joint position sense). DCM is caused by dynamic repeated compression of the spinal cord from degenerative arthritis of the cervical spine.[2] Proposed mechanisms include axonal stretch-associated injury[2] and spinal cord ischemia from compression of larger vessels and impaired microcirculation.[3,4] Surgery to decompress and stabilize the spine often is advocated for severe or progressive symptoms, with mixed results. Approximately two-thirds of patients improve with surgery, and surgery is not successful in 15% to 30% of cases.[5] More than 112,400 cervical spine operations for degenerative spondylosis are performed annually in the United States (100% increase over the past decade),[6] with DCM accounting for nearly 20% of cervical spine operations in the United States.[7] Annual hospital charges for DCM surgery exceed $2 billion per year.[6] In addition, DCM is associated with substantial postsurgical outpatient expenses (eg, physician visits, imaging, physical therapy, medications).

The surgical treatment of DCM is accomplished by either an anterior approach or a posterior approach in most cases. Decompression of the spinal canal to a diameter of at least 12 mm with restoration of cerebrospinal fluid pulsation around the spinal cord parenchyma is the goal regardless of approach. Remarkably, this has not changed over the past 50 years, although there has been greater usage of posterior cervical laminoplasty in the past decade. In some circumstances, both anterior and posterior approaches are used, particularly when a correction of cervical deformity

Disclosure Statement: The author has no relationship with any commercial company that has direct financial interest in the subject matter or materials discussed.
Department of Neurosurgery, Alan and Jacqueline Stuart Spine Center, Lahey Hospital and Medical Center, Tufts University School of Medicine, 41 Mall Road, Burlington, MA 01805, USA
E-mail address: zoher.ghogawala@lahey.org

Neurosurg Clin N Am 29 (2018) 83–89
https://doi.org/10.1016/j.nec.2017.09.005
1042-3680/18/© 2017 Elsevier Inc. All rights reserved.

is thought to be essential for addressing myelopathy. This article focuses on anterior approaches. There are essentially 4 types of anterior approaches:

- Anterior corpectomy and fusion
- Anterior cervical discectomy and fusion
- Multilevel oblique corpectomy without fusion
- Cervical arthroplasty

There is considerable debate about the advantages of anterior approaches to the cervical spine versus posterior approaches. In general, patients with 2 to 3 levels of cervical spondylosis with cord compression are ideal candidates for anterior surgery. In addition, patients with kyphosis are generally best treated with anterior surgery. Preoperative kyphosis greater than 13°, according to one study, is associated with poorer disease-specific outcome (measured using modified Japanese Orthopaedic Association [JOA]) when the posterior laminoplasty approach is used compared with an anterior approach.[8] In another study, patients with preoperative intramedullary signal changes on MRI had significantly greater improvement following ventral decompression compared with dorsal approaches.[9]

ANTERIOR CORPECTOMY AND FUSION

Corpectomy is an ideal surgical approach when there is significant ventral compression of the spinal cord from the dorsal aspect of the vertebral body that would not likely be addressed with discectomy above and below the vertebral body. An example of a patient with spinal cord compression at the C5-C6 and C6-C7 level is shown in **Fig. 1** along with the postdecompression image showing anterior C6 corpectomy. The technique for performing anterior cervical corpectomy has been described by Cooper and others.[10,11]

Early experience with multilevel corpectomy and fusion for the treatment of multilevel cervical spondylosis was associated with significant complications. There were several reports of graft migration failures and associated fusion complications.[12,13] **Fig. 2** demonstrates an example of cage dislodgement with fracture of the rostral vertebral body just 3 months after anterior corpectomy. According to one study published in 1992, multilevel corpectomy was associated with a 29.3% rate of complications.[14] Many surgeons now back up an anterior corpectomy construct with multilevel posterior lateral mass fixation to "protect" the anterior construct (**Fig. 3**). Another viable option is the use of various hybrid anterior procedures that combine anterior corpectomy with anterior discectomy with fusion. This approach may reduce the number of corpectomies required and might augment overall stability, possibly reducing the need for a backup posterior fixation procedure.[15,16]

MULTILEVEL ANTERIOR CERVICAL DISCECTOMY AND FUSION

Many surgeons use multilevel anterior cervical discectomy and fusion (ACDF) when there is multilevel cervical spondylosis and when the disc-osteophyte appears to be focal and therefore removable without corpectomy. Multilevel discectomy and fusion with plating has been described.[17,18] It is possible to remove significant

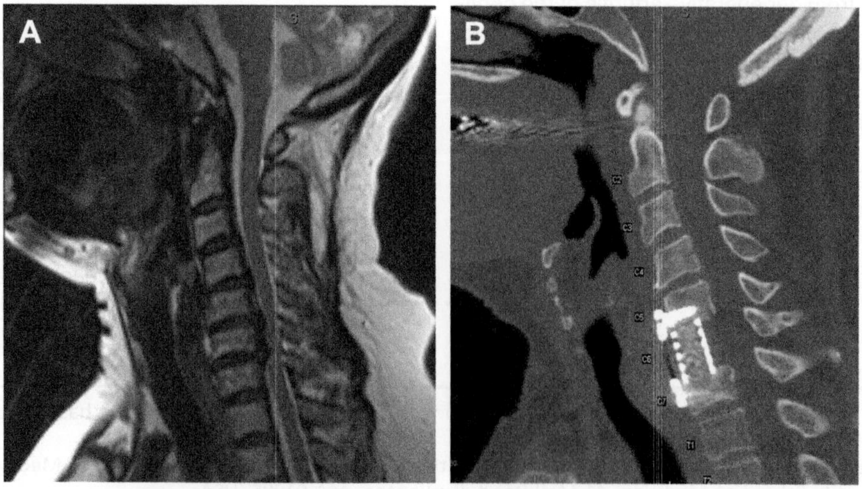

Fig. 1. (*A*) Preoperative sagittal T2-weighted MRI with ventral compression at C5-C6 and C6-C7. (*B*) Postoperative sagittal computed tomography (CT) reconstructed image showing anterior C6 corpectomy with cage placement with anterior cervical plating and fixation.

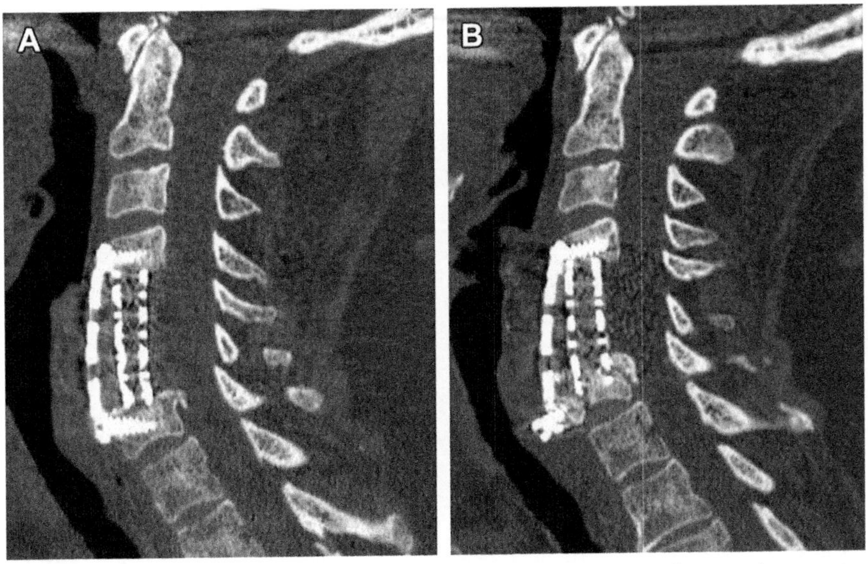

Fig. 2. (*A*) Sagittal reconstructed CT image depicting C5 and C6 corpectomy with cage placement and anterior plating with fixation. (*B*) Sagittal reconstructed CT image 3 months postoperatively showing subsidence of cage into C7 vertebral body with anterior migration of cervical plate and screws.

osteophyte with the ACDF approach. In addition, many surgeons can correct cervical kyphosis using multiple lordotic grafts (**Fig. 4**). One of the concerns with multilevel cervical discectomy is that the fusion rate decreases as the number of levels increases.

MULTILEVEL OBLIQUE CORPECTOMY WITHOUT FUSION

Several groups have described their experience with the technique of multilevel oblique corpectomies for the treatment of DCM over the past 10 to 15 years.[19,20] The approach allows anterolateral access to the cervical spinal canal without destabilizing the spinal column. The approach has been described in detail by George and colleagues.[21] In brief, the vertebral bodies are drilled obliquely toward the opposite posterolateral corner to decompress the spinal canal with less than 50% vertebral body removal and control of the vertebral artery. Special care is taken to avoid damage to the sympathetic chain, which lies on the longus colli muscle. Long-term stability with the use of multilevel oblique corpectomy has

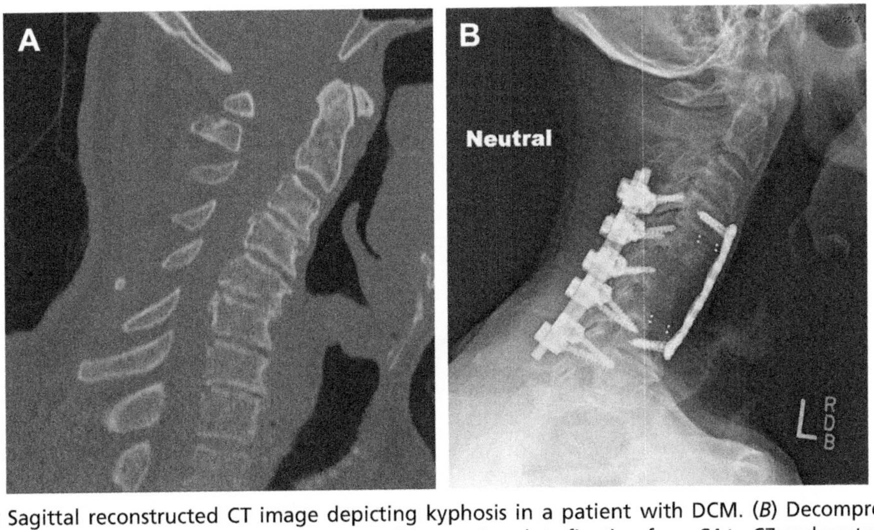

Fig. 3. (*A*) Sagittal reconstructed CT image depicting kyphosis in a patient with DCM. (*B*) Decompression and correction of kyphosis with C5 and C6 corpectomy with anterior plate fixation from C4 to C7 and posterior lateral mass fixation at C4, C5, and C6 with C7 and T1 pedicle screws.

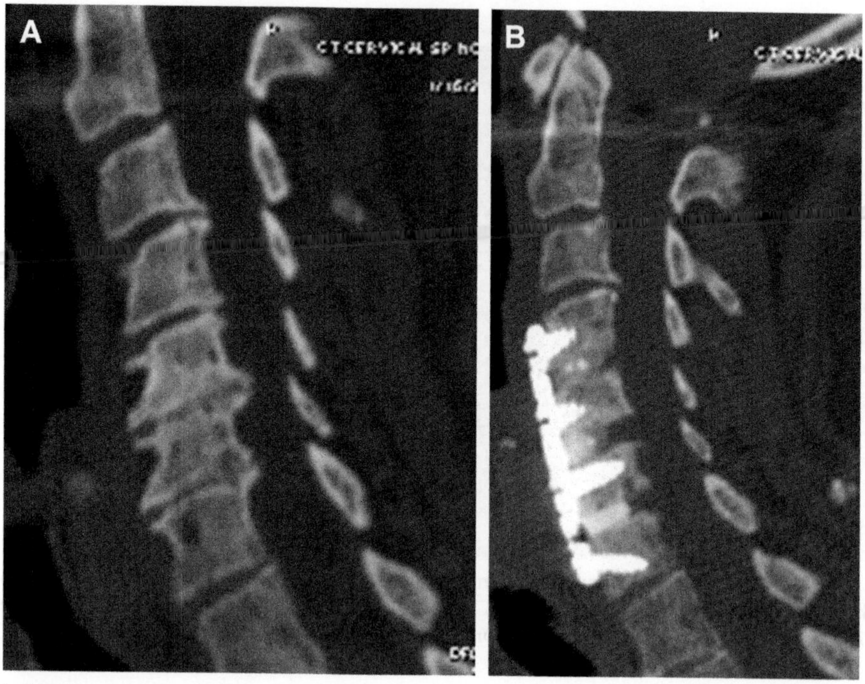

Fig. 4. (*A*) Sagittal reconstructed CT image depicting multilevel cervical spondylosis with significant bony osteophytes at C6-C6 and C6-C7. (*B*) Sagittal reconstructed postoperative CT image demonstrating restoration of cervical lordosis with multilevel cervical discectomy and fusion at C4-C5, C5-C6, and C6-C7 with anterior cervical plating and fixation.

been demonstrated by Chibbaro and colleagues[22] in a prospective study of 268 patients with DCM with mean follow-up of 4 years.

MULTILEVEL CERVICAL ARTHROPLASTY

Relatively less information is available comparing multilevel cervical arthroplasty with other anterior approaches to treating cervical myelopathy. A case series of 72 patients with DCM treated with 1-level or 2-level cervical arthroplasty demonstrated satisfactory results using validated outcomes with 3 years of follow-up.[23] More recently, single-level cervical arthroplasty was compared with single-level ACDF for DCM with comparable patient-reported outcome results, although there were problems with prosthesis migration in 11.7% of arthroplasty cases.[24] There is a need for more prospective comparative studies examining cervical arthroplasty versus anterior cervical fusion for the treatment of multilevel DCM. Until more comparative studies are available, the use of multilevel cervical arthroplasty for DCM should be approached with great caution. Cervical arthroplasty might be more ideal in patients with soft disc pathology. Most patients with DCM have significant disc degenerative changes with reduction of physiologic motion that might not be optimal for cervical arthroplasty. Larger studies with long-term follow-up would be essential to determine the safety and effectiveness of multilevel cervical arthroplasty.

QUALITY OF LIFE OUTCOMES

Both disease-specific and general health-related quality of life (HR-QOL) tools have been used extensively in the literature to assess the comparative effectiveness of treatments for DCM. The modified JOA scale (17-point maximum score) has been frequently used and has been shown, in many studies, to improve by 2.5 to 4.0 points after surgery for DCM.[25–27] DCM has an enormous impact on HR-QOL. A Veterans Administration study found that patients with DCM had a mean physical component summary score of the SF-36 HR-QOL that was more than 2 SDs lower than age-adjusted means for healthy adults.[28] Surgery for DCM consistently demonstrates improvement in HR-QOL after surgery, including patients with mild symptoms.[26] There is some evidence that anterior approaches are associated with less pain and greater QOL compared with posterior approaches. We found this to be the case in a nonrandomized study comparing multilevel ACDF with posterior laminectomy and lateral mass fixation and fusion.[29] A multicenter randomized controlled trial (RCT) comparing anterior versus posterior surgery for DCM has recently been sponsored by PCORI (Patient Centered Outcomes Research Institute).[30] Results from this trial might provide valuable data regarding the comparative outcomes for anterior surgical approaches for treating DCM.

ECONOMIC CONSIDERATIONS

Anterior approaches are often associated with less pain and shorter length of hospital stay. In addition, ventral surgery has been reported to result in lower adjusted 5-year reoperation rates than dorsal surgery (12.1% vs 17.7%).[31] It is therefore not surprising that anterior approaches are associated with lower hospital costs compared with posterior approaches. One study used state administrative data and found that dorsal fusion surgery for DCM was associated with 62% greater hospital charges compared with anterior surgery.[31] We also found this to be the case in a prospective multicenter study.[29]

COMPLICATIONS

Another study also used the Nationwide Inpatient Sample (from 1993 to 2002; 58,115 admissions) to compare complication rates between ventral and dorsal fusion procedures for DCM. This retrospective analysis identified a complication rate of 11.9% for ventral surgery and 16.4% for dorsal fusion surgery.[32] The recently completed AO Spine North America Cervical Spondylotic Myelopathy studies found 1 or more perioperative complications in 11%, 19%, and 37% of patients who underwent anterior-only, posterior-only, or combined anterior-posterior procedures, respectively.[33] A higher rate of wound infection was observed in patients who underwent posterior-only versus anterior-only approaches (4.7% vs 0.6%). Combined anterior-posterior approaches resulted in a higher rate of dysphagia (21.1%) than anterior-only (2.3%) and posterior-only (0.9%) approaches. Surgical approach was not associated with the incidence of C-5 radiculopathy.[33]

Two types of surgical complications are commonly observed after operations for treating DCM: dysphagia (difficulty with swallowing: more common after anterior surgery) and C5 nerve root paresis (temporary, but occasionally permanent, weakness of the shoulder: seen after both anterior and posterior surgery but more commonly after dorsal surgery). Edwards and colleagues[34] reported a 31% rate of persistent dysphagia or dysphonia (hoarseness) after ventral surgery and noted that this complication is often underreported. Published rates of C5 paresis range from 12% (ventral procedures) to 30% (dorsal procedures).[35] This complication often is disabling for several months and might be related to traction on the C5 root caused by spinal cord shift after decompression.[36] Administrative hospital discharge databases are not likely to capture these complication rates accurately nor can they estimate complication severity or impact on a patient's quality of life.[7] Prospective studies are required to provide reliable postoperative complication rate data and assess the impact of these complications on patients' lives.

There has been considerable interest in techniques to minimize the incidence and magnitude of postoperative dysphagia after anterior cervical spine surgery. Reducing retractor time has been shown to reduce the incidence of dysphagia in a study of 51 patients.[37] In this study, reduction of endotracheal tube cuff to 20 mm Hg during retraction was associated with improved patient comfort and reduction of retractor time was associated with less dysphagia.[37] It is possible that wide soft tissue release during the approach to the cervical spine might reduce the tension on retractors and reduce dysphagia. Perioperative steroids and reduction of plate thickness might also be modifiable factors that may reduce postoperative dysphagia.[38,39]

SUMMARY

DCM is the most common cause of spinal cord dysfunction in the world. Anterior cervical approaches are effective in treating the symptoms of DCM; however, complications and reoperations are prevalent after these surgical approaches have been performed. Prospective comparative studies including the recently funded RCT comparing anterior and posterior approaches might provide useful comparative information regarding outcomes and complications following surgery for DCM. Further comparative studies are also necessary to evaluate the comparative effectiveness of multilevel cervical arthroplasty versus other approaches for the treatment of DCM.

REFERENCES

1. Young WF. Cervical spondylotic myelopathy: a common cause of spinal cord dysfunction in older persons. Am Fam Physician 2000;62(5):1064–70, 1073.
2. Henderson FC, Geddes JF, Vaccaro AR, et al. Stretch-associated injury in cervical spondylotic

myelopathy: new concept and review. Neurosurgery 2005;56(5):1101–13 [discussion: 1101–13].
3. al-Mefty O, Harkey HL, Marawi I, et al. Experimental chronic compressive cervical myelopathy. J Neurosurg 1993;79(4):550–61.
4. Baron EM, Young WF. Cervical spondylotic myelopathy: a brief review of its pathophysiology, clinical course, and diagnosis. Neurosurgery 2007;60(1 Supp1 1):S35–41.
5. Rowland LP. Surgical treatment of cervical spondylotic myelopathy: time for a controlled trial. Neurology 1992;42(1):5–13.
6. Patil PG, Turner DA, Pietrobon R. National trends in surgical procedures for degenerative cervical spine disease: 1990-2000. Neurosurgery 2005; 57(4):753–8 [discussion: 753–8].
7. Wang MC, Chan L, Maiman DJ, et al. Complications and mortality associated with cervical spine surgery for degenerative disease in the United States. Spine 2007;32(3):342–7.
8. Suda K, Abumi K, Ito M, et al. Local kyphosis reduces surgical outcomes of expansive open-door laminoplasty for cervical spondylotic myelopathy. Spine 2003;28(12):1258–62.
9. Suri A, Chabbra RP, Mehta VS, et al. Effect of intramedullary signal changes on the surgical outcome of patients with cervical spondylotic myelopathy. Spine J 2003;3(1):33–45.
10. Cooper PR. Anterior cervical vertebrectomy: tips and traps. Neurosurgery 2001;49(5):1129–32.
11. Douglas AF, Cooper PR. Cervical corpectomy and strut grafting. Neurosurgery 2007;60(1 Supp1 1): S137–42.
12. Sasso RC, Ruggiero RA Jr, Reilly TM, et al. Early reconstruction failures after multilevel cervical corpectomy. Spine 2003;28(2):140–2.
13. Wang JC, Hart RA, Emery SE, et al. Graft migration or displacement after multilevel cervical corpectomy and strut grafting. Spine 2003;28(10):1016–21 [discussion: 1021–2].
14. Yonenobu K, Hosono N, Iwasaki M, et al. Laminoplasty versus subtotal corpectomy. A comparative study of results in multisegmental cervical spondylotic myelopathy. Spine 1992;17(11):1281–4.
15. Liu Y, Yu KY, Hu JH. Hybrid decompression technique and two-level corpectomy are effective treatments for three-level cervical spondylotic myelopathy. J Zhejiang Univ Sci B 2009;10(9):696–701.
16. Ashkenazi E, Smorgick Y, Rand N, et al. Anterior decompression combined with corpectomies and discectomies in the management of multilevel cervical myelopathy: a hybrid decompression and fixation technique. J Neurosurg Spine 2005;3(3):205–9.
17. Stewart TJ, Schlenk RP, Benzel EC. Multiple level discectomy and fusion. Neurosurgery 2007;60(1 Supp1 1):S143–8.
18. Brodke DS, Zdeblick TA. Modified Smith-Robinson procedure for anterior cervical discectomy and fusion. Spine 1992;17(10 Suppl):S427–30.
19. Rocchi G, Caroli E, Salvati M, et al. Multilevel oblique corpectomy without fusion: our experience in 48 patients. Spine 2005;30(17):1963–9.
20. Kiris T, Kilincer C. Cervical spondylotic myelopathy treated by oblique corpectomy: a prospective study. Neurosurgery 2008;62(3):674–82 [discussion: 674–82].
21. George B, Gauthier N, Lot G. Multisegmental cervical spondylotic myelopathy and radiculopathy treated by multilevel oblique corpectomies without fusion. Neurosurgery 1999;44(1):81–90.
22. Chibbaro S, Mirone G, Makiese O, et al. Multilevel oblique corpectomy without fusion in managing cervical myelopathy: long-term outcome and stability evaluation in 268 patients. J Neurosurg Spine 2009;10(5):458–65.
23. Fay LY, Huang WC, Wu JC, et al. Arthroplasty for cervical spondylotic myelopathy: similar results to patients with only radiculopathy at 3 years' follow-up. J Neurosurg Spine 2014;21(3):400–10.
24. Shi S, Zheng S, Li XF, et al. Comparison of 2 Zero-Profile Implants in the treatment of single-level cervical spondylotic myelopathy: a preliminary clinical study of cervical disc arthroplasty versus fusion. PLoS One 2016;11(7):e0159761.
25. Chiles BW 3rd, Leonard MA, Choudhri HF, et al. Cervical spondylotic myelopathy: patterns of neurological deficit and recovery after anterior cervical decompression. Neurosurgery 1999;44(4):762–9 [discussion: 769–70].
26. Fehlings MG, Barry S, Kopjar B, et al. Anterior versus posterior surgical approaches to treat cervical spondylotic myelopathy: outcomes of the prospective multicenter AOSpine North America CSM study in 264 patients. Spine 2013;38(26):2247–52.
27. Tetreault L, Nouri A, Kopjar B, et al. The minimum clinically important difference of the modified Japanese Orthopaedic Association scale in patients with degenerative cervical myelopathy. Spine 2015;40(21):1653–9.
28. King JT Jr, McGinnis KA, Roberts MS. Quality of life assessment with the medical outcomes study short form-36 among patients with cervical spondylotic myelopathy. Neurosurgery 2003;52(1):113–20 [discussion: 121].
29. Ghogawala Z, Martin B, Benzel EC, et al. Comparative effectiveness of ventral vs dorsal surgery for cervical spondylotic myelopathy. Neurosurgery 2011; 68(3):622–30 [discussion: 630–1].
30. Ghogawala Z, Benzel EC, Heary RF, et al. Cervical spondylotic myelopathy surgical trial: randomized, controlled trial design and rationale. Neurosurgery 2014;75(4):334–46.

31. King JT Jr, Abbed KM, Gould GC, et al. Cervical spine reoperation rates and hospital resource utilization after initial surgery for degenerative cervical spine disease in 12,338 patients in Washington State. Neurosurgery 2009;65(6):1011–22 [discussion: 1022–3].
32. Boakye M, Patil CG, Santarelli J, et al. Cervical spondylotic myelopathy: complications and outcomes after spinal fusion. Neurosurgery 2008;62(2):455–61 [discussion: 461–2].
33. Fehlings MG, Smith JS, Kopjar B, et al. Perioperative and delayed complications associated with the surgical treatment of cervical spondylotic myelopathy based on 302 patients from the AO Spine North America cervical spondylotic myelopathy study. J Neurosurg Spine 2012;16(5):425–32.
34. Edwards CC 2nd, Karpitskaya Y, Cha C, et al. Accurate identification of adverse outcomes after cervical spine surgery. J Bone Joint Surg Am 2004;86-A(2): 251–6.
35. Bose B, Sestokas AK, Schwartz DM. Neurophysiological detection of iatrogenic C-5 nerve deficit during anterior cervical spinal surgery. J Neurosurg Spine 2007;6(5):381–5.
36. Saunders RL. On the pathogenesis of the radiculopathy complicating multilevel corpectomy. Neurosurgery 1995;37(3):408–12 [discussion: 412–3].
37. Ratnaraj J, Todorov A, McHugh T, et al. Effects of decreasing endotracheal tube cuff pressures during neck retraction for anterior cervical spine surgery. J Neurosurg 2002;97(2 Suppl):176–9.
38. Chin KR, Eiszner JR, Adams SB Jr. Role of plate thickness as a cause of dysphagia after anterior cervical fusion. Spine 2007;32(23):2585–90.
39. Adenikinju AS, Halani SH, Rindler RS, et al. Effect of perioperative steroids on dysphagia after anterior cervical spine surgery: a systematic review. Int J Spine Surg 2017;11:9.

Laminectomy with or Without Fusion to Manage Degenerative Cervical Myelopathy

Fahad H. Abduljabbar, MBBS, FRCSC[a,b],
Alisson R. Teles, MD[c], Rakan Bokhari, MBBS[d],
Michael Weber, MD, FRCSC[a],
Carlo Santaguida, MD, FRCSC[d,*]

KEYWORDS

• Cervical laminectomy • Cervical myelopathy • Cervical spondylosis • Decompression
• Laminectomy • Kyphosis

KEY POINTS

- Posterior decompression is generally recommended in patients with multilevel cervical stenosis with preserved cervical lordosis.
- Successful treatment of multilevel degenerative cervical myelopathy (DCM) requires adequate decompression, restoration of the normal curvature, and reconstruction of the cervical stability.
- Fixed cervical kyphosis is a contraindication for a posterior-only approach.
- Laminectomy alone may put DCM patients at higher risk of postlaminectomy kyphosis and axial neck pain.

Degenerative cervical myelopathy (DCM) is among the most common causes of cervical spinal cord dysfunction in the elderly.[1] It results from spondylotic changes and ossification of the spinal ligaments, leading to compression of neural structures and subsequent spinal cord dysfunction. As the population ages, the demand for these surgeries will keep rising. A thorough knowledge of the advantages and limitations of the different surgical treatments is essential for decision-making.[2]

Cervical laminectomy was the first procedure described for the management of degenerative cervical spine disease. It provided validation to the hypothesis that alleviating neural compression will result in clinical improvement in these patients. The procedure has since been found to have a high incidence of postoperative instability that necessitated the modifications to this procedure and the development of alternatives, including fusion.[3]

HISTORICAL OVERVIEW

Spine surgery for cervical degenerative disc disease has been described since the earlier half of the twentieth century. The initial fear of inducing significant postoperative instability status postdecompression alone was not realized and the procedure gained increased popularity. Many investigators reported

Disclosure Statement: No funds were received in support of this work. No benefits in any form have been or will be received from a commercial party related directly or indirectly to the subject of this article.
[a] Department of Orthopedic Surgery, McGill University Health Centre, Montreal, 1003 Decarie Boulevard, Quebec H4A 0A9, Canada; [b] King Abdulaziz University Hospital, PO box 80125, Jeddah, Saudi Arabia; [c] Department of Clinical Neurosciences–Neurosurgery, University of Calgary, Calgary, 1403 29 Street NW Calgary, Alberta T2N 2T9, Canada; [d] Department of Neurology and Neurosurgery, McGill University Health Centre, Montreal, Quebec, Canada
* Corresponding author. 109-3801 rue Universite, Montreal, Quebec H3A 2B4, Canada.
E-mail address: carlo.santaguida@mcgill.ca

Neurosurg Clin N Am 29 (2018) 91–105
https://doi.org/10.1016/j.nec.2017.09.017
1042-3680/18/© 2017 Elsevier Inc. All rights reserved.

the clinical success of laminectomy for DCM[4–22] (**Table 1**). In the early twentieth century, many of these investigators did not pay any attention to the radiological failure in the form of postlaminectomy kyphosis.[4–6,8,10,11] The initial impression that this procedure was well tolerated changed as long-term follow-up of these patients was obtained. It became clear that this procedure was marred by an unacceptably high rate of kyphosis, approaching 20%, and subsequent pain and neurologic deterioration as the spinal cord draped and compressed against the kyphosing spine.[15,17,23]

Improved understanding of spinal biomechanics, along with the continued innovation in surgical access and reconstruction provided, a growing list of operative strategies to decompress the cervical spine while maintaining its alignment. The earliest was provided by the description of the anterior cervical approach. This allowed spine surgeons to address cervical compressive myelopathy and radiculopathy without disrupting the posterior tension band.[3]

Modifications to the posterior approach were also developed to compensate for the destabilizing effect of posterior element resection. Laminoplasty was 1 such modification to preserve the posterior elements popularized in East Asia in the 1970s.[24] This procedure retains the posterior bony elements with their attached ligaments and musculature in the hopes of maintaining segmental mechanical integrity.[25] Another strategy is the instrumentation of the destabilized segment, currently performed most commonly with polysegmental lateral mass screws. This results in a rigid construct that resists the kyphotic forces and allows for maintenance of sagittal alignment with long-term follow-up.[17] Stand-alone laminectomies have, therefore, been generally abandoned in contemporary spine practice.[2]

DEFINITIONS

Laminectomy, as currently practiced, is the removal of the spinous processes with interposed interspinous and supraspinous ligaments; the laminae; and, in varying extent, the facet joints and capsules. This is followed by resection of the ligamentum flavum, until decompression and exposure of the thecal sac is obtained.

Posterior access to the spinal column is through a median approach bisecting the ligamentum nuchae, which exploits an avascular plane between the posterior paraspinal muscles. Exposure of the bony structures is done by stripping the musculature Sharpey fibers from their bony attachments via electrocautery in a subperiosteal fashion.[26] Laminectomies can then be supplemented with posterior instrumentation. This frequently consists of lateral mass screws that span the destabilized segments.[2,17]

In contrast, laminoplasty preserves the laminae and ligaments, but instead obtains expansion of the spinal canal by remodeling the lamina. This procedure posteriorly displaces the laminae, increasing spinal canal size, and fixes them in the new position while preserving the integrity of spinal ligaments and muscle attachments. Motion is, therefore, preserved in the operated motion segments. This procedure was developed to reduce the risk of postoperative kyphosis by maintaining the osteoligamentous tension band. Remodeling of the lamina is obtained via several techniques that include the initially described Z-plasty, the open door, and the French door, among other modifications.[27]

ANTERIOR VERSUS POSTERIOR APPROACHES TO THE CERVICAL SPINE

It is critical to optimize a surgery that is best suited for a patient's pathologic findings. The objectives of surgery should include an adequate neural decompression, while respecting the normal spinal alignment, all while minimizing complications and disruption to local anatomy.

Deciding on the optimal approach for the myelopathic patient requires taking multiple factors into consideration. Large retrospective and prospective studies did not reveal any approach to be clearly superior when compared with others.[2,28–30] In addition, the very large number of variations in procedures and differing compressive etiologic factors across populations creates a very heterogeneous mix of patients who are difficult to pool.[2]

The anterior spinal approach allows direct access to anterior compressive pathologic findings, as well as allows for correction of any significant kyphotic deformity. It also seems to be the surgical corridor that carries the lower risk for surgical site infection and that results in less postoperative pain compared with a posterior approach.[28] The drawbacks are the need to dissect between important neurovascular and aerodigestive structures with occasional access-related complications, such as hoarseness and dysphagia,[28] particularly in the elderly. Also, there is the high risk of dural tear with CSF leak after surgery for ossified posterior longitudinal ligament (OPLL).[28]

The risk of complications with anterior approaches increases with the number of operated levels.[2,31] This led to the general preference for posterior surgery when encountering pathologic findings extending for 3 or more segments.[2] Posterior approaches offer quick access that can be readily extended should the need arise, but they

Table 1
Summary of studies reporting outcomes for laminectomy surgery for degenerative cervical myelopathy

Authors	Study Design	Location	Number of Subjects	Clinical Outcome	Radiologic Outcome	Follow-up (y)	Complications
Stoops & King,[4] 1965	Retrospective cohort	United States	42	33% marked improvement 50% definite improvement 17% unchanged 5 persistent neurologic deficit	NR	(1–6)	6 wound complications
Crandall & Batzdorf,[5] 1966	Retrospective cohort	United States	62	22% excellent outcome 9% improved 30% no change 39% worse	NR	(1–10)	8 neurologic deficits
Epstein et al,[6] 1969	Retrospective cohort	United States	57	13 excellent outcome 26 good 4 fair 6 unchanged 5 poor	NR	3.5 (1–8)	NR
Bishara,[7] 1971	Retrospective cohort	United Kingdom	59	56% improvement at 5-y follow-up 51% at 10-y follow-up	No instability or postlaminectomy kyphosis	10 (5–20)	NR
Jenkins,[9] 1973	Case series	United Kingdom	5	4 walk without an aid 1 uses an aid	No kyphosis	15.6 (12–17)	NR
Fager,[8] 1973	Retrospective cohort	United States	35	24 improved 9 unchanged 2 worse	NR	(1–7)	5 transient neurologic deficit 1 wound infection
Gorter,[10] 1976	Retrospective cohort	Netherlands	58	29 improved 13 unchanged 16 worse	NR	(2.4–5.9)	NR

(*continued on next page*)

Table 1
(continued)

Authors	Study Design	Location	Number of Subjects	Clinical Outcome	Radiologic Outcome	Follow-up (y)	Complications
Casotto & Buoncristiani,[11] 1981	Retrospective cohort	Italy	44	46% excellent 34% fair 11% poor	NR	(6 mo–8 y)	NR
Miyazaki & Kirita,[12] 1986	Retrospective cohort	Japan	155	82% overall improvement 7% unchanged 11% worse	17% postlaminectomy kyphosis	1	NR
Mikawa et al,[13] 1987	Retrospective cohort	Japan	64 (DCM or OPLL)	NR	Kyphotic deformity in 9 (12.5%)	7 (2–23)	NR
Snow & Weiner,[14] 1993	Retrospective cohort	United States	90	77% improved 13% unchanged 10% deteriorated	No comment on long-term follow-up radiographs	(6 mo–4 y)	1 pulmonary embolus 1 epidural abscess
Kato et al,[16] 1998	Retrospective cohort	Japan	44 (OPLL)	JOA RR: 44.2% +/– 37.8 after 1 y 42.9% +/– 39.5 after 5 y 32.8% +/–45.5 after 10 y	Postoperative progression of OPLL in 70% Postoperative progression of kyphotic deformity in 47%	14.1	1 postoperative hematoma 1 dural tear 3 intraoperative hemiplegic-type spinal cord injury
Guigui et al,[15] 1998	Retrospective cohort	France	58	65% mean JOA RR 8 mean preoperative JOA 14 mean postoperative JOA	31% postlaminectomy deformity (6 kyphotic, 5 meandering, 5 straight)	3.6 (2–10)	Instability required reoperation in 3 subjects
Kaptain et al,[17] 2000	Retrospective cohort	United Kingdom	46	Nurick outcome score: 13 (29%) of 45 improved 19 (42%) of 45 remained unchanged	Kyphosis developed in 30% who had straight preoperative alignment and in only 14% of subjects with preoperative lordosis	4	NR

Hansen-Schwartz et al,[18] 2003	Retrospective cohort	Denmark	27	74% satisfied or fairly satisfied	45% were kyphotic	7.7 + 0.6 y	1 C6 nerve root palsy 1 postoperative mortality
Cho et al,[19] 2008	Retrospective cohort	Korea	14 (OPLL)	43% mean JOA RR	CI decreased significantly postoperatively (*P*<.002)	41 m (26–28m)	1 epidural hematoma 3 Transient C5 palsies
Li et al,[21] 2015	Retrospective cohort	China	91	68.4% mean JOA RR	CI decreased significantly from 20.8 ± 2.1–11.5 ± 1.8 Cervical ROM at C2–7 decreased from 42.7° to 20.4°	12.1 (10–13.5)	1 neurologic deterioration from recurrent stenosis 2 CSF leaks
Laiginhas et al,[20] 2015	Retrospective cohort	Portugal	57	mJOA (13.0 vs 14.7, *P*<.001) EMS (13.6 vs 15.4, *P*<.001) scores Lower MDI score (9.3 vs 5.7, *P*<.001)	Mean postoperative CI was 19.3 1 (2%) kyphosis at long-term follow-up	6 (3.5–12)	3 transient postoperative C5 radiculopathies
van Geest et al,[22] 2015	Retrospective cohort	Netherlands	77	mJOA: 13.3 (6–17; 2.5) EMS: 14.5 (8–18; 2.3) Nurick: 1.8 (0–5; 1.3)	Incidence of kyphosis and segmental instability 15% and 18%, respectively, occurred almost exclusively if preoperative lordosis <20°	8.4 (3.8–15.8)	19 reoperations 12 persistent compression 5 kyphosis (reoperations)

The neurologic recovery rate was calculated using the Hirabayashi method (postoperative JOA score–preoperative score)/(17–preoperative score) × 100%. Recovery rates were graded as follows: 75%, excellent; 50% to 74%, good; 25% to 49%, fair; and 25%, poor. Neck disability index (NDI): 0–4, no disability; 5–14, mild disability; 15–24, moderate disability; 25–34, severe disability; >35, complete disability.

Abbreviations: CI, curvature index; CSF, cerebrospinal fluid; EMS, the European Myelopathy Score; JOA, Japanese Orthopedic Association; MDI, Myelopathy Disability Index; mJOA, modified Japanese Orthopedic Association; OPLL, ossified posterior longitudinal ligament; NR, not reported; ROM, range of motion; RR, recovery rate.

do not allow significant kyphotic deformity correction or sufficient access to resect anteriorly located pathologic findings.[2,32]

BIOMECHANICS IN THE DEGENERATING CERVICAL SPINE

The cervical spine carries the weight of the skull and its contents through their articulation at the occipitoatlantal joint. This load distribution is dictated by the cranial center of gravity and the lordotic configuration of the cervical spine.[33,34]

In the normal lordotic spine, most loadbearing is distributed to the posterior elements. As the cervical intervertebral discs degenerate and lose height, the segment gradually loses its normal lordosis. As a result, the cranial center of gravity shifts more anteriorly and a larger share of the axial load is borne by the anterior columns.[34–36] This exerts more force on the intervertebral discs, further accelerating disc degeneration.[35] The nature of forces exerted on the posterior elements (the facet joints and ligaments) also change from compression to tension. Ligaments and paraspinal muscles, the so-called tension band, are subjected to increasing tension as they try to maintain lordosis.[34,35] The ensuing ligamentous and facet capsular hypertrophy contributes to stenosis of the cervical canal.[35] This strain is also believed to underlie some of the axial pain experienced by these patients.[34,35,37]

EFFECTS OF LAMINECTOMY ON SPINE BIOMECHANICS

Several studies have described the effects of laminectomies on spinal stability.[17,23,38–41] Although laminectomies do not seem to cause immediate instability, their removal is not without consequences. Clinical and biomechanical studies have displayed how the different components of a posterior decompression can affect spinal mechanics.

Nowinski and colleagues[39] have shown that stability is adversely affected with progressively increasing facetectomy. This effect was seen with as little as 25% facet resection. It has also been shown that spinal stability is progressively affected as the number of laminae resected is increased.[38,42] Laminar resection not only affects spinal stability but was shown to alter axial loadbearing across the cervical vertebral body in the anterior column.[40]

In addition to the bony disruption, surgery also affects the neck extensors by detaching them during the subperiosteal dissection performed for exposure. The effects of this disruption are greatest at the upper and lower attachment sites of the tension band, which correspond to C2 and C7.[41,43] It has also been shown in cranial surgeries that subperiosteal dissection with electrocautery can induce muscular atrophy.

It is, therefore, not surprising that this procedure is associated with a significant incidence of postoperative kyphosis. This is particularly expected in patients predisposed to develop this complication, which include younger patients, those with preoperative loss of lordosis, those with tumors which require wide enough exposures, as well as patients receiving a high dose of radiation to the operative field.[17,38,42]

SURGICAL TRENDS FOR THE TREATMENT OF DEGENERATIVE CERVICAL MYELOPATHY

During the past decade, there were tremendous changes in health care delivery, surgical technology, and patient care needs. Patil and colleagues[44] used a nationwide inpatient sample database and showed that: posterior fusions were sharply increasing, rising from 0.3% of procedures (1291 procedures) to 3.8% of procedures (4265 procedures) over the decade. By contrast, nonfusion decompressions declined sharply from 70.5% of procedures in 1990 (41,272 procedures) to 24.6% of procedures in 2000 (27,611 procedures). In a survey with 30 experienced spine surgeons from different academic institutions in North America regarding the procedure of choice for posterior approach in DCM, only 7% reported laminectomy alone, 23% laminoplasty, and 70% laminectomy and fusion.[45] In a study of 286 patients included in the AOSpine Cervical Spondylotic Myelopathy (CSM) studies who had posterior-only approaches, only 20 (7%) were treated with laminectomy alone, 100 received (35%) laminoplasty, and 166 (58%) laminectomy and fusion.[30]

DECISION-MAKING BETWEEN LAMINECTOMY AND LAMINECTOMY PLUS FUSION

Several studies have demonstrated that both anterior or posterior approaches are similarly effective and safe when the approach is chosen based on factors such as ventral versus dorsal compression, cervical sagittal alignment, and focal versus diffuse compression.[46,47] Posterior decompression is generally recommended in patients with multilevel cervical stenosis with preserved cervical lordosis. Fixed cervical kyphosis is a relative contraindication for posterior-only approaches.[48]

Cervical laminectomy was historically the most popular posterior operation for DCM. However, the potential complications related to this procedure, such as postoperative cervical deformity (**Figs. 1** and **2**), segmental instability (**Fig. 3**), and

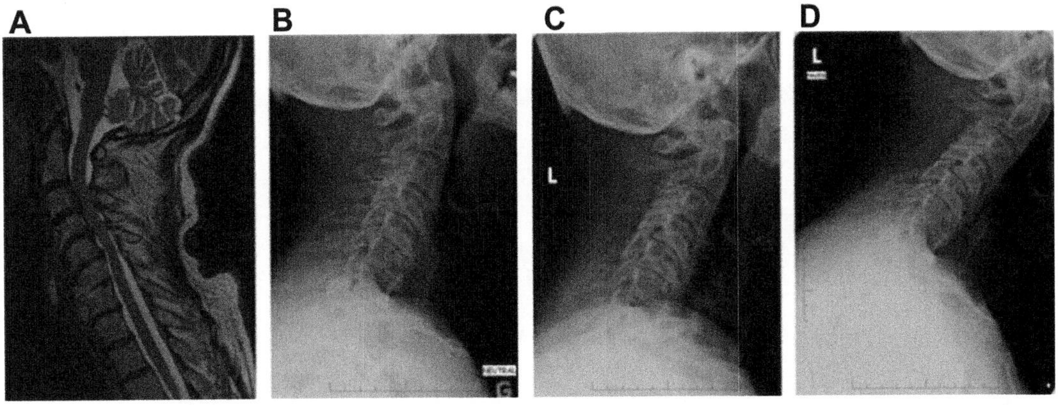

Fig. 1. A 64-year-old man presenting with degenerative cervical myelopathy secondary to multilevel cervical stenosis (*A, B*). The patient was submitted to C3-C5 laminectomies and developed postlaminectomy kyphosis and severe neck pain. Postoperative radiographs at 6 weeks (*C*) and 6 months (*D*) showing progressive cervical kyphosis.

recurrent stenosis due to extradural scar formation (**Fig. 4**), have led to the development and increased popularity of laminoplasty and laminectomy with instrumented fusion over the last decades.[2]

It is recognized that postoperative epidural scarring forms a laminectomy membrane that partially originates from muscle on dural contact. Any form of barrier between the muscle and dura aids in

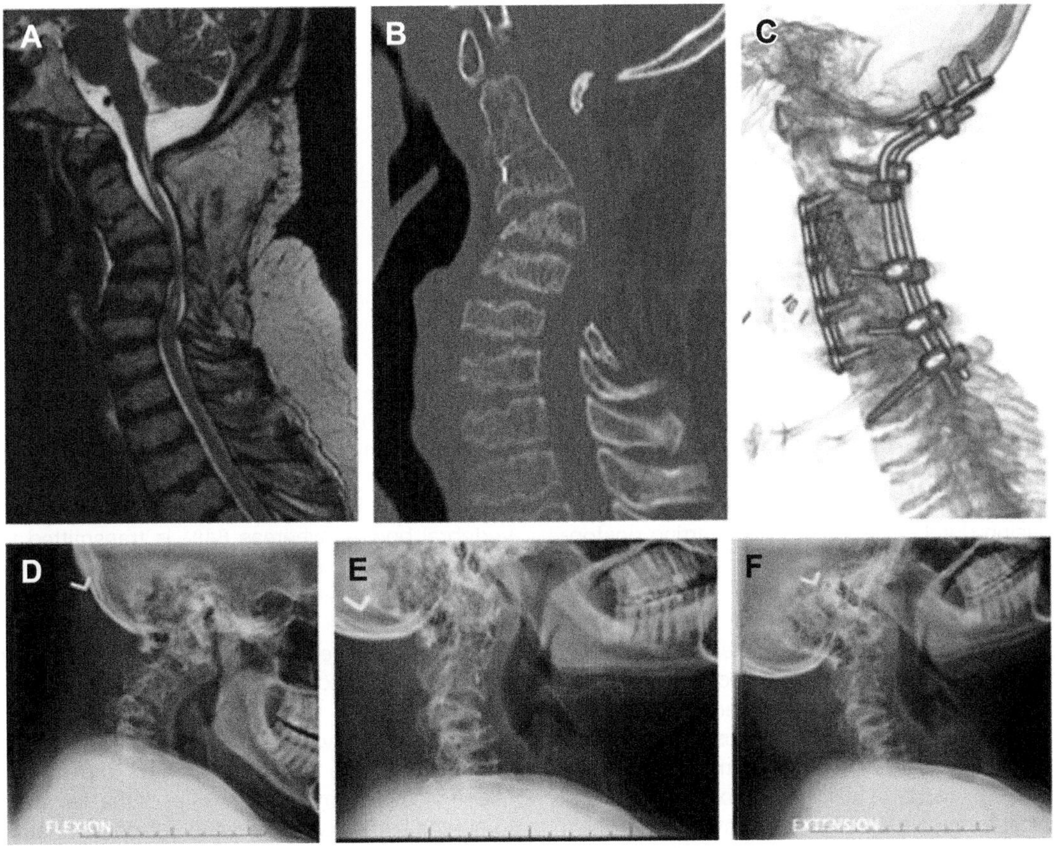

Fig. 2. A 41-year-old man diagnosed with Morquio syndrome underwent C2-C5 laminectomies 2 years before to treat cervical myelopathy. The patient presented with severe neck pain and progressive myelopathy secondary to postlaminectomy kyphosis (*A, B, D–F*). He underwent revision surgery and deformity correction via C4-C5 corpectomies and occiput T1-instrumented fusion with good clinical and radiological results (*C*).

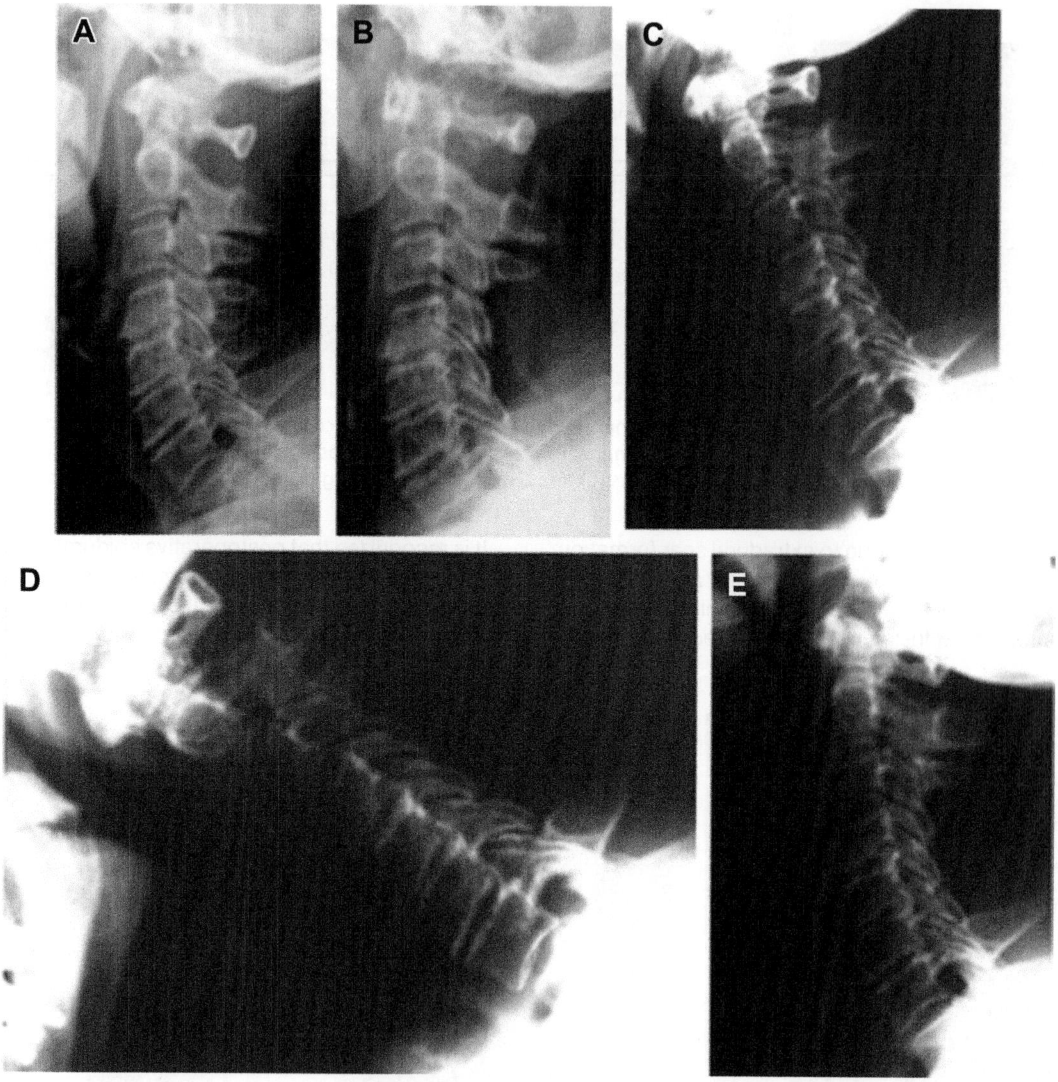

Fig. 3. A 67-year-old woman with degenerative cervical myelopathy and preserved cervical lordosis (*A*) was treated with C4-C6 laminectomies. Postoperative radiographs at 2 days (*B*) and 4 months (*C*) demonstrating progressive loss of cervical lordosis and C3-C4 instability in the flexion (*D*) and extension (*E*) views.

reducing dural constriction from scarring postoperatively.[49,50] Increased tensile forces in the posterior spine musculature from loss of lordosis may lead to more scar formation or even dynamic compression of neural elements. Theoretically, immobilization of the spine reduces dynamic compression from scar and the addition of hardware prevents extensive dural-muscle contact.

The possibility of restenosis from epidural scarring may dissuade surgeons from stand-alone laminectomy procedures; however, the main reason to add instrumentation is to diminish the risk of development of postoperative cervical kyphotic deformity or instability. The cervical spine transmits 36% of compressive loads through the vertebral bodies, whereas 64% is transmitted to the posterior elements.[36,51] In this sense, removal of the posterior tension band can result in a progressive increase in the compressive loads on the discs and vertebral bodies, resulting in anterior wedge compression and kyphosis. Several biomechanical studies have demonstrated increased mobility after cervical laminectomy, which could contribute to late cervical deformity and clinical failure.[52–56] The more extensive is the laminectomy, the higher is the potential for postoperative hypermobility. In the classic study by Kumaresan and colleagues,[52] facet resection of more than 50% resulted in increased segmental motion and intervertebral disc stress. In addition, surgical

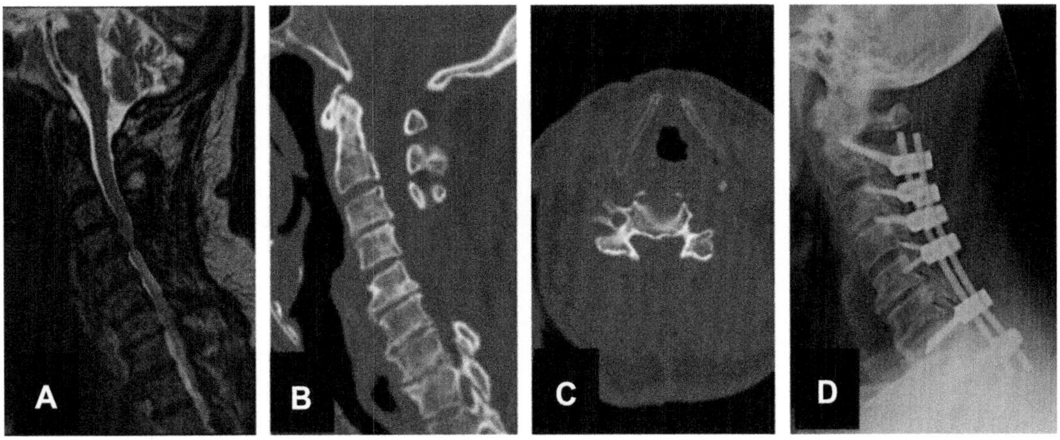

Fig. 4. Case of recurrent symptomatic stenosis 15 years following cervical decompression. The patient became progressively nonambulatory with loss of hand function over a 2-year period. The compression was entirely due to a thick scar under tension. (*A*) T2-weighted sagittal MRI demonstrating multilevel compression and cord signal change. (*B, C*) Sagittal and axial CT (C4-5) demonstrating a wide decompression. (*D*) Radiograph demonstrating postoperative instrumentation following revision surgery.

trauma can result in denervation and atrophy of the neck extensor muscles, contributing to the development of deformity.

The first studies that documented postlaminectomy kyphosis in DCM reported incidences ranging from 14% to 47%.[13,15,17,49,57–59] The identified risk factors associated with cervical deformity after laminectomy alone were presence of a straight or kyphotic spine; wide laminectomies; young patients with neck hypermobility; laminectomies, including C2; and crossing the cervicothoracic junction (C7 laminectomy). As the kyphotic deformity progresses, the spinal cord may become progressively draped over the posterior vertebral body, resulting in flattening of small feeding vessels to the cord and increased longitudinal cord tension caused by the tethering effect of the dentate ligaments and cervical roots. The combination of spinal cord tension and ischemia results in direct neuronal injury and myelopathy.[60] In addition to neurologic deterioration, patients with loss of cervical alignment may have worsening neck pain secondary to facet joint disruption.[61]

Notably, several groups have recently reported good long-term clinical and radiological outcomes with laminectomy alone in selected patients with DCM.[20–22,62–64] These studies reported lower incidences of postlaminectomy kyphosis. Bartels and colleagues[65] published a small randomized clinical trial comparing 9 subjects receiving laminectomy and 9 laminectomy and instrumented fusion for DCM. They did not find difference in the neurologic outcome or quality of life between the groups at an average follow-up of 18.3 ($\pm$ 8.9) months. These results suggest that laminectomy alone may be safe and effective in patients with preserved cervical lordosis and a stable cervical spine, without preoperative spinal instability, in whose decompression would not involve the facet joints, C2 lamina, or the cervicothoracic junction (C7). On the other hand, patients who develop iatrogenic cervical deformity requiring surgical correction present with a significant decline in health-related quality of life[66] and surgical treatment is associated with high morbidity and mortality.[67] Thus, (1) instrumented fusion should be performed in patients with any risk factor for cervical instability and kyphosis and (2) close clinical and radiological follow-up should be performed in patients undergoing laminectomy alone for DCM. Only 3 studies compared laminectomy with laminectomy and fusion for DCM[61,65,68] (**Table 2**). Du and colleagues[61] showed that the laminectomy group is more prone to postlaminectomy kyphosis and subsequent axial neck pain. Another 4 studies looked at the clinical and radiological outcome for laminectomy and fusion for DCM[30,69–71] (**Table 3**), which demonstrated largely favorable outcomes.

A distinct form of postlaminectomy deformity includes the dropped head syndrome, which is a flexible deformity correctable with passive neck extension. This deformity is not caused by structural changes of the cervical spine, although the muscle weakness may eventually contribute to cervical instability and accelerate degenerative changes. This complication has been reported acutely after cervical laminectomy or few months later and it is proposed mechanism is cervical muscle extension weakness.[72,73] Arnts and Bartels[73] estimated a 0.87% incidence of flexible

Table 2
Summary of studies comparing laminectomy to laminectomy and fusion for degenerative cervical myelopathy

Authors	Study Design	Location	Number of Subjects or Interventions	Clinical Outcome	Radiologic Outcome	Follow-up (y)	Complications
Bartels et al,[65] 2017	Randomized prospective	Netherlands	18 (DCM) 9 (LC) 9 (LF) Mean age: 73.4 ± 5.4	mJOA difference: 0.41 (P = .597)	C2-C7 angle: LC group 19 ± 15 LF 8 ± 8	1.8 ± 8.9 m	NR
Du et al,[61] 2013	Retrospective cohort	China	LC (30) (21 men, 9 women) Mean age: 56.2 (43–74)	RR: 1 excellent, 25 good, 4 fair JOA score RR: 56.55 ± 9.39% NDI: 14.07 76.7% axial symptoms	Loss of CI (%) 3.20 ± 0.88 P<.05	9.4 (7.6–11.7)	NR
			LF (32) (23M/9 F) Mean age: 55.9 (40–72)	RR: excellent 11, good in 21 JOA score RR 70.54 ± 12.80 P<.001 NDI: 4.97 Only 37.5% had axial symptoms	CI (%) 1.22 ± 0.72 P = .34	8.9 (7.2–11.5)	NR
Hamanishi & Tanaka,[68] 1996	Retrospective cohort	Japan	LC (35) Mean age: 66.1 ± 9.4	JOA score RR: 50.8 ± 30.2	1 postoperative kyphosis progression	3.5 (1–10)	Temporary motor paresis in 1 subject 1 instability 2 postlaminectomy kyphosis
			LF (34) Mean age: 58.4 ± 11.7	JOA score RR: 51.2 ± 23.8	2 postoperative Kyphosis		Temporary motor paresis in 1 subject 7 pseudoarthrosis

The RR was calculated using the Hirabayashi method (postoperative JOA score–preoperative score)/(17–preoperative score) × 100%. Recovery rates were graded as follows: 75%, excellent; 50% to 74%, good; 25% to 49%, fair; and 25%, poor. NDI: 0–4, no disability; 5–14, mild disability; 15–24, moderate disability; 25–34, severe disability; >35, complete disability.

Abbreviations: LC, laminectomy; LF, laminectomy and fusion; NDI, neck disability index.

Table 3
Summary of studies reporting laminectomy and fusion for degenerative cervical myelopathy

Authors	Study Design	Location	Number of Subjects	Clinical Outcome	Radiologic Outcome	Follow-up (y)	Complications
Fehlings et al,[30] 2017	Prospective cohort	Multicenter	166 (DCM)	Nurick grades improved by 1.18 (95% CI: 0.92–1.44) $P = .0770$ mJOA scores improved by 2.39 (95% CI: 1.91–2.86) $P = .0069$ NDI, 10.45 (95% CI: 7.13, 13.77) P value .2039	5 postoperative kyphosis	2	1 hardware failure 4 C5 radiculopathy 4 adjacent segment degeneration
Chen et al,[71] 2009	Retrospective cohort	China	83 (OPLL) (64 men and 19 women) average age: 56.4 y	RR grade: 59 (71.1%) good (RR ≥50%), and 24 (28.9%) subjects poor (RR<50%) JOA score RR: 11.1%–87.5%, with a mean of 62.4 ± 13.2%	Cervical lordosis in good prognosis group: 16.1 ± 1.5 and 10.4 ± 1.3 in the poor prognosis group $P<.01$	4.8 (4.0–6.5)	10 nerve root palsies (7 C5 palsy, 2 C6 palsy and 1 C7 palsy) 3 hematomas Screw pullout in 3 cases
Houten & Cooper,[70] 2003	Retrospective cohort	United States	38 (DCM or OPLL)	Mean mJOA scores improved from 12.9 preoperatively to 15.58 postoperatively ($P<.0001$)	No difference between the mean preoperative CI of 3.6 (range 10–21) & the mean CI at last follow-up of 3.7 (range 9.4–24.3)	2.5 (6m-100 m)	4 unilateral screw back-out and 1 bilateral screw back-out 1 screw misplacement (revised) 1 C5 nerve root palsy, which recovered
Kumar et al,[69] 1999	Retrospective cohort	United States	25 (DCM) 17 men and 8 women (mean age, 60 y; range 33–79 y)	Myelopathy grades using a modification of the method presented by Harsh: 20 subjects (80%) experienced good outcomes (myelopathy grade IIIA or better and hand function). 5 subjects (20%) poor (1 of which was grade IIIA but with poor hand function)	There was no progressive kyphosis and no instability during the follow-up period	3.9 (2–6.8)	1 epidural hematoma

The neurologic recovery rate was calculated using the Hirabayashi method (postoperative JOA score–preoperative score)/(17–preoperative score) × 100%. Recovery rates were graded as follows: 75%, excellent; 50% to 74%, good; 25% to 49%, fair; and 25%, poor. NDI: 0–4, no disability; 5–14, mild disability; 15–24, moderate disability; 25–34, severe disability; >35, complete disability.

Abbreviations: 95% CI, confidence interval; CI, curvature index.

dropped head deformity following cervical laminectomy. Although rare, this complication can severely affect a patient's quality of life because of inability to maintain horizontal gaze and potential for neurologic deterioration.

Controversy exists about whether laminoplasty may or may not prevent postoperative kyphosis in DCM resulting in better long-term outcomes.[62,64,74] From a biomechanical perspective, both laminectomy alone and laminoplasty require wide muscle dissection and ligamentous structures transected; however, the facet joints usually need to be exposed in laminoplasty because the implants are fixed to the lateral mass and lamina. Recently, new modalities of laminectomy have been described to reduce the potential for cervical deformity and instability. In 2002, Shiraishi[75] described the skip cervical laminectomy for DCM, which involves preservation of selected spinous process and the laminectomies or partial laminectomies are restricted to the levels of greatest compression, theoretically reducing the risk of postoperative deformity. Some studies have demonstrated similar clinical outcomes comparing skip laminectomies and laminoplasty.[76–78] In addition, some groups have reported the use of minimally invasive techniques involving a parasagittal muscle-splitting approach with tubular retractors to accomplish posterior spinal cord decompression.[79–81] Larger comparative studies are necessary to assess the efficacy and safety of these procedures.

The role of fusion in patients presenting with chronic neck pain remains controversial. Prevalence of axial symptoms after posterior cervical surgery varies from 7% to 58% and it seems to be lower after instrumented fusion in comparison with motion-preserved approaches.[82] Thus, in patients with preoperative neck pain, instrumented fusion should be considered. Another potential benefit compared with simple decompression is the regression of anterior disc-osteophyte complex observed after laminectomy and fusion, which provides another mechanism of spinal cord decompression.[83]

Potential complications related to instrumented-fusion compared with simple decompression include higher infection rates, misplaced cervical screws requiring reoperation, or vascular injury pseudoarthrosis and adjacent segment disease. However, the overall complication rate for laminectomy and fusion was not statistically different from the laminoplasty cohort in the AOSpine CSM studies.[30] Regarding the incidence of C5 nerve root palsy after posterior procedures, Basaran and Kaner[84] summarized the current literature, according to different procedures, as 0% to 16% in laminoplasty (mean incidence 5.88%), 1.7% to 25% in laminectomy and fusion (mean incidence 10.59%), and 0% to 16% in laminectomy alone (mean incidence 3.62%). However, recent international multicenter study reported rates of 2.41% in cervical laminectomy and fusion versus 3% in laminoplasty.[30]

SUMMARY

A posterior surgical approach to treat DCM is generally recommended in patients with multilevel cervical stenosis with preserved cervical lordosis. Fixed cervical kyphosis is a relative contraindication for a posterior-only approach. Laminectomy and fusion is an effective surgical option at improving clinical disease severity, functional status, quality of life, and preservation of sagittal alignment in patients with DCM. Laminectomy alone may be safe and effective in highly selected patients who have a stiff cervical spine, preserved cervical lordosis, and no radiographic evidence of spinal instability. Stand-alone laminectomy procedures require careful attention to not violate the facet joints and the C2 and C7 muscle attachments. Patients undergoing stand-alone laminectomies should be counseled of the potential for postprocedure kyphosis and made aware of surgical alternatives during the informed consent process.

REFERENCES

1. Young WF. Cervical spondylotic myelopathy: a common cause of spinal cord dysfunction in older persons. Am Fam Physician 2000;62(5): 1064–70, 1073.
2. Wilson JR, Tetreault LA, Kim J, et al. State of the art in degenerative cervical myelopathy: an update on current clinical evidence. Neurosurgery 2017; 80(3s):S33–45.
3. Denaro V, Di Martino A. Cervical spine surgery: an historical perspective. Clin Orthop Relat Res 2011; 469(3):639–48.
4. Stoops WL, King RB. Chronic myelopathy associated with cervical spondylosis: its response to laminectomy and foramenotomy. JAMA 1965;192:281–4.
5. Crandall PH, Batzdorf U. Cervical spondylotic myelopathy. J Neurosurg 1966;25(1):57–66.
6. Epstein JA, Carras R, Lavine LS, et al. The importance of removing osteophytes as part of the surgical treatment of myeloradiculopathy in cervical spondylosis. J Neurosurg 1969;30(3):219–26.
7. Bishara SN. The posterior operation in treatment of cervical spondylosis with myelopathy: a long-term follow-up study. J Neurol Neurosurg Psychiatry 1971;34(4):393–8.

8. Fager CA. Results of adequate posterior decompression in the relief of spondylotic cervical myelopathy. J Neurosurg 1973;38(6):684–92.
9. Jenkins DH. Extensive cervical laminectomy. Long-term results. Br J Surg 1973;60(11):852–4.
10. Gorter K. Influence of laminectomy on the course of cervical myelopathy. Acta Neurochir (Wien) 1976; 33(3–4):265–81.
11. Casotto A, Buoncristiani P. Posterior approach in cervical spondylotic myeloradiculopathy. Acta Neurochir (Wien) 1981;57(3–4):275–85.
12. Miyazaki K, Kirita Y. Extensive simultaneous multisegment laminectomy for myelopathy due to the ossification of the posterior longitudinal ligament in the cervical region. Spine (Phila Pa 1976) 1986; 11(6):531–42.
13. Mikawa Y, Shikata J, Yamamuro T. Spinal deformity and instability after multilevel cervical laminectomy. Spine (Phila Pa 1976) 1987;12(1):6–11.
14. Snow RB, Weiner H. Cervical laminectomy and foraminotomy as surgical treatment of cervical spondylosis: a follow-up study with analysis of failures. J Spinal Disord 1993;6(3):245–50 [discussion: 250-1].
15. Guigui P, Benoist M, Deburge A. Spinal deformity and instability after multilevel cervical laminectomy for spondylotic myelopathy. Spine 1998;23(4):440–7.
16. Kato Y, Iwasaki M, Fuji T, et al. Long-term follow-up results of laminectomy for cervical myelopathy caused by ossification of the posterior longitudinal ligament. J Neurosurg 1998;89(2):217–23.
17. Kaptain GJ, Simmons NE, Replogle RE, et al. Incidence and outcome of kyphotic deformity following laminectomy for cervical spondylotic myelopathy. J Neurosurg 2000;93(2 Suppl):199–204.
18. Hansen-Schwartz J, Kruse-Larsen C, Nielsen CJ. Follow-up after cervical laminectomy, with special reference to instability and deformity. Br J Neurosurg 2003;17(4):301–5.
19. Cho WS, Chung CK, Jahng TA, et al. Post-laminectomy kyphosis in patients with cervical ossification of the posterior longitudinal ligament: does it cause neurological deterioration? J Korean Neurosurg Soc 2008;43(6):259–64.
20. Laiginhas AR, Silva PA, Pereira P, et al. Long-term clinical and radiological follow-up after laminectomy for cervical spondylotic myelopathy. Surg Neurol Int 2015;6:162.
21. Li Z, Xue Y, He D, et al. Extensive laminectomy for multilevel cervical stenosis with ligamentum flavum hypertrophy: more than 10 years follow-up. Eur Spine J 2015;24(8):1605–12.
22. van Geest S, de Vormer AM, Arts MP, et al. Long-term follow-up of clinical and radiological outcome after cervical laminectomy. Eur Spine J 2015; 24(Suppl 2):229–35.
23. Yasuoka S, Peterson HA, Laws ER Jr, et al. Pathogenesis and prophylaxis of postlaminectomy deformity of the spine after multiple level laminectomy: difference between children and adults. Neurosurgery 1981;9(2):145–52.
24. Hirabayashi K, Watanabe K, Wakano K, et al. Expansive open-door laminoplasty for cervical spinal stenotic myelopathy. Spine 1983;8(7):693–9.
25. Kode S, Gandhi AA, Fredericks DC, et al. Effect of multilevel open-door laminoplasty and laminectomy on flexibility of the cervical spine: an experimental investigation. Spine 2012;37(19):E1165–70.
26. Lu JJ. Cervical laminectomy: technique. Neurosurgery 2007;60(1 Supp1 1):S149–53.
27. Patel CK, Cunningham BJ, Herkowitz HN. Techniques in cervical laminoplasty. Spine J 2002;2(6): 450–5.
28. Wang T, Tian XM, Liu SK, et al. Prevalence of complications after surgery in treatment for cervical compressive myelopathy: a meta-analysis for last decade. Medicine 2017;96(12):e6421.
29. Yoon ST, Hashimoto RE, Raich A, et al. Outcomes after laminoplasty compared with laminectomy and fusion in patients with cervical myelopathy: a systematic review. Spine 2013;38(22 Suppl 1):S183–94.
30. Fehlings MG, Santaguida C, Tetreault L, et al. Laminectomy and fusion versus laminoplasty for the treatment of degenerative cervical myelopathy: results from the AOSpine North America and International prospective multicenter studies. Spine J 2017;17(1):102–8.
31. Liu X, Min S, Zhang H, et al. Anterior corpectomy versus posterior laminoplasty for multilevel cervical myelopathy: a systematic review and meta-analysis. Eur Spine J 2014;23(2):362–72.
32. Wu TK, Wang BY, Meng Y, et al. Multilevel cervical disc replacement versus multilevel anterior discectomy and fusion: a meta-analysis. Medicine 2017; 96(16):e6503.
33. Ames CP, Blondel B, Scheer JK, et al. Cervical radiographical alignment: comprehensive assessment techniques and potential importance in cervical myelopathy. Spine (Phila Pa 1976) 2013;38(22 Suppl 1):S149–60.
34. Scheer JK, Tang JA, Smith JS, et al. Cervical spine alignment, sagittal deformity, and clinical implications: a review. J Neurosurg Spine 2013;19(2):141–59.
35. Shedid D, Benzel EC. Cervical spondylosis anatomy: pathophysiology and biomechanics. Neurosurgery 2007;60(1 Supp1 1):S7–13.
36. Pal GP, Sherk HH. The vertical stability of the cervical spine. Spine (Phila Pa 1976) 1988;13(5):447–9.
37. Chan WC, Sze KL, Samartzis D, et al. Structure and biology of the intervertebral disk in health and disease. Orthop Clin North Am 2011;42(4):447–64, vii.
38. Katsumi Y, Honma T, Nakamura T. Analysis of cervical instability resulting from laminectomies for removal of spinal cord tumor. Spine (Phila Pa 1976) 1989;14(11):1171–6.

39. Nowinski GP, Visarius H, Nolte LP, et al. A biomechanical comparison of cervical laminaplasty and cervical laminectomy with progressive facetectomy. Spine (Phila Pa 1976) 1993;18(14):1995–2004.
40. Ozgur BM, Florman JE, Lew SM, et al. Laminectomy contributes to cervical spine deformity demonstrated by holographic interferometry. J Spinal Disord Tech 2003;16(1):51–4.
41. Zhang P, Shen Y, Zhang YZ, et al. Preserving the C7 spinous process in laminectomy combined with lateral mass screw to prevent axial symptom. J Orthopaedic Sci 2011;16(5):492–7.
42. Sciubba DM, Chaichana KL, Woodworth GF, et al. Factors associated with cervical instability requiring fusion after cervical laminectomy for intradural tumor resection. J Neurosurg Spine 2008;8(5):413–9.
43. Sakaura H, Hosono N, Mukai Y, et al. Preservation of muscles attached to the C2 and C7 spinous processes rather than subaxial deep extensors reduces adverse effects after cervical laminoplasty. Spine 2010;35(16):E782–6.
44. Patil PG, Turner DA, Pietrobon R. National trends in surgical procedures for degenerative cervical spine disease: 1990-2000. Neurosurgery 2005; 57(4):753–8 [discussion: 753–8].
45. Manzano GR, Casella G, Wang MY, et al. A prospective, randomized trial comparing expansile cervical laminoplasty and cervical laminectomy and fusion for multilevel cervical myelopathy. Neurosurgery 2012;70(2):264–77.
46. Fehlings MG, Barry S, Kopjar B, et al. Anterior versus posterior surgical approaches to treat cervical spondylotic myelopathy: outcomes of the prospective multicenter AOSpine North America CSM study in 264 patients. Spine (Phila Pa 1976) 2013; 38(26):2247–52.
47. Lawrence BD, Jacobs WB, Norvell DC, et al. Anterior versus posterior approach for treatment of cervical spondylotic myelopathy: a systematic review. Spine (Phila Pa 1976) 2013;38(22 Suppl 1):S173–82.
48. Winestone JS, Farley CW, Curt BA, et al. Laminectomy, durotomy, and piotomy effects on spinal cord intramedullary pressure in severe cervical and thoracic kyphotic deformity: a cadaveric study. J Neurosurg Spine 2012;16(2):195–200.
49. Ishida Y, Suzuki K, Ohmori K, et al. Critical analysis of extensive cervical laminectomy. Neurosurgery 1989;24(2):215–22.
50. LaRocca H, Macnab I. The laminectomy membrane. Studies in its evolution, characteristics, effects and prophylaxis in dogs. J Bone Joint Surg Br 1974; 56B(3):545–50.
51. Raynor RB, Pugh J, Shapiro I. Cervical facetectomy and its effect on spine strength. J Neurosurg 1985; 63(2):278–82.
52. Kumaresan S, Yoganandan N, Pintar FA, et al. Finite element modeling of cervical laminectomy with graded facetectomy. J Spinal Disord 1997;10(1): 40–6.
53. Kode S, Kallemeyn NA, Smucker JD, et al. The effect of multi-level laminoplasty and laminectomy on the biomechanics of the cervical spine: a finite element study. Iowa Orthop J 2014;34:150–7.
54. Hong-Wan N, Ee-Chon T, Qing-Hang Z. Biomechanical effects of C2-C7 intersegmental stability due to laminectomy with unilateral and bilateral facetectomy. Spine (Phila Pa 1976) 2004;29(16):1737–45 [discussion: 1746].
55. Subramaniam V, Chamberlain RH, Theodore N, et al. Biomechanical effects of laminoplasty versus laminectomy: stenosis and stability. Spine (Phila Pa 1976) 2009;34(16):E573–8.
56. Zdeblick TA, Zou D, Warden KE, et al. Cervical stability after foraminotomy. A biomechanical in vitro analysis. J Bone Joint Surg Am 1992;74(1):22–7.
57. Batzdorf U, Batzdorff A. Analysis of cervical spine curvature in patients with cervical spondylosis. Neurosurgery 1988;22(5):827–36.
58. Matsunaga S, Sakou T, Nakanisi K. Analysis of the cervical spine alignment following laminoplasty and laminectomy. Spinal Cord 1999;37(1):20–4.
59. Ryken TC, Heary RF, Matz PG, et al. Cervical laminectomy for the treatment of cervical degenerative myelopathy. J Neurosurg Spine 2009;11(2):142–9.
60. Breig A, el-Nadi AF. Biomechanics of the cervical spinal cord. Relief of contact pressure on and overstretching of the spinal cord. Acta Radiol Diagn (Stockh) 1966;4(6):602–24.
61. Du W, Wang L, Shen Y, et al. Long-term impacts of different posterior operations on curvature, neurological recovery and axial symptoms for multilevel cervical degenerative myelopathy. Eur Spine J 2013;22(7):1594–602.
62. Nurboja B, Kachramanoglou C, Choi D. Cervical laminectomy vs laminoplasty: is there a difference in outcome and postoperative pain? Neurosurgery 2012;70(4):965–70 [discussion: 970].
63. Lee SE, Chung CK, Jahng TA, et al. Long-term outcome of laminectomy for cervical ossification of the posterior longitudinal ligament. J Neurosurg Spine 2013;18(5):465–71.
64. Bartels RH, van Tulder MW, Moojen WA, et al. Laminoplasty and laminectomy for cervical sponydylotic myelopathy: a systematic review. Eur Spine J 2015; 24(Suppl 2):160–7.
65. Bartels RH, Groenewoud H, Peul WC, et al. Lamifuse: results of a randomized controlled trial comparing laminectomy with and without fusion for cervical spondylotic myelopathy. J Neurosurg Sci 2017;61(2):134–9.
66. Smith JS, Line B, Bess S, et al. The health impact of adult cervical deformity in patients presenting for surgical treatment: comparison to United States population norms and chronic disease states based

on the EuroQuol-5 dimensions questionnaire. Neurosurgery 2017;80(5):716–25.
67. Passias PG, Horn SR, Jalai CM, et al. Comparative analysis of peri-operative complications between a multicenter prospective cervical deformity database and the nationwide inpatient sample database. Spine J 2017 [pii:S1529-9430(17)30210-3].
68. Hamanishi C, Tanaka S. Bilateral multilevel laminectomy with or without posterolateral fusion for cervical spondylotic myelopathy: relationship to type of onset and time until operation. J Neurosurg 1996;85(3):447–51.
69. Kumar VG, Rea GL, Mervis LJ, et al. Cervical spondylotic myelopathy: functional and radiographic long-term outcome after laminectomy and posterior fusion. Neurosurgery 1999;44(4):771–7 [discussion: 777–8].
70. Houten JK, Cooper PR. Laminectomy and posterior cervical plating for multilevel cervical spondylotic myelopathy and ossification of the posterior longitudinal ligament: effects on cervical alignment, spinal cord compression, and neurological outcome. Neurosurgery 2003;52(5):1081–7 [discussion: 1087–8].
71. Chen Y, Guo Y, Chen D, et al. Long-term outcome of laminectomy and instrumented fusion for cervical ossification of the posterior longitudinal ligament. Int Orthop 2009;33(4):1075–80.
72. Fast A, Thomas MA. The "baseball cap orthosis": a simple solution for dropped head syndrome. Am J Phys Med Rehabil 2008;87(1):71–3.
73. Arnts H, Bartels RH. Flexible dropped head deformity following laminectomy for cervical spondylotic myelopathy: a case series and review of literature. Spine J 2016;16(10):e721–4.
74. Suk KS, Kim KT, Lee JH, et al. Sagittal alignment of the cervical spine after the laminoplasty. Spine (Phila Pa 1976) 2007;32(23):E656–60.
75. Shiraishi T. Skip laminectomy–a new treatment for cervical spondylotic myelopathy, preserving bilateral muscular attachments to the spinous processes: a preliminary report. Spine J 2002;2(2):108–15.
76. Yukawa Y, Kato F, Ito K, et al. Laminoplasty and skip laminectomy for cervical compressive myelopathy: range of motion, postoperative neck pain, and surgical outcomes in a randomized prospective study. Spine (Phila Pa 1976) 2007;32(18):1980–5.
77. Shiraishi T, Fukuda K, Yato Y, et al. Results of skip laminectomy-minimum 2-year follow-up study compared with open-door laminoplasty. Spine (Phila Pa 1976) 2003;28(24):2667–72.
78. Sivaraman A, Bhadra AK, Altaf F, et al. Skip laminectomy and laminoplasty for cervical spondylotic myelopathy: a prospective study of clinical and radiologic outcomes. J Spinal Disord Tech 2010;23(2):96–100.
79. Hur JW, Kim JS, Shin MH, et al. Minimally invasive posterior cervical decompression using tubular retractor: the technical note and early clinical outcome. Surg Neurol Int 2014;5:34.
80. Dahdaleh NS, Wong AP, Smith ZA, et al. Microendoscopic decompression for cervical spondylotic myelopathy. Neurosurg Focus 2013;35(1):E8.
81. Vergara P. Minimally invasive microscopic posterior cervical decompression: simple, safe, and effective. J Neurol Surg A Cent Eur Neurosurg 2017;78(5):440–5.
82. Wang M, Luo XJ, Deng QX, et al. Prevalence of axial symptoms after posterior cervical decompression: a meta-analysis. Eur Spine J 2016;25(7):2302–10.
83. Ashana AO, Cohen JR, Evans B, et al. Regression of anterior disk-osteophyte complex following cervical laminectomy and fusion for cervical spondylotic myelopathy. Clin Spine Surg 2017;30(5):E609–14.
84. Basaran R, Kaner T. C5 nerve root palsy following decompression of cervical spine with anterior versus posterior types of procedures in patients with cervical myelopathy. Eur Spine J 2016;25(7):2050–9.

History and Evolution of Laminoplasty

Yoshitaka Hirano, MD[a,*], Yukoh Ohara, MD[b], Junichi Mizuno, MD, PhD[b], Yasunobu Itoh, MD, PhD[c]

KEYWORDS

- Degenerative cervical myelopathy • Ossified posterior longitudinal ligament • Multisegmental lesion
- Posterior decompression • Expansive laminoplasty • Evolution of surgical procedure
- Recent advance in implants

KEY POINTS

- Expansive laminoplasty for degenerative cervical myelopathy and ossified longitudinal ligament is reviewed, focusing on the history of the surgical procedure.
- Laminoplasty was developed by Japanese orthopedic surgeons from the 1970s to 1980s to overcome adverse conditions related to laminectomy.
- Recent laminoplasty techniques offer less invasive maneuvers to obtain better functional outcome, but every operation is carried out based on the unchanged initial concept.
- Complications related to laminoplasty and some potential solutions are introduced, with some literature review.
- Modifications of the surgical techniques and development of new implants are also discussed.

INTRODUCTION

Surgical treatment of degenerative cervical myelopathy and ossified posterior longitudinal ligament (OPLL) is intended to release the spinal cord from cord-compressing pathology, by either direct removal of the cord-compressing lesion through the anterior approach or indirect decompression of the spinal cord through the posterior approach. Laminectomy has been the main method of the posterior approach, and has become safer with the development of high-speed drills. However, surgical outcomes have been significantly affected by the complications of postlaminectomy kyphosis (25%) and anterior subluxation (40%) even in patients with cervical radiculopathy.[1] Late neurologic deterioration caused by local epidural scar formation, the so-called laminectomy membrane, may also occur. Laminoplasty was developed by Japanese orthopedic surgeons from the 1970s to the 1980s to overcome these problems with conventional laminectomy. Since then, laminoplasty has been accepted as one of the standard techniques for posterior decompression among Japanese spine surgeons. Recently, laminoplasty has been associated with less invasive maneuvers to the posterior cervical muscle structures that reduce axial neck pain and obtain better functional outcome, but every operation is carried out based on the unchanged initial concept.

Disclosure: The authors report no conflict of interest concerning the materials or methods used in this study or the finding specified in this article.

[a] Spine Section, Department of Neurosurgery, Southern TOHOKU Research Institute for Neuroscience, 7-115 Yatsuyamada, Koriyama, Fukushima 963-8563, Japan; [b] Department of Spine and Peripheral Nerve Surgery, Shin-Yurigaoka General Hospital, 255 Tsuko, Furusawa, Asao-ku, Kawasaki, Kanagawa 215-0026, Japan; [c] Department of Neurosurgery, Tokyo General Hospital, 3-15-2 Egoda, Nakano-ku, Tokyo 165-8906, Japan
* Corresponding author.
E-mail address: mth10yhirano@flute.ocn.ne.jp

Neurosurg Clin N Am 29 (2018) 107–113
https://doi.org/10.1016/j.nec.2017.09.019
1042-3680/18/© 2017 Elsevier Inc. All rights reserved.

Here the development and 45-year history of cervical laminoplasty is described, and its evolution is discussed with some literature review. Some recent attempts to improve the surgical results are also discussed, focusing on less-invasive maneuvers to the posterior muscle structures and the development of implants.

Z-SHAPED LAMINOPLASTY

The original concept of cervical laminoplasty was based on extensive simultaneous multisegmental laminectomy for cervical OPLL, as initially described by Miyazaki and Kirita in 1968, and reported in 1986.[2] This technique starts with attenuation of the laminae, and laminotomy in the midline with the drill. Then the lateral gutters are formed until the laminae are bent and elevated. The remaining laminar edges are finally removed with scissors. Expeditious and simultaneous elevation of the multiple laminae is considered to be important to prevent localized posterior shift of the spinal cord after decompression, which may cause postoperative neurologic deterioration. Based on this concept of extensive simultaneous multisegmental decompression, several surgical procedures without resection of the elevated laminae were introduced in the following 15 years.

The first expansive laminoplasty was described by Oyama and colleagues[3] in 1973 as "expansive Z-shaped laminoplasty." The attenuated laminae are cut into Z-shape and elevated for suturing on the midline (**Fig. 1**). The posterior spinal canal is reconstructed to prevent scar formation over the dural surface, which is also expected to minimize reduction of spinal stability. The introduction of the high-speed automated surgical burr was important in establishing this procedure.[4]

EN BLOC LAMINOPLASTY

En bloc laminectomy in which laminotomies are carried out bilaterally along the lateral margin of the spinal canal to separate laminae from the articular processes was introduced by Tsuji.[5] This procedure has been the principal technique for extensive multisegmental posterior decompression since 1978. This technique was modified to en bloc laminoplasty by reflecting the laminae as a flap to permit floating over the dural surface, without fixing sutures or bone grafting.[6] This technique was further modified to stabilize the laminar flap using bone blocks and wire ligatures to achieve stable and thorough decompression of the spinal canal.[7] Open-door laminoplasty (described later) was developed based on this modified technique of en bloc laminoplasty.[8]

Another modification of en bloc laminoplasty by a Japanese neurosurgeon involved insertion of hydroxyapatite (HA) beads between the cut surfaces of the laminae.[9] Because of the complexity and pitfalls in the surgical maneuvers, this procedure is no longer included as a standard treatment option.

OPEN-DOOR LAMINOPLASTY

Unilateral open-door laminoplasty was introduced by Hirabayashi and coworkers in 1977,[10–12] and continues to be one of the standard techniques for posterior decompression of the cervical spine (**Fig. 2**). Gutters are created with the high-speed drill at the junction between the articular processes and the laminae. The gutters on the dominant side of the symptoms are cut completely to achieve laminotomy, and the spinous processes and the laminae are displaced laterally to the hinges of the gutters on the opposite side. The spinal canal is enlarged by opening the posterior bony elements, and the laminae are kept open with three or four sutures on the facet capsule on the hinge side.[12] The benefits of these procedures are to allow simultaneous decompression of multiple segments, and to preserve the posterior muscle structures that prevent postoperative

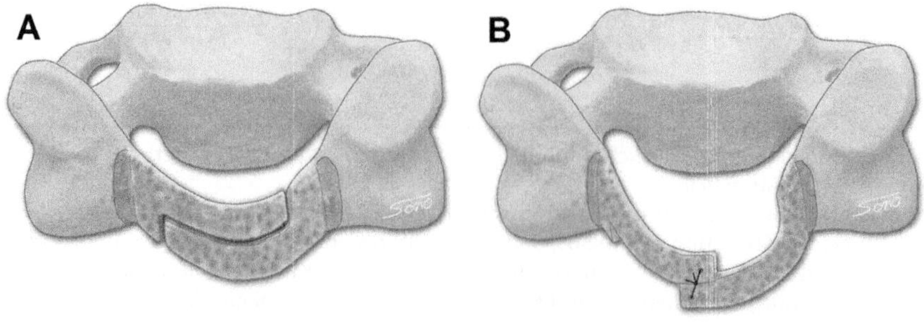

Fig. 1. Surgical diagrams of Z-shaped laminoplasty. (*A*) Laminae are attenuated with the drill, and Z-shaped laminotomies are formed in each lamina. (*B*) Split laminae are elevated and sutured to reconstruct the expanded spinal canal.

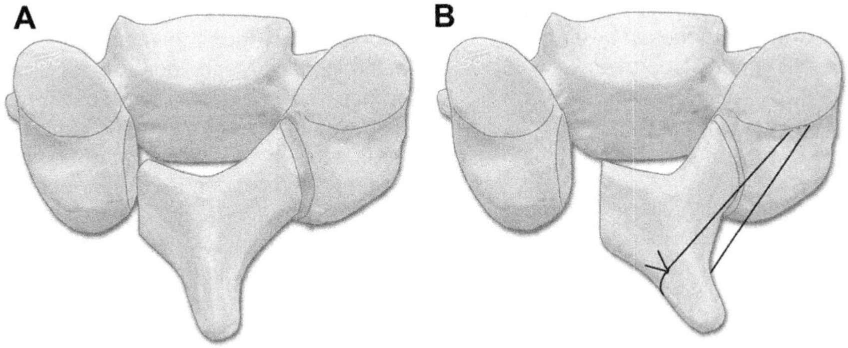

Fig. 2. Surgical diagrams of Hirabayashi unilateral open-door laminoplasty. (*A*) Bony gutters are drilled bilaterally at the lateral margins of the laminae, and the bone completely removed on one side while preserving the inner cortex as hinges on the other side. (*B*) Spinal canal is enlarged by opening the posterior bony elements, and the laminae are kept open with sutures on the facet capsule on the hinge side.

progression of cervical kyphosis and segmental instability.[13] The original technique had two shortcomings: loss of increased sagittal diameter, and time-consuming complexity of the canal reconstruction.[14] Various implants, such as HA[15,16] and titanium miniplates with or without allografts,[14,17,18] have been used to maintain postoperative sagittal diameter. These implants are also involved in the early stabilization of the opened laminae.

DOUBLE-DOOR LAMINOPLASTY

Spinous process splitting double-door laminoplasty is another important development of cervical laminoplasty described by Kurokawa and coworkers in 1982 (**Fig. 3**).[19] With subsequent improvements in techniques and implants by many spine surgeons, this procedure has become one of the principal techniques of cervical laminoplasty today. After exposure from the spinous processes to the medial border of the facet joints, the high-speed drill with a small burr of 1.5 to 2.0 mm in diameter is introduced to carry out midline laminotomy. Lateral gutters are created bilaterally at the junction between the articular processes and laminae. These maneuvers allow symmetric opening of both sides of the laminae with hinges at the bilateral gutters, and adequate decompression is confirmed. The tips of the spinous processes are used as spacers between the opened laminae to maintain the enlarged spinal canal. Iliac bone grafts, HA spacers of various shapes and sizes,[18,20,21] and small metal plates[19] are often used as alternatives to keep the laminae open.

For the spinous process splitting procedure, a new maneuver of midline laminotomy with a threaded wire saw of 0.54 mm in diameter (T-saw) to achieve shorter operating time and less blood loss was developed by Tomita and colleagues.[22] Special care has to be taken to prevent further damage to the spinal cord when passing

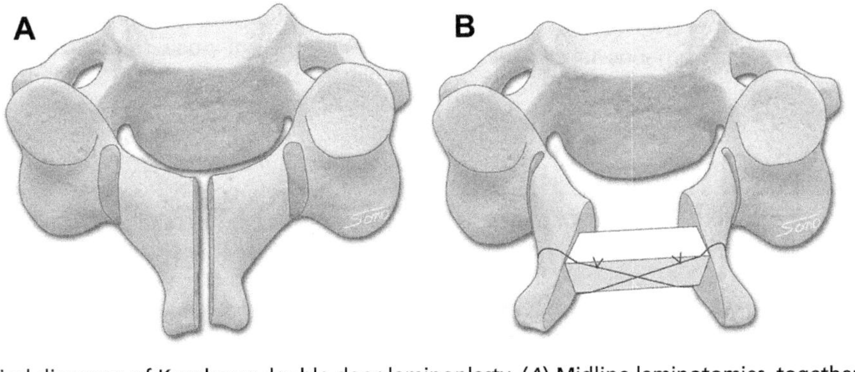

Fig. 3. Surgical diagrams of Kurokawa double-door laminoplasty. (*A*) Midline laminotomies, together with splitting of the spinous processes on the midline, are carried out first. The lateral margins of the laminae are drilled to form hinge gutters. (*B*) Laminae are elevated bilaterally to achieve enlargement of the spinal canal. Artificial spacers, such as hydroxyapatite, are usually required to keep the laminae open.

the wire into the spinal canal, especially in patients with severe canal stenosis caused by large OPLL.[4] There is some risk of dural laceration.

PROBLEMS AND COMPLICATIONS RELATED TO LAMINOPLASTY

Common complications arising from cervical laminoplasty are axial neck pain, C5 nerve root palsy, development of kyphosis, and epidural hematoma. These problems often occur focally compared with anterior decompression and fusion, and are considered to be major disadvantages of the posterior approach.

Axial Neck Pain

Axial neck pain is an intractable form of pain around the neck and shoulder, and often persists as a major concern for several years after laminoplasty, even in patients with excellent neurologic recovery.[23] Its incidence has been reported to be 60% to 80%,[23,24] but the cause has not yet been clarified. Several interventions to reduce this unfavorable condition have been introduced, including early start of isometric muscle exercise, and avoiding use of orthosis. However, modifications of the surgical procedure are considered more important in the reduction of axial neck pain.

Preservation of the paraspinal muscle structures is important to reduce axial neck pain and maintain cervical alignment.[25] Dissection of the muscles attached to the C2 and C7 spinous processes is related to the development of axial neck pain.[26,27] Shiraishi and Yato[28] developed a novel technique to preserve all muscular attachments to the C2 spinous process, intended to reduce axial neck pain and prevent postoperative malalignment. An anatomic study by Ono and colleagues[29] revealed that the rhomboideus minor, the serratus posterior superior, and the splenius capitis are preserved if the C7 spinous process is not resected for laminoplasty. Following these studies, Japanese spine surgeons tend to avoid manipulation of the C2 and C7 spinous processes during laminoplasty if possible.

C5 Nerve Root Palsy

Postoperative paresis of the upper extremity was first reported by Scoville and Stoops in 1961 as a neurologic complication of cervical laminectomy.[30,31] Most of those patients presented with weakness of the deltoid muscle and sensory disturbance in the C5 territory. Postoperative C5 nerve root palsy has since been recognized as occurring exclusively as a postoperative complication of posterior cervical decompression surgery. Reports of postoperative C5 palsy have become more common during the development of laminoplasty techniques and subsequent widespread implementation. Most patients develop C5 palsy within a week of surgery, but the onset varies from 2 to 4 weeks in a limited number of cases. The reported incidence of postoperative C5 palsy is 4.6% on average, 5.3% in unilateral open-door laminoplasty, and 4.3% in double-door laminoplasty.[32] The incidence of this complication is slightly higher in patients with OPLL (8.3%) than in patients with cervical spondylotic myelopathy (5.6%), but its occurrence is not related to either surgical procedures or disease etiology. C5 palsy has also occurred after anterior cervical decompression and fusion, but the reported incidence, 4.3% on average, is slightly lower than for posterior approaches.[32]

The pathogenesis of postoperative C5 palsy is not fully understood, but several hypotheses have been proposed: (1) inadvertent injury to the nerve root during surgery, (2) tethering phenomenon in which consecutive shifting of the spinal cord causes nerve root traction, (3) spinal cord ischemia caused by decreased blood supply from the radicular artery, (4) segmental spinal cord disorder, and (5) reperfusion injury of the spinal cord.[32] Consequent to the unclear and varied proposed mechanisms of pathogenesis, no specific treatments for this condition have been established. The prognosis for postoperative C5 nerve root palsy is generally good, and complete resolution of the symptoms is expected within several months. However, patients with severe motor deficits of the deltoid muscle (muscle power of 2/V or less on manual muscle testing) take a longer period for full recovery.[4]

Development of Kyphosis

Unlike laminectomy, laminoplasty was expected to reconstruct the posterior elements of the spine to prevent postoperative development of kyphosis. However, Hukuda and colleagues[33] reported that 28% of patients developed kyphosis within 5 years postoperatively, a similar incidence to laminectomy (30%). Even within a series of patients with early postoperative cervical range of motion exercises, 7.2% developed kyphosis.[34] Cervical kyphosis may be a result of a protective physiologic mechanism to increase the spinal canal volume as a response to compression of the spinal cord.[8] The degree of repair in the semispinalis cervicis is suggested to affect postoperative cervical alignment,[26] and muscle-preserving procedures are considered important.

Epidural Hematoma

Postoperative epidural hematoma is another major complication of cervical laminoplasty, which commonly occurs within 48 hours of surgery. Reported incidence of epidural hematoma following laminoplasty is 0.44%,[35] and preoperative administration of anticoagulants, excessive epidural bleeding during surgery, and high blood pressure are major risk factors. Because delayed diagnosis and reoperation are associated with poor recovery, surgeons should be aware of the risk of postoperative neurologic deterioration, and early removal of the hematoma is recommended.

TECHNIQUES FOR MUSCLE PRESERVATION

The original procedures of cervical laminoplasty included detachment of the muscles from the posterior elements of the spine, and such maneuvers are considered to have negative effects on axial neck pain and postoperative kyphotic deformity. Skip laminectomy and the technique for muscle-preserving double-door laminoplasty (TEMPL) developed by Shiraishi and coworkers[28,36–38] represent one of the major attempts to overcome these problems. TEMPL requires minimum resection of the muscle attachment to the cervical spine, and is applicable to various posterior cervical spine surgeries. This procedure preserves the attachments of the semispinalis cervicis and multifidus muscles to the cervical spinous processes, and limits damage to the attachments of the interspinous and rotator muscles. The outcomes of TEMPL support positive effects on pain management, preservation of motion and alignment, and TEMPL is adopted by many spine surgeons today. A study on deep extensor muscle volume at 2 years postoperatively showed significantly larger muscle volume after TEMPL (88% of preoperative volume) compared with conventional laminoplasty (56%).[39]

Kim and coworkers[40] further investigated methods to reconstitute the cervical musculature, and developed a technique called myoarchitectonic spinolaminoplasty. This technique starts with cutting the spinous processes along the midline, then cutting them off from the laminae without severing the muscular attachments before exposing the laminae. The attachments of the semispinalis cervicis, multifidus, interspinalis, and rotator muscles are fully preserved. After double-door laminoplasty with HA spacers, the bone-muscle flaps are affixed to the spinous processes of the HA spacers. Outcomes showed positive effects on preservation of the volume and function of the nuchal musculature, and significant reduction of postoperative axial neck pain and shoulder strain. The concept of the myoarchitectonic spinolaminoplasty has been widely accepted as a methodology for reducing surgical invasion.

DEVELOPMENT OF INSTRUMENTS

Another major disadvantage of cervical laminoplasty is the complicated surgical procedures compared with other spine surgeries. Takayasu and coworkers[41] developed a simple double-door laminoplasty in which HA spacers and titanium screws are secured to preserve the posterior supporting elements, such as the nuchal ligament and the supraspinous and interspinous ligaments. In the conventional procedure of laminoplasty, HA spacers are secured to the spinous process with wires or nylon sutures.[7,18,40] This modified technique with titanium screws is easier with shorter

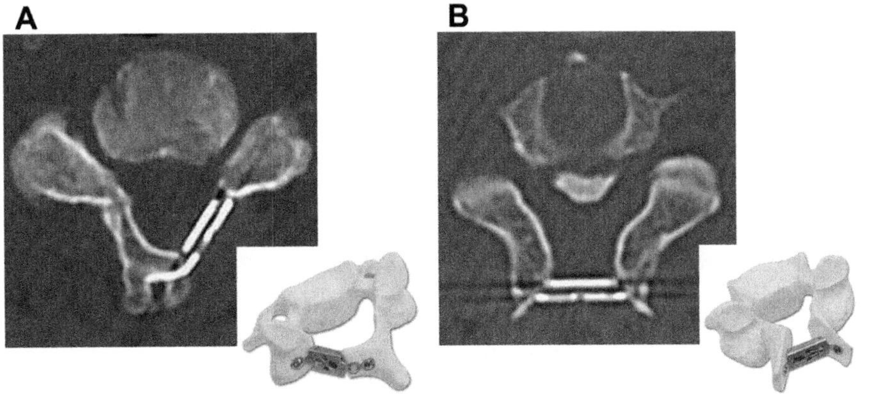

Fig. 4. Laminoplasty Basket (Ammtec, Tokyo, Japan) used for open-door laminoplasty (*A*) and double-door laminoplasty (*B*). Illustrations are shown together with axial computed tomographic scans obtained 1 year postoperatively. The basket component of the implant is filled with artificial bone compound made of collagen fibers and hydroxyapatite (Refit, Hoya Technosurgical, Tokyo, Japan) with the intention of full reconstruction of the laminae by osteoconduction.

operating time, and a biomechanical study proved greater strength in fixation compared with the conventional procedure.

However, HA spacers have the disadvantages of lower plasticity and implant-related complications, such as breakage of the implant and difficulty in fixation with the sutures resulting in loosening of the spacers.[42–44] Tani and coworkers[45] developed a new box-shaped titanium spacer, the Laminoplasty Basket (Ammtec, Tokyo, Japan), to compensate for these disadvantages of HA implants. The Laminoplasty Basket has several advantages. The malleability is sufficient to fit any condition of the elevated laminae, so it can be used for either open-door or double-door laminoplasty (**Fig. 4**). Unlike HA, this titanium basket carries less risk of implant failure. A biomechanical study proved stronger stabilization force compared with fixation with titanium miniplates.[46] The Laminoplasty Basket can also promote bone conduction through the basket component. Above all, the surgical procedure using the Laminoplasty Basket is simple, and shorter operating time and less surgical invasiveness are expected.

SUMMARY

This article provides a brief review of the techniques of cervical laminoplasty including the origins and subsequent advances. The authors pay tribute to the founders of this standard technique in modern spine surgery. With further evolution in techniques, tools, and implants, expansive laminoplasty is expected to achieve better outcomes with less surgical invasiveness in patients with degenerative cervical myelopathy and cervical OPLL.

ACKNOWLEDGMENTS

The authors express their sincere gratitude to Mr Shunji Ono for his technical support in preparing surgical diagrams.

REFERENCES

1. Herkowitz HN. A comparison of anterior cervical fusion, cervical laminectomy, and cervical laminoplasty for the surgical management of multiple level spondylotic radiculopathy. Spine (Phila Pa 1976) 1988;13:774–80.
2. Miyazaki K, Kirita Y. Extensive simultaneous multisegment laminectomy for myelopathy due to the ossification of the posterior longitudinal ligament in the cervical region. Spine (Phila Pa 1976) 1986;11:531–42.
3. Oyama M, Hattori S, Moriwaki N, et al. A new method of cervical laminectomy. Chubu Nippon Seikeigeka Saigaigeka Gakkai Zasshi 1973;16:792–4 [in Japanese].
4. Ito M, Nagahama K. Laminoplasty for cervical myelopathy. Glob Spine J 2012;2:187–94.
5. Tsuji H. En-bloc laminectomy. Seikeigeka 1978;29: 1755–61 [in Japanese].
6. Tsuji H. Laminoplasty for patients with compressive myelopathy due to so-called spinal canal stenosis in cervical and thoracic regions. Spine (Phila Pa 1976) 1982;7:28–34.
7. Itoh T, Tsuji H. Technical improvements and results of laminoplasty for compressive myelopathy in the cervical spine. Spine (Phila Pa 1976) 1985;10:729–36.
8. Kurokawa R, Kim P. Cervical laminoplasty: the history and the future. Neurol Med Chir (Tokyo) 2015; 55:529–39.
9. Koyama T, Handa J. Cervical laminoplasty using apatite beads as implants. Experiences in 31 patients with compressive myelopathy due to developmental canal stenosis. Surg Neurol 1985;24:663–7.
10. Hirabayashi K. Expansive open-door laminoplasty for cervical spondylotic myelopathy. Jpn J Surg 1978;32:1159–63 [in Japanese].
11. Hirabayashi K, Miyakawa J, Satomi K, et al. Operative results and postoperative progression of ossification among patients with ossification of cervical posterior longitudinal ligament. Spine (Phila Pa 1976) 1981;6:354–64.
12. Hirabayashi K, Watanabe K, Wakano K, et al. Expansive open-door laminoplasty for cervical spinal stenotic myelopathy. Spine (Phila Pa 1976) 1983;8: 693–9.
13. Satomi K, Nishu Y, Kohno T, et al. Long-term follow-up studies of open-door expansive laminoplasty for cervical stenotic myelopathy. Spine (Phila Pa 1976) 1994;19:507–10.
14. Shaffrey CI, Wiggins GC, Piccirilli CB, et al. Modified open-door laminoplasty for treatment of neurological deficits in younger patients with congenital spinal stenosis: analysis of clinical and radiological data. J Neurosurg 1999;90(2 Suppl):170–7.
15. Tani S, Isoshima A, Nagashima H, et al. Laminoplasty with preservation of posterior cervical elements: surgical technique. Neurosurgery 2002;50:97–102.
16. Kihara S, Umebayashi T, Hoshimaru M. Technical improvements and results of open-door expansive laminoplasty with hydroxyapatite implants for cervical myelopathy. Neurosurgery 2005;57(4 Suppl): 348–56.
17. O'Brien MF, Peterson D, Casey AH, et al. A novel technique for laminoplasty augmentation of spinal canal area using titanium miniplate stabilization: a computerized morphometric analysis. Spine (Phila Pa 1976) 1996;21:474–84.
18. Itoh Y, Nakagawa H, Mizuno J. Minimally invasive expansive laminoplasty. In: Mummaneni P, Kanter AS, Wang MY, et al, editors. Cervical spine surgery: current trends and challenges. Boca Raton: CRC Press; 2013. p. 415–32.

19. Kurokawa T, Tsuyama N, Tanaka H, et al. Enlargement of spinal canal by sagittal splitting of spinous processes. Bessatsu Seikeigeka 1982;2:234–40 [in Japanese].
20. Hase H, Watanabe T, Hirasawa Y, et al. Bilateral open laminoplasty using ceramic laminas for cervical myelopathy. Spine (Phila Pa 1976) 1991;16:1269–76.
21. Kubo S, Goel VK, Yang SJ, et al. Biomechanical evaluation of cervical open-door laminoplasty using hydroxyapatite spacer. Spine (Phila Pa 1976) 2003;28:227–34.
22. Tomita K, Kawahara N, Toribatake Y, et al. Expansive midline T-saw laminoplasty (modified spinous process-splitting) for the management of cervical myelopathy. Spine (Phila Pa 1976) 1998;23:32–7.
23. Hosono N, Yonenobu K, Ono K. Neck and shoulder pain after laminoplasty: a noticeable complication. Spine (Phila Pa 1976) 1996;21:1969–73.
24. Kawaguchi Y, Kanamori M, Ishihara H, et al. Axial symptoms after en-bloc cervical laminoplasty. J Spinal Disord 1999;24:1023–8.
25. Kato M, Nakamura H, Konishi S, et al. Effect of preserving paraspinal muscles on postoperative axial pain in the selective cervical laminoplasty. Spine (Phila Pa 1976) 2008;33:E455–9.
26. Iizuka H, Shimizu T, Tateno K, et al. Extensor musculature of the cervical spine after laminoplasty: morphologic evaluation by coronal view of the magnetic resonance image. Spine (Phila Pa 1976) 2001;26:2220–6.
27. Takeuchi K, Yokoyama T, Aburakawa S, et al. Axial symptoms after cervical laminoplasty with C3 laminectomy compared with conventional C3-C7 laminoplasty: a modified laminoplasty preserving the semispinalis cervicis inserted into axis. Spine (Phila Pa 1976) 2005;30:2544–9.
28. Shiraishi T, Yato Y. New double-door laminoplasty procedure for the axis to preserve all muscular attachments to the spinous process: technical note. Neurosurg Focus 2002;12(1):E9.
29. Ono A, Tonosaki Y, Yokoyama T, et al. Surgical anatomy of the nuchal muscles in the posterior cervicothoracic junction: significance of the preservation of the C7 spinous process in cervical laminoplasty. Spine (Phila Pa 1976) 2008;33:E349–54.
30. Scoville WB. Cervical spondylosis treated by bilateral facetectomy and laminectomy. J Neurosurg 1961;18:423–8.
31. Stoops WL. Neural complication of cervical spondylosis; their response to laminectomy and foraminotomy. J Neurosurg 1961;19:986–99.
32. Sakaura H, Hosono N, Mukai Y, et al. C5 palsy after decompression surgery for cervical myelopathy. Spine (Phila Pa 1976) 2003;28:2447–51.
33. Hukuda S, Ogata M, Mochizuki T, et al. Laminectomy versus laminoplasty for cervical myelopathy: brief report. J Bone Joint Surg Br 1988;70:325–6.
34. Machino M, Yukawa Y, Hida T, et al. Cervical alignment and range of motion after laminoplasty: radiological data from more than 500 cases with cervical spondylotic myelopathy and a review of the literature. Spine (Phila Pa 1976) 2012;37:E1243–50.
35. Aono H, Ohwada T, Hosono N, et al. Incidence of postoperative symptomatic epidural hematoma in spinal decompression surgery. J Neurosurg Spine 2011;15:202–5.
36. Shiraishi T, Fukuda K, Yato Y, et al. Results of skip laminectomy: minimum 2-year follow-up study compared with open-door laminoplasty. Spine (Phila Pa 1976) 2003;28:2667–72.
37. Shiraishi T, Yato Y, Yoshida H, et al. New double-door laminoplasty procedures to preserve the muscular attachments to the spinous processes including the axis. Eur J Orthop Surg Traumatol 2002;12:175–80.
38. Shiraishi T, Kato M, Yato Y, et al. New techniques for exposure of posterior cervical spine through intermuscular planes and their surgical application. Spine (Phila Pa 1976) 2012;37:E286–96.
39. Kotani Y, Abumi K, Ito M, et al. Minimum 2-year outcome of cervical laminoplasty with deep extensor muscle-preserving approach: impact on cervical spine function and quality of life. Eur Spine J 2009;18:663–71.
40. Kim P, Murata H, Kurokawa R, et al. Myoarchitectonic spinolaminoplasty: efficacy in reconstituting the cervical musculature and preserving biomechanical function. J Neurosurg Spine 2007;7:293–304.
41. Takayasu M, Takagi T, Nishizawa T, et al. Bilateral open-door cervical expansive laminoplasty with hydroxyapatite spacers and titanium screws. J Neurosurg 2002;96(1 Suppl):22–8.
42. Ono A, Yokoyama T, Numasawa T, et al. Dural damage due to a loosened hydroxyapatite intraspinous spacer after spinous process-splitting laminoplasty. Report of two cases. J Neurosurg Spine 2007;7:230–5.
43. Kanemura A, Doita M, Iguchi T, et al. Delayed dural laceration by hydroxyapatite spacer causing tetraparesis following double-door laminoplasty. J Neurosurg Spine 2008;8:121–8.
44. Kaito T, Hosono N, Makino T, et al. Postoperative displacement of hydroxyapatite spacers implanted during double-door laminoplasty. J Neurosurg Spine 2009;10:551–6.
45. Tani S, Suetsuna F, Mizuno J, et al. New titanium spacer for cervical laminoplasty: initial clinical experience. Technical note. Neurol Med Chir (Tokyo) 2010;50:1132–6.
46. Nagashima H, Yuge K, Taniyama R, et al. Stress distribution and construct stability in an experimental cervical open-door laminoplasty model–three-dimensional finite element analysis. Spinal Surg 2013;27:139–44 [in Japanese].

Significant Predictors of Outcome Following Surgery for the Treatment of Degenerative Cervical Myelopathy

A Systematic Review of the Literature

Lindsay Tetreault, PhD[a,b,*], Lisa M. Palubiski, MSc[b], Michael Kryshtalskyj[c], Randy K. Idler, MSc[b], Allan R. Martin, MD, PhD[a,c], Mario Ganau, MD, PhD, FACS[a], Jefferson R. Wilson, MD, PhD[d], Mark Kotter, MD, MPhil, PhD[e], Michael G. Fehlings, MD, PhD, FRCSC[a,c]

KEYWORDS

• Degenerative cervical myelopathy • Prediction • Surgery • Outcomes • Clinical predictors

KEY POINTS

- Several high-quality prospective studies have emerged that have evaluated important clinical predictors of surgical outcomes in patients with degenerative cervical myelopathy.
- Based on this review, patients with a longer duration of symptoms and more severe preoperative myelopathy are likely to have worse surgical outcomes.
- Similar to the review published by Tetreault and colleagues (2015), there is little consensus in the literature as to whether age is a significant predictor of surgical outcome.
- Smoking status and presence of comorbidities may be significant predictors of outcome.

INTRODUCTION

Degenerative cervical myelopathy (DCM) is a progressive, degenerative spine condition and the most common cause of spinal cord impairment worldwide.[1] The natural history of this disease dictates that 20% to 60% of patients with symptoms of myelopathy will deteriorate over time if not managed surgically.[2] The anatomic goals of surgical intervention include removing the compressive pathology, increasing the space available for the spinal cord, and stabilizing the vertebral column. These structural changes help to prevent further neurologic decline and often translate to improvements in functional impairment, disability, and quality of life.

A recent systematic review of the literature was conducted to synthesize the current evidence on outcomes following surgery. The key result from this review was that surgical intervention results in significant improvements in (modified) Japanese

Disclosure: The authors have no conflicts of interest to disclose.
[a] Department of Neurosurgery, Toronto Western Hospital, Toronto, ON, Canada; [b] Graduate Entry Medicine, University College Cork, Cork, Ireland; [c] University of Toronto, Toronto, ON, Canada; [d] Department of Neurosurgery, St. Michael's Hospital, Toronto, ON, Canada; [e] Cambridge University, Cambridge, UK
* Corresponding author. Department of Neurosurgery, Toronto Western Hospital, Toronto, ON, Canada.
E-mail address: lindsay.tetreault89@gmail.com

Neurosurg Clin N Am 29 (2018) 115–127
https://doi.org/10.1016/j.nec.2017.09.020
1042-3680/18/© 2017 Elsevier Inc. All rights reserved.

Orthopedic Association (mJOA) scores in the short, medium, and long term. Furthermore, the extent of these improvements can be predicted by preoperative disease and patient characteristics; specifically, there is low evidence that the odds of achieving an mJOA score of 16 or greater are associated with duration of symptoms and myelopathy severity.

Several other factors may be relevant in assessing a patient's likely outcome, including age, symptomatology, neurologic signs, comorbidities, and imaging features. In 2012, Tetreault and colleagues[3] summarized results from studies discussing important clinical predictors of surgical outcome; this review indicated that a longer duration of symptoms and more severe myelopathy are associated with worse scores on the mJOA or JOA. However, several high-quality prognostic studies have emerged since this publication that may influence these conclusions and add to our understanding of outcome prediction. It was therefore the objective of this study to update the systematic review of the literature conducted by Tetreault and colleagues[3] and address the following key question: In patients with DCM, what are the most important clinical predictors of surgical outcome?

METHODS

Eligibility Criteria

A "PPO" table was constructed to outline the target patient population, prognostic variables of interest, and outcome (**Table 1**).

Patient population

This article targeted studies involving adult patients (>18 years) with cervical myelopathy secondary to spondylosis (cervical spondylotic myelopathy [CSM]), disk herniation, ossification of the posterior longitudinal ligament (OPLL), congenital stenosis, and/or subluxation. All patients were treated surgically and followed postoperatively. Studies were excluded if they included patients with traumatic spinal cord injury, thoracic or lumbar myelopathy, tumor, infection, radiculopathy, or other nondegenerative forms of myelopathy.

Prognostic variables

This article focused on studies that evaluated the predictive value of various clinical factors, such as age, duration of symptoms, preoperative myelopathy severity, and gender.

Outcomes

Outcome was evaluated using measures of functional impairment, disability, and health-related quality of life, including the mJOA, Nurick score, 30-m timed walking test, Neck Disability Index (NDI), and Short Form-36 (SF-36).

Study Characteristics

This article focused on studies that used multivariate analyses to evaluate the association between various clinical factors and surgical outcome. The following types of studies were excluded from each review: review articles, letters, editorials, commentaries, meeting abstracts, and books; those with fewer than 15 patients; and animal or biomechanical studies.

Information Sources

A systematic search of MEDLINE, MEDLINE in Process, EMBASE, and/or Cochrane Central Register of Controlled Trials was conducted to identify relevant studies.

Search Strategy

We developed a search strategy with a librarian who specializes in neuroscience research. The strategy was first developed in MEDLINE and then appropriately modified for the other databases. It was reviewed thoroughly by 2 researchers to ensure accuracy and to confirm that all disease-related synonyms were included. We used the following search terms to search all databases: Cervical Myelopathy AND Surgery or Postoperative AND Prediction/Prognosis AND observational studies.

Only studies on humans and written in English were considered for inclusion, with no other limits applied.

Data Extraction and Synthesis

The following data were extracted from each included article: study design; patient sample and characteristics, including diagnosis and treatment administered; clinical and nonclinical factors evaluated; outcome assessment tool; and results of association, including odds ratios (ORs), confidence intervals (CIs), and *P* values.

Risk of Bias in Individual Studies

The class of evidence for each article was rated (Class I, II, III, IV) using criteria outlined by the *Journal of Bone and Joint Surgery* for prognostic studies and modified to encompass both methodological quality and risk of bias. Prognostic studies included in this article were all cohort studies and were assessed based on whether patients were at a similar time point in their disease/treatment, the rate of follow-up, and whether the analysis controlled for important confounders.

Table 1
Inclusion and exclusion criteria

	Inclusion Criteria	Exclusion Criteria
Patient population	• Age ≥18 • Cervical myelopathy secondary to spondylosis, disk herniation, ossification of the posterior longitudinal ligament, congenital stenosis, subluxation and/or deformity • Treated surgically • Follow-up postoperatively	• Patients with traumatic spinal cord injury, thoracic or lumbar myelopathy, tumor, infection, radiculopathy or other nondegenerative forms of myelopathy • Patients treated nonoperatively
Prognostic variables	• Age • Duration of symptoms • Baseline severity score • Neurologic signs • Symptomatology • Comorbidities • Smoking status • Drug and alcohol use • Medications • Gender • Race • Disease progression • Onset of disease	• Imaging factors • Surgical factors
Outcomes	• Functional outcomes ([modified] Japanese Orthopedic Association score, Nurick score, 30-m walking test, 10-s step test) • Disability outcomes (Neck Disability Index) • Health-related quality of life (Short Form-36)	• Patient satisfaction • Independent walking • Subjective neurologic status

Reporting

The systematic reviews were formatted based on the Preferred Reporting Items for Systematic Reviews and Meta-Analyses statement.

RESULTS

Study Selection

The initial electronic search yielded a total of 1677 citations. An updated search identified an additional 2532 citations published from 2011 to May 2017. After initial review of abstracts and titles, 2367 articles were excluded because (1) they studied patients without degenerative myelopathy; (2) they were not prognostic studies; (3) patients were not treated surgically or there was no follow-up; (4) only the predictive value of imaging factors was assessed; (5) there was no distinction between patients with cervical myelopathy and those with cervical radiculopathy; and/or (6) they were not in English. After full-text review, 98 studies were further excluded because they did not meet our inclusion criteria. A total of 67 studies conducted a multivariate analysis to evaluate the predictive value of various clinical factors.

Study Characteristics

We identified 67 studies (24 prospective, 43 retrospective) discussing significant clinical predictors of surgical outcome. Sample sizes ranged from 20 to 743 surgical patients. All patients were diagnosed with some form of DCM, with most presenting with either CSM or OPLL. Fifty-eight studies assessed age as a predictor, 52 evaluated preoperative myelopathy severity, and 45 reported on duration of symptoms. Various outcome measures were used across the studies, with the mJOA/JOA score or recovery rate reported the most frequently ($n = 53$), followed by the Nurick grade ($n = 17$).

Risk of Bias

We critically appraised the 67 studies that conducted a multivariate analysis. Of these, 13 were classified as level I, 19 as level II, and 35 as level

III. Most studies were level III evidence because they were retrospective cohort studies with unreported follow-up rates or follow-up rates less than 80%. The 11 prospective studies did not have a complete follow-up (<80%) and were downgraded from level I to level II evidence. In each study, patients were at similar points in the course of their disease or treatment and were followed long enough for outcomes to occur. In addition, all analyses accounted for other prognostic factors.

Are There Clinical Factors That Can Predict Surgical Outcome?

The results from the 67 studies included in our review are summarized in Appendices 1 and 2.

Age

Two studies aimed to directly identify whether age was an independent predictor of outcome.[4,5] In the study by Nakashima and colleagues,[4] "elderly" patients (≥65 years) exhibited worse outcomes on the mJOA and Nurick scores compared with "younger" patients (<65 years), even following adjustment for relevant confounders. In contrast, age was not significantly associated with NDI, SF-36 Physical Component Score (PCS), or SF-36 Mental Component Score (MCS). A second study by Son and colleagues[5] demonstrated no significant differences in JOA recovery rate or final JOA scores between patients aged ≥65 years versus younger than 65 years.

Modified Japanese Orthopedic Association or Japanese Orthopedic Association recovery rate Several studies evaluated the association between mJOA or JOA recovery rate and age. Recovery rate was calculated using the following equation developed by Hirabayashi and colleagues[6] (postoperative mJOA/JOA − preoperative mJOA/JOA)/(18/17 − preoperative mJOA/JOA) × 100%.

Thirteen studies established cutoffs for JOA recovery rate to distinguish between "excellent" or "good" and "fair" or "poor" outcomes: (1) greater than 50%, less than 50%[7–18]; (2) greater than 75%, less than 75%[19]; and (3) greater than 20%, less than 20%.[20] A fourteenth study by Chen and colleagues[21] defined 4 groups based on the JOA recovery rate: "excellent" as ≥75%, "good" as 50% to 74%, "fair" as 25% to 49%, and "poor" as less than 25%. Four studies reported that older age is significantly associated with a reduced likelihood of achieving a JOA recovery rate greater than 50%.[9–11,14] A fifth study by Kim and colleagues[17] demonstrated that the interaction between diabetes and old age increases a patient's risk of a poor surgical outcome (OR 2.21, 95% CI 1.15–4.23, $P = .04$).

Seven other studies did not identify a significant relationship between categories of JOA recovery rate and age.[7,8,13,15,16,19,21]

Modified Japanese Orthopedic Association or Japanese Orthopedic Association scores Eight studies reported that older patients have a less favorable surgical outcome based on either the mJOA or JOA recovery rate.[12,18,22–27] Of these, 4 developed regression equations relating a combination of significant clinical and imaging variables to recovery rate; all included age as an important predictor of outcome.[22–25] In contrast, 10 studies failed to identify a significant association between age and JOA recovery rate.[28–37] In the study by Koyanagi and colleagues,[34] patients were divided into 3 groups depending on whether their primary diagnosis was CSM, OPLL, or cervical disk herniation (CDH). Based on univariate analysis, age was significantly correlated with JOA recovery rate in patients with OPLL and CDH but not in patients with CSM; however, in multivariate analysis, age was deemed an insignificant predictor of recovery rate in all 3 forms of DCM. Furthermore, Yeh and colleagues[37] identified a significant correlation between age and recovery rate ($r = -0.25$, $P<.05$) in univariate but not multivariate analysis.

Twelve studies used postoperative or change in mJOA or JOA as the primary outcome measure. Of these, 8 reported an insignificant association between age and surgical outcome.[25,30,33,38–42] In contrast, studies by Su and colleagues,[43] Furlan and colleagues,[44] and Floeth and colleagues[45] identified age as a significant predictor of either postoperative JOA or mJOA or change in JOA scores. Furthermore, age was included as a predictor in a regression model constructed by Morio and colleagues[24] using a continuous JOA score as the outcome variable.

Three additional studies by Tetreault and colleagues[46–48] identified that older patients have a decreased likelihood of achieving a score ≥16 or a minimum clinically important difference (MCID) on the mJOA.

Nurick score Several studies used Nurick as an outcome measure: (1) change in Nurick ≥1 versus less than 1; (2) change in Nurick; and/or (3) "cure" defined as a score of 0 (or 1). Of these, 3 studies identified an association between age and surgical outcomes.[44,49,50] In the study by Vedantam and colleagues,[49] age ≤40 years was the only significant independent predictor of a Nurick grade change ≥1 (OR 3.1, $P = .03$); age, however, was not predictive of a "cure" (ie, a Nurick grade of

0 or 1). This association was also identified by Suri and colleagues[50]: patients in the younger than 40 age group were 2.17 times more likely to exhibit improvement on the Nurick than patients aged 40 to 60 years ($P<.001$). Finally, a third study by Furlan and colleagues[44] confirmed a significant association between Nurick score at 1 year and age ($P = .015$). In contrast, 7 studies reported age as an insignificant predictor of outcome.[51–57]

Other Single studies reported a nonsignificant association between age and the Oswestry Disability Index (ODI),[58] the lower limb component of the Japanese Orthopedic Association Cervical Myelopathy Evaluation Questionnaire (JOACMEQ-L),[10] and the Berg Balance Scale.[44] Age was identified as a significant predictor of NDI, SF-36 PCS, and recovery rate on the Neurosurgical Cervical Spine Scale (NCSS) by single studies.[59–61]

Preoperative myelopathy severity

Modified Japanese Orthopedic Association or Japanese Orthopedic Association recovery rate Twelve studies defined cutoffs for JOA recovery rate: (1) greater than 50%, less than 50%; (2) greater than 20%, less than 20%; (3) greater than 75%, less than 75%; and (4) ≥75%, 50% to 74%, 25% to 49% and less than 25%. Of these, 9 failed to identify an association between JOA recovery rate and preoperative myelopathy severity.[7,10,11,13,14,16,17,20,21] In contrast, in a study by Gao and colleagues,[8] patients with a preoperative JOA score ≤9 were 4.84 times more likely to exhibit a "fair" recovery rate (<50%) than those with a preoperative JOA score greater than 9 ($P = .003$). Similarly, studies by Shin and colleagues[19] and Naruse and colleagues[15] reported that a lower preoperative JOA score was associated with decreased odds of recovering greater than 75% (OR 1.34, $P = .036$) or ≥50% (OR 1.64, $P = .0019$) on the JOA score, respectively.

Eighteen studies discussed the association between JOA or mJOA recovery rate and preoperative myelopathy severity. Six studies demonstrated that patients with milder myelopathy experience a higher JOA or mJOA recovery rate than those with more severe disease.[22,23,25,27,30,36] Two studies, by Kim and colleagues[29] and Sun and colleagues,[62] identified a significant association between preoperative JOA and recovery rate in univariate but not multivariate analysis. A study by Yeh and colleagues[37] indicated that preoperative Nurick scores and sensory function in the upper extremities section of the JOA score are strong predictors of JOA recovery rate. In contrast, 9 studies reported no association between preoperative myelopathy severity and JOA or mJOA recovery rate.[18,24,26,28,31–35]

Results were significantly different when the primary outcome was postoperative or change in mJOA or JOA scores instead of recovery rate. All 10 studies reported a significant association between preoperative myelopathy severity and surgical outcomes.[24,25,30,33,38–40,42,44,63]

Two studies by Tetreault and colleagues[47,48] indicated that patients with a higher preoperative mJOA score were more likely to achieve a score ≥16 or ≥12 on the mJOA. A third study by Tetreault and colleagues[46] reported no association between preoperative myelopathy severity and exhibiting an MCID on the mJOA between preoperative and postoperative visits.

Nurick Nine studies evaluated the association between preoperative myelopathy severity and surgical outcomes as evaluated by the Nurick classification system. In the studies by Kusin and colleagues,[51,53] preoperative Nurick score was significantly predictive of change in Nurick score. Furlan and colleagues[44] also identified that patients with a lower and milder Nurick score have a better surgical outcome.

Studies by Pumberger and colleagues,[54] Vedantam and colleagues,[49] and Rajshekhar and Kumar[57] evaluated important predictors of Nurick improvement as well as achieving a "cure," defined as a postoperative Nurick score of 0 (or 1). In general, Pumberger and colleagues[54] reported that patients with a lower Nurick grade are significantly more likely to achieve a postoperative Nurick grade of 0, ≤1, or ≤2 than those with a Nurick grade of 4. Vedantam and colleagues[49] indicated that preoperative Nurick scores are significantly associated with achieving a "cure" (OR 0.23, $P<.001$) but not with improving by ≥1 grade (OR 1.4, $P = .10$). Finally, patients with a preoperative Nurick score of 4 were 8.6 more likely to be "cured" than those with a score of 5.[57] Preoperative severity score, however, was not a significant predictor of "improvement" on the Nurick. A fourth study by Sarkar and colleagues[64] indicated that patients with a preoperative Nurick grade of 1 or 2 are 4.14 times more likely to improve by ≥1 point than patients with a preoperative Nurick grade of 3, 4, or 5.

Two studies indicated no association between preoperative Nurick score and surgical outcomes.[55,56]

Other Single studies reported significant associations between preoperative and postoperative ODI,[58] SF-36 PCS,[60] NDI[60] and Berg Balance Scale.[44] In a study by Wilson and colleagues,[59] postoperative NDI was significantly related to preoperative NDI but not to preoperative mJOA. Finally, single studies reported that preoperative myelopathy severity was not predictive of NCSS recovery[61] rate or JOACMEQ-L.[10]

Duration of symptoms

Modified Japanese Orthopedic Association or Japanese Orthopedic Association recovery rate Twelve studies defined cutoffs for JOA recovery rate: (1) greater than 50%, less than 50%; (2) greater than 20%, less than 20%; and (3) ≥75%, 50% to 74%, 25% to 49%, and less than 25%. Five studies identified duration of symptoms as an important predictor of outcome; specifically, patients with a longer duration of symptoms were less likely to achieve a JOA recovery rate of greater than 50%.[8–10,13,14] In a sixth study, by Yamazaki and colleagues,[16] duration of symptoms was a significant predictor of an "excellent" recovery (≥50%) in patients aged ≥65 years, but not in those younger than 65 years. Two additional studies identified an association between duration of symptoms and outcomes in univariate but not multivariate analysis.[12,21]

Twelve studies evaluated the relationship between duration of symptoms and JOA or mJOA recovery rate. Of these, 9 identified duration of symptoms as a significant predictor of outcome,[22–24,26,30–32,34,35] whereas 4 failed to identify a significant association.[25,27,36,62]

Nine studies reported the association between postoperative or change in mJOA or JOA scores and duration of symptoms. Of these, 3 included duration of symptoms in a clinical prediction model.[24,30,40] Two additional studies identified that a longer duration of symptoms was associated with worse improvements in JOA scores at 12 months in univariate but not multivariate analysis.[41,45] Four studies indicated that duration of symptoms is an insignificant predictor of outcome as evaluated by change in mJOA, mJOA or JOA scores.[25,31,38,44]

Three additional studies by Tetreault and colleagues[46–48] identified that patients with a longer duration of symptoms have a decreased likelihood of achieving a score ≥16, ≥12, or an MCID on the mJOA.

Nurick Eight studies evaluated the association between Nurick score and duration of symptoms. In a study by Pumberger and colleagues,[54] patients with a longer duration of symptoms have reduced odds of recovering to a Nurick grade of 2 or less (OR 0.96, P = .004), 1 or less (OR 0.97, P = .004). or to a score of 0 (OR 0.97, P = .035). Rajshekhar and Kumar[57] reported that patients with a duration of symptoms ≤12 months were 4.8 times more likely to improve and 14.0 times more likely to be "cured" following surgery than patients with a duration of symptoms longer than 12 months. In addition, according to Suri and colleagues[50] and Kusin and colleagues,[52] patients with a longer duration of symptoms were less likely to exhibit improvement on the Nurick. Four studies identified no relationship between duration of symptoms and Nurick outcome.[44,49,53,56]

Other Single studies reported a significant association between duration of symptoms and ODI[58] and NCSS recovery rate.[61] Furlan and colleagues[44] identified that duration of symptoms is not predictive of outcome using the Berg Balance Scale.

Smoking status

Twelve studies evaluated the predictive value of smoking status. Variations of outcomes included JOA recovery rate, improvement on the Nurick, a postoperative mJOA ≥16 or ≥12, NDI, and SF-36 PCS.[8,9,28,37,46–48,51–53,59,60]

The study by Kusin and colleagues[53] aimed to determine whether tobacco use attenuates benefits of early decompressive surgery. Based on their results, tobacco use was significantly associated with smaller improvements in Nurick score, whether categorized by pack-years (OR 0.91, P<.0001) or packs per day (OR 0.60, P<.0001). An earlier study by Kusin and colleagues[52] identified a significant negative correlation between pack-years, packs per day, and improvements in Nurick scores.

Results from the AOSpine North America and International studies have also identified smoking status as an important predictor of outcome. In studies by Tetreault and colleagues,[46–48] patients who smoked were less likely to achieve a score ≥16 on the mJOA (ref = nonsmoking: relative risk [RR] 0.78, P = .0056; OR 0.46, P = .043) or an MCID on this scale (ref = nonsmoking: RR 0.84, P = .0043). In a subanalysis of patients with severe myelopathy (mJOA <12), smoking status was not predictive of a mJOA score ≥12 at 1-year follow-up.[48] Finally, in the study by Wilson and colleagues,[59] smoking status was a significant predictor of NDI.

Four other studies indicated no relationship between smoking status and surgical outcomes as evaluated by JOA recovery rate.[8,9,28,37] The study by Oichi and colleagues[60] did not report their results of association between smoking status and outcomes.

Comorbidities

Several studies have evaluated the impact of a patient's preoperative health status on surgical outcomes; unfortunately, the lack of standardization of comorbidity definitions prevents the synthesis of the evidence.

A study by Oichi and colleagues[60] investigated the predictive validity of the Charlson Comorbidity Index (CCI) and the Self-administered Comorbidity Questionnaire (SCQ), both of which incorporate the relative severities of several preexisting conditions. Based on their results, a lower SCQ was associated with greater postoperative SF-36 PCS ($P<.05$) and NDI ($P<.001$) scores; back pain was the most relevant component of this comorbidity scoring system. In contrast, CCI was not associated with either the SF-36 PCS or NDI.

According to Furlan and colleagues,[44] the number of *International Classification of Diseases, Ninth Revision* (ICD-9) codes was a significant predictor of mJOA at 1-year follow-up; this variable, however, was not associated with the Nurick or Berg Balance Scales. CCI was also not a significant predictor of outcome in this study. Tetreault and colleagues[46,48] developed a comorbidity scoring system that incorporates both number and severity of preexisting disease; this score was associated with achieving an mJOA ≥16 (RR 0.93, $P = .0067$) as well as an MCID on the mJOA (RR 0.97, $P = .035$ on univariate analysis; not significant on multivariate analysis).

Single studies identified no association between hypertension, hyperlipidemia, and coronary artery disease and JOA recovery rate.[9,37] Furthermore, studies by Tetreault and colleagues[46–48] indicated that respiratory, gastrointestinal, renal, neurologic, endocrine, and rheumatologic disease are not important predictors of achieving an mJOA ≥16, mJOA ≥12, or an MCID on the mJOA.

Diabetes Fourteen studies evaluated the association between diabetes and postoperative outcomes using a variety of assessment tools: JOA or mJOA scores, Nurick classification, NDI, and SF-36.[7,9,11,13,14,17,28,37,51–53,56,65,66]

Five studies reported a significant relationship between diabetes and outcomes. In the study by Machino and colleagues,[9] HbA1c levels (ref ≥6.5%: OR 2.82, $P = .044$) and duration of diabetes (ref ≥10 years: OR 2.24, $P = .041$) were predictive of achieving a JOA recovery rate ≥50%, but fasting blood glucose levels were not (ref ≥150 mg/dL: OR 0.85, $P = .68$). Kim and colleagues[17] determined that patients with diabetes were 2.92 times more likely to have an unfavorable outcome (JOA recovery rate <50%) than those without; the OR of this association increased to 4.01 if the patient also smoked. Three additional studies confirmed an association between improvement in Nurick score and diabetes.[51,53,56] Furthermore, in a subanalysis, Kusin and colleagues[51] identified a strong correlation between average perioperative glucose levels and decreasing improvements on Nurick scores.

The other 9 studies failed to identify a relationship between diabetes and surgical outcomes.[7,11,13,14,28,37,52,65,66]

Psychiatric comorbidities Six studies evaluated the impact of depression and other psychiatric disorders on surgical outcomes.[37,46–48,67,68] In the AOSpine studies, among North American patients, the presence of depression or bipolar disorders was significantly associated with decreased odds of achieving an mJOA ≥16 (ref = absence: OR 0.33, $P = .0035$) and smaller improvements on the NDI, SF-36 PCS, and SF-36 MCS.[47,67] Interestingly, in an analysis involving patients from international centers, the presence of psychiatric disorders was not a significant predictor of outcome.[48]

In a study by Zong and colleagues,[68] patients with continuous depression had smaller change scores on the mJOA, Visual Analog Scale, and NDI than those classified as having a normal mood. In contrast, there were no significant differences between these groups with respect to the Beck Depression Inventory score. Finally, although significant in univariate analysis, depression was not associated with JOA recovery rate in a multivariate analysis by Yeh and colleagues.[37]

Gender

Twenty-eight studies evaluated the impact of gender on a variety of outcome measures, including JOA recovery rate,[8–11,13–15,18–20,28,37,62] mJOA recovery rate,[25] postoperative or change in mJOA or JOA scores,[25,39,42–44,46–48] Nurick grade,[44,51–56] NDI,[59,60] SF-36 PCS,[60] Berg Balance Scale,[44] and JOACMEQ-L.[10]

Of these, only 3 reported a significant association between gender and surgical outcomes.[10,59,60] Specifically, in the study by Nakashima and colleagues,[10] men were more likely to achieve improvements on JOA scores (significant in univariate but not multivariate analysis) and an "effective" rating on the JOACMEQ-L (ref = female: hazard ratio 3.78, $P = .019$). In contrast, Wilson and colleagues[59] determined that female gender was associated with increased neck disability at follow-up. Finally, although the study by Oichi and colleagues[60] identified gender as an important predictor of SF-36 PCS, it did not specify whether men or women have superior outcomes.

Signs and symptoms

Six studies discussed the predictive value of various signs and symptoms.[22,46–48,54,63] In a univariate analysis conducted by Pumberger and colleagues,[54] there were no significant differences in the frequency of radiculopathy or neck pain between the "improvement" (improvement on Nurick by ≥1 grade) and "nonimprovement" groups.

Tetreault and colleagues[46–48] evaluated important predictors of achieving an MCID or a score ≥16 or ≥12 on the mJOA. In univariate analysis, patients were less likely to exhibit (1) an MCID on the mJOA if they had upgoing plantar responses, lower limb spasticity, or broad-based unstable gait[46]; (2) an mJOA score ≥16 if they had clumsy hands, impaired gait, bilateral arm paresthesia, general weakness, corticospinal motor deficits, hyperreflexia, upgoing plantar responses, or lower limb spasticity[47,48]; and (3) an mJOA score ≥12 if they had hyperreflexia or lower limb spasticity.[48] In multivariate analysis, the significant predictors of outcome were impaired gait (mJOA ≥16), lower limb spasticity (mJOA ≥12), and broad-based unstable gait (change in mJOA ≥ MCID).

In a fifth study, by Zhang and colleagues,[22] a positive Babinski sign was significantly correlated with JOA recovery rate and was included in the final regression equation. Finally, Chiles and colleagues[63] reported that hand wasting was predictive of postoperative and change in mJOA scores but spastic gait was not associated with either.

Diagnosis

Seven studies evaluated whether type of myelopathy was predictive of surgical outcome.[19,43,54,57,61,63,69] Of these, 5 compared patients with and without OPLL (ie, with other forms of DCM),[19,43,54,57,69] 1 assessed NCSS recovery rates in patients with OPLL, CSM, or CDH,[61] and a final study evaluated differences in outcome between patients with CSM and those with soft disk herniation.[63]

According to Rajshekhar and Kumar,[57] patients with CSM were 5.3 times more likely to exhibit improvement on the Nurick score than those with myelopathy secondary to OPLL ($P = .02$). There was, however, no significant association between disease diagnosis (CSM or OPLL) and achieving a "cure" or a score of 0 or 1 on the Nurick. In contrast, 4 studies reported that OPLL was not a significant predictor of surgical outcomes.[19,43,54,69] In the study by Park and colleagues,[61] NCSS recovery rates were not significantly different among patients with OPLL, CSM, and CDH. Finally, patients with soft disk herniation had a better postoperative mJOA and change in mJOA than patients diagnosed with CSM.[63]

Body mass index

Six studies assessed the predictive value of body mass index using a variety of outcome measures: JOA recovery rate,[9,13,14,28] Nurick,[54] and NDI.[59] Of these, 5 reported that body mass index is not significantly associated with surgical outcomes.[9,13,14,28,54] In a fifth study, by Wilson and colleagues,[59] NDI scores at 1-year were, on average, 4.5 points higher for overweight patients and 5.7 points higher for obese patients compared with patients of normal weight. Furthermore, the odds of achieving the MCID for the NDI were significantly reduced (ref = normal weight: OR 0.5) in obese patients. This study failed to identify an association between body mass index and SF-36 PCS, SF-36 MCS, and mJOA.

Others

Two studies by Floeth and colleagues[41,45] identified that preoperative deterioration during the 3 months leading up to study enrollment (acute or progressive myelopathy) was significantly correlated with a favorable outcome in univariate but not multivariate analysis.

A single study by Sadhu and Ahn[70] identified a significant negative correlation between cocaine use and improvement on the Nurick grade ($r = -0.45$, $P = .044$). Three studies by Kusin and colleagues[51–53] also included cocaine use in their multiple regression analysis; however, specific associations between this variable and outcome were not recorded.

Single studies identified no association between surgical outcomes and anticoagulant or antiplatelet use,[9] race,[71] and American Society of Anesthesiologists Physical Status.[20]

DISCUSSION

This systematic review aimed to synthesize existing evidence related to important predictors of surgical outcome. This knowledge is valuable in a clinical setting and can be used to facilitate shared decision making, appropriately manage patients' expectations, and counsel concerned patients as to potential treatment options.

Based on this review, patients with a longer duration of symptoms are likely to have worse surgical outcomes. The rationale behind this finding is that patients with a longer disease duration may experience irreversible damage due to the pathophysiological events that accompany mechanical compression of the spinal cord. Specifically, chronic cord compression results in ischemia, disruption of the blood spinal cord barrier, neuroinflammation, and apoptosis of the neurons and oligodendrocytes; these changes ultimately cause demyelination, axonal degeneration of the corticospinal tracts, scarring, and cavitation.[2,72] Furthermore, a longer duration of compression and period of hypoxia may amplify the ischemia reperfusion injury that results from restoration of tissue blood flow after long periods of ischemia.[73] Further research is required to (1) define the threshold duration of symptoms beyond which there is a negative impact on outcome; and (2) evaluate whether there is an interaction between preoperative myelopathy severity and duration of symptoms when assessing surgical outcomes.

This review also identified preoperative myelopathy severity score as an important predictor of outcome. This association, however, was dependent on the type of assessment tool used to evaluate outcome. For example, most studies failed to identify a relationship between preoperative JOA score and JOA recovery rate; this is likely because the equation for recovery rate already incorporates a patient's preoperative JOA score. Similarly, Tetreault and colleagues[46] reported an insignificant association between preoperative mJOA and the likelihood of achieving an MCID on the mJOA; however, this study defined different values for the MCID based on preoperative myelopathy severity (MCID = 1 for mild patients [mJOA = 15–17]; MCID = 2 for moderate patients [mJOA = 12–14]; and MCID = 3 for severe patients). In contrast, most studies using JOA, Nurick, or mJOA as the primary outcome measure identified preoperative myelopathy severity as an important predictor of outcome.

Similar to the review published by Tetreault and colleagues,[3] there is little consensus in the literature as to whether age is a significant predictor of surgical outcome. Although most surgeons will not discriminate on the basis of age, they should be aware that the elderly may not be able to translate neurologic improvement to functional recovery as well as their younger patients. Potential explanations for this discrepancy include (1) the elderly experience age-related changes in their spinal cord, including a decrease in γ-motor neurons, number of anterior horn cells, and number of myelinated fibers in the corticospinal tracts and posterior funiculus; (2) because DCM is a progressive disease, older patients are likely to have more substantial degenerative pathology and may require a more complex surgery; (3) older patients have reduced physiologic reserves and are more likely to have unassociated comorbidities that may affect outcome; and (4) the elderly may not be able to conduct all activities on a certain functional scale because of these comorbidities (eg, walking time may be affected by osteoarthritis).[40,74–77] Despite differences in functional recovery, Nakashima and colleagues[4] indicated that there were no significant differences between an elderly ($\geq$65 years) and younger (<65 years) group with respect to disability and quality-of-life outcomes. When managing elderly patients, we recommend that surgeons consider a patient's physiologic age instead, evaluate all potential comorbidities, and develop treatment strategies on a case-to-case basis.

In this review, a number of studies identified smoking as an important predictor of surgical outcome. In previous clinical studies, smoking has been associated with poor wound healing, decreased bone density, impaired fracture healing, prolonged ventilation time, and increased rates of pseudoarthrosis and perioperative complications.[47,52,78–81] Preclinically, using animal models, nicotine treatment resulted in necrosis and hyalinization of the nucleus pulposus; stenosis of and a decreased number of vascular bulbs; and enlargement of vascular endothelial cells.[82] Furthermore, smoking can increase the permeability of the blood spinal cord barrier, aggravate edema, decrease glutathione levels, and ultimately reinforce oxidative damage.[2,52,53,83,84] These changes, along with the fact that nicotine is a potent vasoconstrictor, can amplify the hypoxic conditions caused by cord compression. Finally, nicotine may worsen the severity of the ischemia reperfusion injury, resulting in suboptimal outcomes.[85–88] Based on the existing evidence, it is unclear whether outcomes improve following smoking cessation; future research should investigate this question.

The 2 most common comorbidities discussed in the literature are diabetes and psychiatric disorders. There is a lack of consensus as to whether diabetes is an important predictor of surgical outcomes. Diabetic patients may exhibit abnormalities in their spinal cord and peripheral nerves, such as infarcts, demyelination, atrophy, and softening of the posterior columns.[89] Furthermore, diabetes may induce a state of chronic inflammation, impair angiogenesis, and amplify the hypoxic conditions due to associated microvascular and macrovascular disease.[90] Complications associated with diabetes, especially peripheral neuropathy, may impair a patient's postoperative neurologic recovery and functional improvement. Several studies identified depression or other psychiatric disorders as important predictors of outcome. These results corroborate the findings from studies in the lumbar spine, which demonstrated that patients with depression are less likely to return to work, report improvements in pain and functional status or achieve an MCID on the EUroQoL 5-dimensions quality-adjusted life-years index.[67]

Further studies are required to deduce the association between surgical outcomes and body mass index, signs and symptoms, diagnosis, and preoperative deterioration.

Limitations

The current body of evidence has substantially improved since the systematic review published by Tetreault and colleagues[48] in 2015; specifically, several high-quality prospective studies have emerged discussing important predictors of outcome. The limitations to this review include the following: (1) studies were not separated based on length of follow-up; (2) analyses that dichotomized a predictor might have done it differently; and (3) some of the articles with relevant abstracts or titles were excluded because they were not available or in a language other than English.

SUMMARY

Based on the results of this review, patients with a longer duration of symptoms and more severe myelopathy are likely to have worse surgical outcomes. With respect to age, several studies have indicated that elderly patients are less likely to translate neurologic recovery into functional improvements. However, many other studies have failed to identify a significant association between age and outcomes. Finally, smoking status and presence of comorbidities may be important predictors of outcomes.

REFERENCES

1. Nouri A, Tetreault L, Singh A, et al. Degenerative cervical myelopathy: epidemiology, genetics, and pathogenesis. Spine (Phila Pa 1976) 2015;40(12): E675–93.
2. Karadimas SK, Erwin WM, Ely CG, et al. Pathophysiology and natural history of cervical spondylotic myelopathy. Spine 2013;38(22 Suppl 1):S21–36.
3. Tetreault LA, Karpova A, Fehlings MG. Predictors of outcome in patients with degenerative cervical spondylotic myelopathy undergoing surgical treatment: results of a systematic review. Eur Spine J 2015;24(Suppl 2):236–51.
4. Nakashima H, Tetreault LA, Nagoshi N, et al. Does age affect surgical outcomes in patients with degenerative cervical myelopathy? Results from the prospective multicenter AOSpine International study on 479 patients. J Neurol Neurosurg Psychiatry 2016;87(7):734–40.
5. Son DK, Son DW, Song GS, et al. Effectiveness of the laminoplasty in the elderly patients with cervical spondylotic myelopathy. Korean J Spine 2014;11(2): 39–44.
6. Hirabayashi K, Miyakawa J, Satomi K, et al. Operative results and postoperative progression of ossification among patients with ossification of cervical posterior longitudinal ligament. Spine 1981;6(4): 354–64.
7. Fujimori T, Iwasaki M, Okuda S, et al. Long-term results of cervical myelopathy due to ossification of the posterior longitudinal ligament with an occupying ratio of 60% or more. Spine 2014;39(1):58–67.
8. Gao R, Yang L, Chen H, et al. Long term results of anterior corpectomy and fusion for cervical spondylotic myelopathy. PLoS One 2012;7(4):e34811.
9. Machino M, Yukawa Y, Ito K, et al. Risk factors for poor outcome of cervical laminoplasty for cervical spondylotic myelopathy in patients with diabetes. J Bone Joint Surg Am 2014;96(24):2049–55.
10. Nakashima H, Yukawa Y, Ito K, et al. Prediction of lower limb functional recovery after laminoplasty for cervical myelopathy: focusing on the 10-s step test. Eur Spine J 2012;21(7):1389–95.
11. Oichi T, Oshima Y, Taniguchi Y, et al. Cervical anterolisthesis: a predictor of poor neurological outcomes in cervical spondylotic myelopathy patients after cervical laminoplasty. Spine 2016;41(8): E467–73.
12. Sun LQ, Li M, Li YM. Predictors for surgical outcome of laminoplasty for cervical spondylotic myelopathy. World Neurosurg 2016;94:89–96.
13. Zhang JT, Meng FT, Wang S, et al. Predictors of surgical outcome in cervical spondylotic myelopathy: focusing on the quantitative signal intensity. Eur Spine J 2015;24(12):2941–5.
14. Zhang JT, Wang LF, Wang S, et al. Risk factors for poor outcome of surgery for cervical spondylotic myelopathy. Spinal Cord 2016;54(12):1127–31.
15. Naruse T, Yanase M, Takahashi H, et al. Prediction of clinical results of laminoplasty for cervical myelopathy focusing on spinal cord motion in intraoperative ultrasonography and postoperative magnetic resonance imaging. Spine 2009;34(24):2634–41.
16. Yamazaki T, Yanaka K, Sato H, et al. Cervical spondylotic myelopathy: surgical results and factors affecting outcome with special reference to age differences. Neurosurgery 2003;52(1):122–6 [discussion: 126].
17. Kim HJ, Moon SH, Kim HS, et al. Diabetes and smoking as prognostic factors after cervical laminoplasty. J Bone Joint Surg Br 2008;90(11):1468–72.
18. Chen CJ, Lyu RK, Lee ST, et al. Intramedullary high signal intensity on T2-weighted MR images in cervical spondylotic myelopathy: prediction of prognosis with type of intensity. Radiology 2001;221(3): 789–94.
19. Shin JW, Jin SW, Kim SH, et al. Predictors of outcome in patients with cervical spondylotic myelopathy undergoing unilateral open-door laminoplasty. Korean J Spine 2015;12(4):261–6.
20. Hirai T, Yoshii T, Arai Y, et al. A comparative study of anterior decompression with fusion and posterior

decompression with laminoplasty for the treatment of cervical spondylotic myelopathy patients with large anterior compression of the spinal cord. Clin Spine Surg 2017;17:17.
21. Chen GD, Lu Q, Sun JJ, et al. Effect and prognostic factors of laminoplasty for cervical myelopathy with an occupying ratio greater than 50%. Spine 2016; 41(5):378–83.
22. Zhang YZ, Shen Y, Wang LF, et al. Magnetic resonance T2 image signal intensity ratio and clinical manifestation predict prognosis after surgical intervention for cervical spondylotic myelopathy. Spine 2010;35(10):E396–9.
23. Zhang P, Shen Y, Zhang YZ, et al. Significance of increased signal intensity on MRI in prognosis after surgical intervention for cervical spondylotic myelopathy. J Clin Neurosci 2011;18(8):1080–3.
24. Morio Y, Teshima R, Nagashima H, et al. Correlation between operative outcomes of cervical compression myelopathy and MRI of the spinal cord. Spine 2001;26(11):1238–45.
25. Karpova A, Arun R, Davis AM, et al. Predictors of surgical outcome in cervical spondylotic myelopathy. Spine 2013;38(5):392–400.
26. Fujimura Y, Nishi Y, Chiba K, et al. Multiple regression analysis of the factors influencing the results of expansive open-door laminoplasty for cervical myelopathy due to ossification of the posterior longitudinal ligament. Arch Orthop Trauma Surg 1998; 117(8):471–4.
27. Kato Y, Iwasaki M, Fuji T, et al. Long-term follow-up results of laminectomy for cervical myelopathy caused by ossification of the posterior longitudinal ligament. J Neurosurg 1998;89(2):217–23.
28. Kim B, Yoon DH, Shin HC, et al. Surgical outcome and prognostic factors of anterior decompression and fusion for cervical compressive myelopathy due to ossification of the posterior longitudinal ligament. Spine J 2015;15(5):875–84.
29. Kim TH, Ha Y, Shin JJ, et al. Signal intensity ratio on magnetic resonance imaging as a prognostic factor in patients with cervical compressive myelopathy. Medicine (Baltimore) 2016;95(39):e4649.
30. Zhang P, Shen Y, Zhang YZ, et al. Prognosis significance of focal signal intensity change on MRI after anterior decompression for single-level cervical spondylotic myelopathy. Eur J Orthop Surg Traumatol 2012;22(4):269–73.
31. Uchida K, Nakajima H, Takeura N, et al. Prognostic value of changes in spinal cord signal intensity on magnetic resonance imaging in patients with cervical compressive myelopathy. Spine J 2014;14(8):1601–10.
32. Wada E, Yonenobu K, Suzuki S, et al. Can intramedullary signal change on magnetic resonance imaging predict surgical outcome in cervical spondylotic myelopathy? Spine 1999;24(5):455–61 [discussion: 462].
33. Iwasaki M, Okuda S, Miyauchi A, et al. Surgical strategy for cervical myelopathy due to ossification of the posterior longitudinal ligament: part 1: clinical results and limitations of laminoplasty. Spine 2007; 32(6):647–53.
34. Koyanagi T, Hirabayashi K, Satomi K, et al. Predictability of operative results of cervical compression myelopathy based on preoperative computed tomographic myelography. Spine 1993;18(14): 1958–63.
35. Okada Y, Ikata T, Yamada H, et al. Magnetic resonance imaging study on the results of surgery for cervical compression myelopathy. Spine 1993; 18(14):2024–9.
36. Shin JJ, Jin BH, Kim KS, et al. Intramedullary high signal intensity and neurological status as prognostic factors in cervical spondylotic myelopathy. Acta Neurochir (Wien) 2010;152(10):1687–94.
37. Yeh KT, Yu TC, Chen IH, et al. Expansive open-door laminoplasty secured with titanium miniplates is a good surgical method for multiple-level cervical stenosis. J Orthop Surg Res 2014;9:49.
38. Chibbaro S, Benvenuti L, Carnesecchi S, et al. Anterior cervical corpectomy for cervical spondylotic myelopathy: experience and surgical results in a series of 70 consecutive patients. J Clin Neurosci 2006;13(2):233–8.
39. Iwasaki M, Kawaguchi Y, Kimura T, et al. Long-term results of expansive laminoplasty for ossification of the posterior longitudinal ligament of the cervical spine: more than 10 years follow up. J Neurosurg 2002;96(2 Suppl):180–9.
40. Tanaka J, Seki N, Tokimura F, et al. Operative results of canal-expansive laminoplasty for cervical spondylotic myelopathy in elderly patients. Spine 1999; 24(22):2308–12.
41. Floeth FW, Galldiks N, Eicker S, et al. Hypermetabolism in 18F-FDG PET predicts favorable outcome following decompressive surgery in patients with degenerative cervical myelopathy. J Nucl Med 2013;54(9):1577–83.
42. Uchida K, Nakajima H, Sato R, et al. Multivariate analysis of the neurological outcome of surgery for cervical compressive myelopathy. J Orthop Sci 2005;10(6):564–73.
43. Su N, Fei Q, Wang B, et al. Long-term outcomes and prognostic analysis of modified open-door laminoplasty with lateral mass screw fusion in treatment of cervical spondylotic myelopathy. Ther Clin Risk Manag 2016;12:1329–37.
44. Furlan JC, Kalsi-Ryan S, Kailaya-Vasan A, et al. Functional and clinical outcomes following surgical treatment in patients with cervical spondylotic myelopathy: a prospective study of 81 cases. J Neurosurg Spine 2011;14(3):348–55.
45. Floeth FW, Stoffels G, Herdmann J, et al. Prognostic value of 18F-FDG PET in monosegmental stenosis

and myelopathy of the cervical spinal cord. J Nucl Med 2011;52(9):1385–91.
46. Tetreault L, Wilson JR, Kotter MR, et al. Predicting the minimum clinically important difference in patients undergoing surgery for the treatment of degenerative cervical myelopathy. Neurosurg Focus 2016;40(6):E14.
47. Tetreault LA, Kopjar B, Vaccaro A, et al. A clinical prediction model to determine outcomes in patients with cervical spondylotic myelopathy undergoing surgical treatment: data from the prospective, multi-center AOSpine North America study. J Bone Joint Surg Am 2013;95(18):1659–66.
48. Tetreault L, Kopjar B, Cote P, et al. A clinical prediction rule for functional outcomes in patients undergoing surgery for degenerative cervical myelopathy analysis of an international prospective multicenter data set of 757 subjects. J Bone Joint Surg Am 2015; 97(24):2038–46.
49. Vedantam A, Jonathan A, Rajshekhar V. Association of magnetic resonance imaging signal changes and outcome prediction after surgery for cervical spondylotic myelopathy: clinical article. J Neurosurg Spine 2011;15(6):660–6.
50. Suri A, Chabbra RP, Mehta VS, et al. Effect of intramedullary signal changes on the surgical outcome of patients with cervical spondylotic myelopathy. Spine J 2003;3(1):33–45.
51. Kusin DJ, Ahn UM, Ahn NU. The influence of diabetes on surgical outcomes in cervical myelopathy. Spine 2016;41(18):1436–40.
52. Kusin DJ, Ahn UM, Ahn NU. The effect of smoking on spinal cord healing following surgical treatment of cervical myelopathy. Spine (Phila Pa 1976) 2015;40(18):1391–6.
53. Kusin DJ, Li SQ, Ahn UM, et al. Does tobacco use attenuate benefits of early decompression in patients with cervical myelopathy? Spine 2016;41(20): 1565–9.
54. Pumberger M, Froemel D, Aichmair A, et al. Clinical predictors of surgical outcome in cervical spondylotic myelopathy: an analysis of 248 patients. Bone Joint J 2013;95 B(7):966–71.
55. Salem HM, Salem KM, Burget F, et al. Cervical spondylotic myelopathy: the prediction of outcome following surgical intervention in 93 patients using T1- and T2-weighted MRI scans. Eur Spine J 2015; 24(12):2930–5.
56. Choi S, Lee SH, Lee JY, et al. Factors affecting prognosis of patients who underwent corpectomy and fusion for treatment of cervical ossification of the posterior longitudinal ligament: analysis of 47 patients. J Spinal Disord Tech 2005;18(4): 309–14.
57. Rajshekhar V, Kumar CSS. Functional outcome after central corpectomy in poor-grade patients with cervical spondylotic myelopathy or ossified posterior longitudinal ligament. Neurosurgery 2005;56(6): 1279–84.
58. Hoffman H, Lee SI, Garst JH, et al. Use of multivariate linear regression and support vector regression to predict functional outcome after surgery for cervical spondylotic myelopathy. J Clin Neurosci 2015; 22(9):1444–9.
59. Wilson JR, Tetreault LA, Schroeder G, et al. Impact of elevated body mass index and obesity on long-term surgical outcomes for patients with degenerative cervical myelopathy: analysis of a combined prospective dataset. Spine 2017;42(3):195–201.
60. Oichi T, Oshima Y, Takeshita K, et al. Evaluation of comorbidity indices for a study of patient outcomes following cervical decompression surgery: a retrospective cohort study. Spine 2015;40(24):1941–7.
61. Park YS, Nakase H, Kawaguchi S, et al. Predictors of outcome of surgery for cervical compressive myelopathy: retrospective analysis and prospective study. Neurol Med Chir (Tokyo) 2006;46(5):231–8 [discussion: 238–9].
62. Sun LQ, Li YM, Wang X, et al. Quantitative magnetic resonance imaging analysis correlates with surgical outcome of cervical spondylotic myelopathy. Spinal Cord 2015;53(6):488–93.
63. Chiles BW 3rd, Leonard MA, Choudhri HF, et al. Cervical spondylotic myelopathy: patterns of neurological deficit and recovery after anterior cervical decompression. Neurosurgery 1999;44(4):762–9 [discussion: 769–70].
64. Sarkar S, Turel MK, Jacob KS, et al. The evolution of T2-weighted intramedullary signal changes following ventral decompressive surgery for cervical spondylotic myelopathy: clinical article. J Neurosurg Spine 2014;21(4):538–46.
65. Arnold PM, Fehlings MG, Kopjar B, et al. Mild diabetes is not a contraindication for surgical decompression in cervical spondylotic myelopathy: results of the AOSpine North America multicenter prospective study (CSM). Spine J 2014;14(1):65–72.
66. Dokai T, Nagashima H, Nanjo Y, et al. Surgical outcomes and prognostic factors of cervical spondylotic myelopathy in diabetic patients. Arch Orthop Trauma Surg 2012;132(5):577–82.
67. Tetreault L, Nagoshi N, Nakashima H, et al. Impact of depression and bipolar disorders on functional and quality of life outcomes in patients undergoing surgery for degenerative cervical myelopathy. Spine 2017;42(6):372–8.
68. Zong Y, Xue Y, Zhao Y, et al. Depression contributed an unsatisfactory surgery outcome among the posterior decompression of the cervical spondylotic myelopathy patients: a prospective clinical study. Neurol Sci 2014;35(9):1373–9.
69. Nakashima H, Tetreault L, Nagoshi N, et al. Comparison of outcomes of surgical treatment for ossification of the posterior longitudinal ligament versus

other forms of degenerative cervical myelopathy: results from the prospective, multicenter AOSpine CSM-International study of 479 patients. J Bone Joint Surg Am 2016;98(5):370–8.

70. Sadhu A, Ahn NU. Cocaine use and surgical outcomes of cervical spondylotic myelopathy: a retrospective study. Orthopedics 2012;35(11): e1640–3.
71. Nagoshi N, Tetreault LA, Nakashima H, et al. Do Caucasians and East Asians have different outcomes following surgery for the treatment of degenerative cervical myelopathy? Results from the prospective multicenter AOSpine International study. Spine 2016;41(18):1428–35.
72. Karadimas SK, Gatzounis G, Fehlings MG. Pathobiology of cervical spondylotic myelopathy. Eur Spine J 2015;24(Suppl 2):132–8.
73. Karadimas SK, Laliberte AM, Tetreault L, et al. Riluzole blocks perioperative ischemia-reperfusion injury and enhances postdecompression outcomes in cervical spondylotic myelopathy. Sci Transl Med 2015;7(316):316ra194.
74. Terao S, Sobue G, Hashizume Y, et al. Age-related changes of the myelinated fibers in the human corticospinal tract: a quantitative analysis. Acta Neuropathol 1994;88(2):137–42.
75. Terao S, Sobue G, Hashizume Y, et al. Age-related changes in human spinal ventral horn cells with special reference to the loss of small neurons in the intermediate zone: a quantitative analysis. Acta Neuropathol 1996;92(2):109–14.
76. Machino M, Yukawa Y, Hida T, et al. Can elderly patients recover adequately after laminoplasty? A comparative study of 520 patients with cervical spondylotic myelopathy. Spine 2012; 37(8):667–71.
77. Clegg A, Young J, Iliffe S, et al. Frailty in elderly people. Lancet 2013;381(9868):752–62.
78. Hilibrand AS, Fye MA, Emery SE, et al. Impact of smoking on the outcome of anterior cervical arthrodesis with interbody or strut-grafting. J Bone Joint Surg Am 2001;83-A(5):668–73.
79. Yan C, Avadhani NG, Iqbal J. The effects of smoke carcinogens on bone. Curr Osteoporos Rep 2011; 9(4):202–9.
80. Lau D, Chou D, Ziewacz JE, et al. The effects of smoking on perioperative outcomes and pseudarthrosis following anterior cervical corpectomy: clinical article. J Neurosurg Spine 2014;21(4):547–58.
81. Lee JC, Lee SH, Peters C, et al. Adjacent segment pathology requiring reoperation after anterior cervical arthrodesis: the influence of smoking, sex, and number of operated levels. Spine (Phila Pa 1976) 2015;40(10):E571–7.
82. Iwahashi M, Matsuzaki H, Tokuhashi Y, et al. Mechanism of intervertebral disc degeneration caused by nicotine in rabbits to explicate intervertebral disc disorders caused by smoking. Spine (Phila Pa 1976) 2002;27(13):1396–401.
83. Baron EM, Young WF. Cervical spondylotic myelopathy: a brief review of its pathophysiology, clinical course, and diagnosis. Neurosurgery 2007;60(1 Supp1 1):S35–41.
84. Tetreault L, Goldstein CL, Arnold P, et al. Degenerative cervical myelopathy: a spectrum of related disorders affecting the aging spine. Neurosurgery 2015;77(Suppl 4):S51–67.
85. Wang L, Kittaka M, Sun N, et al. Chronic nicotine treatment enhances focal ischemic brain injury and depletes free pool of brain microvascular tissue plasminogen activator in rats. J Cereb Blood flow Metab 1997;17(2):136–46.
86. Lawrence J, Xiao D, Xue Q, et al. Prenatal nicotine exposure increases heart susceptibility to ischemia/reperfusion injury in adult offspring. J Pharmacol Exp Ther 2008;324(1):331–41.
87. Przyklenk K. Nicotine exacerbates postischemic contractile dysfunction of 'stunned' myocardium in the canine model. Possible role of free radicals. Circulation 1994;89(3):1272–81.
88. Ozkan KU, Ozokutan BH, Inanc F, et al. Does maternal nicotine exposure during gestation increase the injury severity of small intestine in the newborn rats subjected to experimental necrotizing enterocolitis. J Pediatr Surg 2005;40(3):484–8.
89. Machino M, Yukawa Y, Ito K, et al. Impact of diabetes on the outcomes of cervical laminoplasty: a prospective cohort study of more than 500 patients with cervical spondylotic myelopathy. Spine 2014; 39(3):220–7.
90. Arinzon Z, Adunsky A, Fidelman Z, et al. Outcomes of decompression surgery for lumbar spinal stenosis in elderly diabetic patients. Eur Spine J 2004;13(1): 32–7.

Neurologic Complications in Managing Degenerative Cervical Myelopathy

Pathogenesis, Prevention, and Management

Taku Sugawara, MD, PhD

KEYWORDS

- Cervical myelopathy • Nonsurgical treatment • Surgery • Neurologic complications

KEY POINTS

- In the nonsurgical treatments of degenerative cervical myelopathy, cervical spine manipulation therapy and cervical traction are at higher risk of causing neurologic complications.
- Surgical treatments of degenerative cervical diseases can injure spinal cord, spinal nerves, cranial nerves, and sympathetic nerve trunk and major vessels and lead to developing neurologic complications.
- Anterior cervical corpectomy and posterior fixation surgery are at higher risk of inducing severe complications than other procedures.

INTRODUCTION

Degenerative cervical myelopathy (DCM) is a common neuropathologic status induced by a compression of the spinal cord due to degenerative changes of the cervical spine, such as spondylotic osteophytes, herniated disks, hypertrophic facet joint, and thickened ligamentum flavum (ossification of the posterior longitudinal ligament [OPLL]).[1–3] The natural history of DCM may manifest as a slow stepwise decline or there may be a long time of quiescence.[3] In a recent systematic review, there is moderate evidence that 20% to 63% of patients with symptomatic myelopathy deteriorate on Japanese Orthopedic Association scale 3 years to 6 years after initial diagnosis.[4,5] Severe stenosis for a long period of time may induce demyelination of nerve fibers and the symptoms are not likely to be improved without a surgical intervention.[3] In contrast, a single prospective randomized study showed that deterioration is rarely seen in the patients younger than 75 years of age with mild myelopathy and there is no superiority of surgical intervention for these patients over nonsurgical treatment.[6] Given the uncertainty regarding the natural history and treatment outcomes, nonsurgical and surgical treatments are both widely performed. This article is focused on the neurologic complications of these interventions for DCM. In addition to the spinal cord, spinal nerve, cranial nerve, and sympathetic nerve complications, vascular injury to cause cerebrovascular ischemia is also discussed (**Table 1**).

Disclosure: There are no conflicts of interest and funding sources.
Department of Spinal Surgery, Research Institute for Brain and Blood Vessels-Akita, 6-10 Senshu-Kubota-Machi, Akita City 010-0874, Japan
E-mail address: sugawara-taku@akita-noken.jp

Neurosurg Clin N Am 29 (2018) 129–137
https://doi.org/10.1016/j.nec.2017.09.008
1042-3680/18/© 2017 Elsevier Inc. All rights reserved.

Table 1
Neurologic complications of nonsurgical and surgical treatments for cervical degenerative disease

Complication	Incidence (%)	Procedures at Higher Risk
Nonsurgical treatments		
Cerebrovascular ischemia	0.01	CSMT
Progression of myelopathy	0.002–0.01	CSMT > cervical traction
Surgical treatments		
C5 palsy	0–30	Posterior fixation/decompression > ACCF > ACDF
RLN injury	1.9–2.7	ACCF > ACDF
SLN injury	1.1–1.3	Anterior surgery
Vertebral artery injury	0.2–4.1	Posterior C1-2 fixation > ACCF > ACDF
Horner syndrome	0.06–0.1	ACCF > ACDF
Iatrogenic spinal cord injury	0.01–0.3	ACCF, posterior fixation/decompression
Hypoglossal nerve injury	<0.01	Anterior surgery, posterior C1-2 fixation
Carotid artery injury	<0.01	Anterior surgery

NEUROLOGIC COMPLICATIONS OF NONSURGICAL MANAGEMENT

Nonsurgical treatment of degenerative cervical diseases includes cervical immobilization with a soft collar, the use of anti-inflammatory and/or muscle relaxants, spinal injections, manipulation therapy, thermal therapy, cervical traction, discouragement of high-risk activities, and an avoidance of risky environment.[6–8] Among these treatments, manipulation therapy is known to cause deterioration of myelopathy and ischemic neurologic complications.[9,10] Although it is less often than manipulation therapy, cervical tractions can also develop neurologic symptoms, such as myelopathy[11] and facial nerve paralysis.[12]

Cerebrovascular Ischemia

Among the nonsurgical treatments discussed previously, cervical spinal manipulation therapy (CSMT) is known to cause cerebrovascular ischemia mainly due to vertebrobasilar artery dissection.[10,13] There are several types of spinal manipulation, and one type is the high-velocity, low-amplitude thrust technique of providing “sharp thrust with velocity” to induce a gap in the joint.[14] Such type of manipulation has been reported to be at higher risk of causing neurologic complications.[10] A review article analyzed 64 cases of previously reported postmanipulation cerebrovascular ischemia and found that the patients were predominantly women with a mean age of 35.8 years and the frequent ischemic symptoms were loss of coordination, dizziness, speech/swallowing dysfunction, visual disturbances, and numbness.[13] Symptoms occurred within 30 minutes of the manipulation in 75% of the patients and within 2 days in 94%. The review concluded that these complications were unpredictable and should be considered inherent and idiosyncratic.[13] Although the incidence of irreversible complication is as low as 0.01% per 1 manipulation therapy,[10] the risk/benefit analyses do not recommend the manipulation therapy in the patients with neurologic symptoms.[15]

Progression of Myelopathy

Progression of myelopathy after CSMT has been reported. A 5-year retrospective study in a single-group practice analyzed complications of cervical manipulation therapy for patients with cervical degenerative disk diseases.[10] Of the 1712 patients who received 1 or more cervical manipulation therapy, 11 (0.6%) suffered worsened myelopathy, including 2 patients with partial Brown-Séquard syndrome. Regarding the 27 patients with cervical disk herniation causing myelopathy, the symptoms worsened in 7 patients, resulting in surgical treatment in all patients. CSMT is generally considered a contraindication for the acute phase of cervical disk herniation; high-velocity technique, especially, is absolutely contraindicated in the patients with cervical myelopathy.[10] The incidence of irreversible complications, including worsened myelopathy, however, is considered to be low (0.002%–0.01% for single CSMT).[10,16] It is less frequent, but cervical traction can also induce myelopathy in the patients with narrow cervical canal.[11]

NEUROLOGIC COMPLICATIONS OF SURGICAL MANAGEMENT FOR DEGENERATIVE CERVICAL MYELOPATHY PATIENTS

A variety of techniques have been developed to improve functional outcomes of DCM, including anterior cervical discectomy and fusion (ACDF), anterior cervical corpectomy and fusion (ACCF), laminoplasty, laminectomy, and laminectomy with fusion.[17] Regarding the complications of surgical treatments to cause neurologic symptoms, the spinal cord, spinal nerves, and vertebral artery can be injured by both anterior and posterior approaches, and cranial nerves, sympathetic nerve trunk, and carotid artery may be affected by anterior approach.[18,19] Not only frequent and major neurologic complications but also rare disabling adverse events are discussed and up-to-date information about the pathogenesis, prevention, and management is reviewed.

Iatrogenic Spinal Cord Injury

Iatrogenic spinal cord injury is a devastating complication after cervical spine surgery and its incidence was reported as 0.02% to 0.3% in large retrospective studies.[20–22] In 5 cases with detailed information in these studies, 3 had corpectomy, 1 had corpectomy and posterior decompression, and 1 had posterior decompression with fusion. Four patients developed quadriplegia and 1 had 1-sided paralysis. Neuromonitoring using somatosensory evoked potentials and transcranial motor evoked potentials (tcMEPs) was useful to detect the neurologic deficits in the cases of good baseline neuromonitoring signals.[21,22] In the study of the patients with DCM, a significant correlation was shown between tcMEP changes and postoperative neurologic deficits, with a sensitivity of 75%, specificity of 98%, positive predictive value of 75%, and negative predictive value of 98%.[23] Several etiologies can be considered, including deterioration of preexisting spinal stenosis by positioning, spinal cord stretch by spinal alignment correction, malposition of spinal instruments or bone grafts, mechanical compression of dural sac, and vascular injury to cause hyperemia or venous congestion, although precise mechanism of myelopathy is unknown. Therefore, there is no standard intraoperative protocol to prevent this complication, but the neuromonitoring should be recommended for all cervical spine surgeries. And in cases of intraoperative alert by neuromonitoring, the surgeons should examine the deviation of the instruments or bone grafts and spinal alignment and maintain the adequate blood pressure.[22]

Vascular Injury and Stroke

Vertebral artery injury by the anterior cervical spine surgery is uncommon, with an incidence of 0.2% to 0.5%, but sometimes results in severe neurologic deficit or death.[24–26] In anterior spine surgery, most of injuries occurred during ACCF but rarely during ACDF.[25] Vertebral artery is located 1 mm to 2 mm laterally from uncovertebral joints and excessive lateral bone removal by the Kerrison bone punch or high-speed drill may result in laceration of vertebral artery. When removing a part of Luschka joints, care should be taken not to expose dural root sleeve more than 5 mm.[27,28] Also, the risk is greater at more cephalad vertebrae during lateral extension of the central decompression procedures, because inter-Luschka distance increases from C3 to C7.[27,29] For the cases that require uncovertebral joints resection, preoperative contrast-enhanced 3-D–CT is mandatory, because there is 2.7% incidence of anomalous, tortuous vertebral artery in cadaver studies[30] and 5.4% in imaging studies.[31]

Vertebral artery injury by the posterior cervical spine surgery is also rare, with an incidence of 0.07% to 4.1%.[25,26,32–34] Posterior instrumentation surgery of upper cervical spine is at the greatest risk of vertebral artery injury.[32,34–36] In particular, the highest incidence at 1.3% to 4.1% was reported for posterior atlantoaxial transarticular screw fixation (Magerl fixation).[26,34] A majority of the injury occurs during screw placement procedures or in the patients with vertebral artery anomalies,[26,32,34,37] and, therefore, it is essential to assess vertebral artery by CT angiography or MR angiography preoperatively to find the vessel anomaly. A multicenter study of 16,582 cervical spine surgery revealed 14 patients had vertebral artery injury and half of them occurred in the patients with anomalous vertebral artery.[37] For screw fixation procedures, intraoperative screw guiding methods by CT-based navigation systems or patient-specific laminar templates may improve the accuracy and safety.[38,39]

Carotid artery injury by the cervical spine surgery is extremely rare and occurred in only 5 patients who underwent anterior surgery.[40–45] Two patients were diagnosed as direct injury—1 was carotid artery dissection and the other was carotid artery injury.[43,44] The rest of the patients suffered stroke due to prolonged carotid artery retraction.[41,42,45] It is not well known that traction of normal carotid artery by retractor causes a significant reduction in blood flow,[46] and prolonged retraction of the normal common carotid artery can induce lethal stroke.[42] Preoperative evaluation of the carotid artery is needed for the patients with a history of previous stroke or carotid artery stenosis, and the surgical approach should be discussed. Intraoperative neuromonitoring may be beneficial to detect the early signs of cerebral ischemia. If a long operation time is expected, retractor blade should be released intermittently to restore blood flow of carotid artery.[40]

Once bleeding form the major vessels occurs intraoperatively, compression of the bleeding point using absorbable gelatin compressed sponges or cottonoids should be tried for temporal hemostasis,[25] and threads or vascular closure staples can be used for repair of arterial wall.[47] When these trials fail, ligation of vertebral artery can be considered, but it may lead to cerebellar/brain stem infarction and the mortality rate is as high as 12%.[48] Alternatively, intravascular surgery using self-expandable stent can be tried to cover the injury site to control bleeding and simultaneously preserve blood flow of vertebral artery.[49]

C5 Palsy

Postoperative C5 palsy has been reported to occur in 0% to 30% of the patients after the cervical spine surgery. The patients present new weakness in the deltoid and biceps brachii muscles, with sensory deficits or pain in the shoulders, in some cases, immediately to 2 months after surgery.[50–53] Injury to the nerve root during surgery, nerve root traction due to the shift of cervical spinal cord after decompression, and spinal cord ischemia and reperfusion injury have been proposed as mechanisms of postoperative C5 palsy, but pathogenesis has not been clarified.[54] Because the etiology of C5 palsy is still unclear, there are no standard preventative measures.

The risk factors have been proposed in many studies. Preoperative diagnosis seems to affect the incidence of C5 palsy. It has been reported that the incidence was 0% to 3% in the patients with cervical disk herniation, 2.8% to 12.1% in those with DCM, and 2.1% to 14% with OPLL.[53,55,56] Another study found a 9.2-fold greater risk of postoperative C5 palsy in OPLL patients compared with those with DCM patients.[57] A multicenter retrospective review of 13,946 cervical spine surgery reported 0% C5 palsy in radiculopathy patients and 5.8% in DCM patients.[53] Taken together, the patients with DCM or OPLL presumably predispose to develop postoperative C5 palsy.

The type and the level of the surgeries also likely affect the incidence of C5 palsy. In anterior cervical surgery, there is higher incidence after ACCF than ACDF, especially when the surgery involves C3-4 and C4-5 segments.[51,52] In a review of 1001 patients who underwent anterior or posterior decompressions, the incidence was reported to be 5.2% overall, 1.6% in anterior surgery, and 8.6% in posterior surgery.[58] Surgery with internal fixation has been reported to increase the risk of C5 palsy.[59–61] Addition of internal fixation to laminoplasty increased the risk 11.6 times greater than the patients with laminoplasty alone.[60]

The treatment of postoperative C5 palsy is not established, but a combination of physical therapy and pain control medication is usually used. In a review article, the overall incidence of C5 palsy after the cervical spine surgery for compression myelopathy was 4.6%, and when C5 palsy is grade 3 to 4 in manual muscle test, 96.4% of the patients recovered fully, whereas only 71% of the patients with initial manual muscle test grade 0 to 2 recovered to the useful level.[52]

Recurrent Laryngeal Nerve Injury

Hoarseness after the anterior cervical spine surgery has been reported as a consequence of recurrent laryngeal nerve (RLN) palsy.[62] Right RLN leaves the vagus nerve and loops under subclavian artery, whereas the left RLN leaves the vagus nerve at the mediastinum and passes over the aorta. After branching from the vagus nerve, the right nerve does not go into the tracheoesophageal groove until it approaches the cricothyroid joint, whereas the left RLN ascends within the tracheoesophageal groove. The right RLN was thought to be easily injured by the right-sided approach of the anterior cervical spine surgery, because it might cross the operative field.[63] The incidence of postoperative hoarseness, however, does not differ by the side of approach. The overall incidence of RLN palsy had been reported as 1.9% to 2.7%,[62,64] but a recent prospective study showed the incidence rates of hoarseness and subclinical laryngoscopic vocal code paralysis were 8.3% and 15.9%, respectively, at 3 to 7 days and 2.5% and 10.8%, respectively, at 3 months after surgery.[65] Initial and persistent RLN palsy occurred much more often than anticipated. As a cause of RLN palsy, compression of the RLN within the endolarynx was suggested in some studies.[66] Endotracheal tube cuff pressure monitoring and periodic release of the retractor may prevent injury to the RLN during anterior cervical spine surgery.[67] In addition, intraoperative laryngeal myographic monitoring is reported to detect RLN injury at the sensitivity of 100% and the specificity of 87%.[68] Treatment of RLN injury includes steroid administration, voice training, and reinnervation, but complete resolution of the symptoms was obtained in only 74% of the patients in a large multicenter study.[69]

Superior Laryngeal Nerve Injury

Vocal cord paresis after anterior cervical spine surgery is usually attributed to RLN injury. Superior laryngeal nerve (SLN) injury also causes vocal cord paresis, with other symptoms including sensory disturbance of larynx, dysphagia, impaired cough reflex, and change in vocal quality.[70,71] SLN is a branch of the vagus nerve, originates at C1-2 level, and descends by the side of pharynx behind the interncal carotid artery, and divides into 2 branches, external SLN and internal SLN, and innervates cricothyroid muscles. External SLN is susceptible to damage during anterior cervical spine surgery. To avoid SLN injury, it is important to dissect the longus colli muscles laterally to place the retractor blades beneath the muscle layer.[71] And myographic monitoring of cricothyroid muscle was reported as effective to identify SLN intraoperatively. A retrospective study reported a 1% incidence of SLN palsy after ACDF.[72] Because the symptoms of SLN injury resemble those of RLN injury, its diagnosis is difficult and requires strobovideolaryngoscopy and laryngeal electromyography[73]; therefore, the incidence may be higher. Treatment of SLN injury is mostly voice therapy to strengthen cricothyroid muscle, but a recovery rate is unclear because of a paucity of the reports.

Hypoglossal Nerve Injury

Hypoglossal nerve palsy is extremely rare and the main symptoms are dysphagia, dysarthria, and tongue deviation.[74] The hypoglossal nerve exits hypoglossal canal and lies next to the vagus nerve above C1-2 level. It travels between the carotid artery and internal jugular vein and courses medially at C2-3, where direct injury may occur during anterior cervical spine surgery.[75] Placement of C1-2 transarticular screw can also injure the hypoglossal nerve in front of C1-2 facet.[76] The hypoglossal nerve palsy mostly occurred after high cervical spine surgery by anterior approach or C1-2 screw fixation by direct injury.[74] Surprisingly, it also occurred after lower laminectomy/laminoplasty,[77,78] not due to direct nerve injury. The investigators of those reports suggested the compression of the nerve against the mandible by neck flexion or stretching the nerve by the endotracheal tube might have caused the nerve injury.[77] In summary, high anterior cervical surgery and C1-2 transarticular screw fixation are at higher risk of this complication. Some of the hypoglossal injury may be prevented by avoiding cervical hyperflexion position and anterior breach of transarticular screws.

Horner Syndrome

Horner syndrome is a well-known clinical entity characterized by pupillary miosis, facial anhydrosis, and ptosis. It possibly occurs after anterior cervical spine surgery by a damage to the cervical sympathetic trunk. The sympathetic trunk lies on the surface of longus colli muscle in a loose fascial layer and it is most frequently damaged at middle/lower cervical levels, where the trunk courses more medial on the muscle by stretching of the muscle or direct injury.[28,79–82] In recent studies of ACDF with more than 1000 cases, the incidence of Horner syndrome is 0.06% to 0.1%.[83–85] There is much higher incidence, however, at 19.1% after oblique corpectomy.[86–91] A majority of postoperative cases of Horner syndrome spontaneously resolved without specific treatment within 6 months, but permanent deficit occurred in approximately a fifth of the affected patients.[85] The risk of the sympathetic trunk injury is reduced by staying midline, and if lateral exposure is needed, the retractors should be placed beneath the longus colli muscle.[83]

Other Neurologic Complications

There are other uncommon but serious complications after cervical spine surgery, such as bilateral phrenic nerve palsy,[92] with an incidence of 0.01% or less. These complications are not included in this article because of the absence of sufficient data.

SUMMARY

There are a variety of neurologic complications with the nonsurgical and surgical treatments for DCM. Ten common or disabling complications are selected, and the incidence, pathogenesis, prevention, and management are reviewed. Among the nonsurgical treatments for DSM, cervical spine manipulation therapy and cervical traction are at higher risk of causing neurologic complications. Surgical treatments for degenerative cervical diseases can injure spinal cord, spinal nerves, cranial nerves, sympathetic nerve trunk, and major vessels to cause neurologic symptoms. Anterior cervical corpectomy and multilevel posterior surgery, especially when accompanied by fixation, are at higher risk of inducing complications than other procedures. Physical therapists and surgeons should be aware of those neurologic complications to select treatment.

REFERENCES

1. Kimura A, Seichi A, Takeshita K, et al. Fall-related deterioration of subjective symptoms in patients with cervical myelopathy. Spine 2017;42(7):E398–403.
2. Epstein N. Diagnosis and surgical management of cervical ossification of the posterior longitudinal ligament. Spine J 2002;2(6):436–49.

3. Matz PG, Anderson PA, Holly LT, et al. The natural history of cervical spondylotic myelopathy. J Neurosurg Spine 2009;11(2):104–11.
4. Fehlings MG, Tetreault L, Hsieh PC, et al. Introduction: degenerative cervical myelopathy: diagnostic, assessment, and management strategies, surgical complications, and outcome prediction. Neurosurg Focus 2016;40(6):E1.
5. Karadimas SK, Erwin WM, Ely CG, et al. Pathophysiology and natural history of cervical spondylotic myelopathy. Spine (Phila Pa 1976) 2013;38(22 Suppl 1):S21–36.
6. Kadanka Z, Mares M, Bednanik J, et al. Approaches to spondylotic cervical myelopathy: conservative versus surgical results in a 3-year follow-up study. Spine (Phila Pa 1976) 2002;27(20):2205–10 [discussion: 2210–1].
7. Rhee JM, Shamji MF, Erwin WM, et al. Nonoperative management of cervical myelopathy: a systematic review. Spine 2013;38(22 Suppl 1):S55–67.
8. Yoshimatsu H, Nagata K, Goto H, et al. Conservative treatment for cervical spondylotic myelopathy. prediction of treatment effects by multivariate analysis. Spine J 2001;1(4):269–73.
9. Sweeney A, Doody C. Manual therapy for the cervical spine and reported adverse effects: a survey of Irish manipulative physiotherapists. Man Ther 2010;15(1):32–6.
10. Malone DG, Baldwin NG, Tomecek FJ, et al. Complications of cervical spine manipulation therapy: 5-year retrospective study in a single-group practice. Neurosurg Focus 2002;13(6):ecp1.
11. van Zagten MS, Troost J, Heeres JG. Cervical myelopathy as complication of manual therapy in a patient with a narrow cervical canal. Ned Tijdschr Geneeskd 1993;137(32):1617–8 [in Dutch].
12. So EC. Facial nerve paralysis after cervical traction. Am J Phys Med Rehabil 2010;89(10):849–53.
13. Haldeman S, Kohlbeck FJ, McGregor M. Unpredictability of cerebrovascular ischemia associated with cervical spine manipulation therapy: a review of sixty-four cases after cervical spine manipulation. Spine 2002;27(1):49–55.
14. Greenmann PE. In: Greenman PE, editor. Principles of manual medicine. 2nd edition. Baltimore (MD): Williams and Wilkins; 1996. p. 99–103.
15. Powell FC, Hanigan WC, Olivero WC. A risk/benefit analysis of spinal manipulation therapy for relief of lumbar or cervical pain. Neurosurgery 1993;33(1): 73–8 [discussion: 78–9].
16. Dabbs V, Lauretti WJ. A risk assessment of cervical manipulation vs. NSAIDs for the treatment of neck pain. J Manipulative Physiol Ther 1995;18(8):530–6.
17. Mummaneni PV, Kaiser MG, Matz PG, et al. Cervical surgical techniques for the treatment of cervical spondylotic myelopathy. J Neurosurg Spine 2009; 11(2):130–41.
18. Tetreault L, Tan G, Kopjar B, et al. Clinical and surgical predictors of complications following surgery for the treatment of cervicalspondylotic myelopathy: results from the multicenter, prospective AOSpine international study of 479 patients. Neurosurgery 2016;79(1):33–44.
19. Fehlings MG, Smith JS, Kopjar B, et al. Perioperative and delayed complications associated with the surgical treatment of cervicalspondylotic myelopathy based on 302 patients from the AOSpine North America cervicalspondylotic myelopathy study. J Neurosurg Spine 2012;16(5):425–32.
20. Flynn TB. Neurologic complications of anterior cervical interbody fusion. Spine 1982;7(6):536–9.
21. Lee JY, Hilibrand AS, Lim MR, et al. Characterization of neurophysiologic alerts during anterior cervical spine surgery. Spine 2006;31(17):1916–22.
22. Daniels AH, Hart RA, Hilibrand AS, et al. Iatrogenic spinal cord injury resulting from cervical spine surgery. Global Spine J 2017;7(1 Suppl):84S–90S.
23. Clark AJ, Ziewacz JE, Safaee M, et al. Intraoperative neuromonitoring with MEPs and prediction of postoperative neurological deficits in patients undergoing surgery for cervical and cervicothoracic myelopathy. Neurosurg Focus 2013; 35(1):E7.
24. Burke JP, Gerszten PC, Welch WC. Iatrogenic vertebral artery injury during anterior cervical spine surgery. Spine J 2005;5(5):508–14 [discussion: 514].
25. Inamasu J, Guiot BH. Vascular injury and complication in neurosurgical spine surgery. Acta Neurochir (Wien) 2006;148(4):375–87.
26. Neo M, Fujibayashi S, Miyata M, et al. Vertebral artery injury during cervical spine surgery: a survey of more than 5600 operations. Spine 2008;33(7): 779–85.
27. Oh SH, Perin NI, Cooper PR. Quantitative three-dimensional anatomy of the subaxial cervical spine: implication for anterior spinal surgery. Neurosurgery 1996;38(6):1139–44.
28. Pait TG, Killefer JA, Arnautovic KI. Surgical anatomy of the anterior cervical spine: the disc space, vertebral artery, and associated bony structures. Neurosurgery 1996;39(4):769–76.
29. Vaccaro AR, Ring D, Scuderi G, et al. Vertebral artery location in relation to the vertebral body as determined by two-dimensional computed tomography evaluation. Spine 1994;19(23):2637–41.
30. Curylo LJ, Mason HC, Bohlman HH, et al. Tortuous course of the vertebral artery and anterior cervical decompression: a cadaveric and clinical case study. Spine 2000;25(22):2860–4.
31. Hong JT, Park DK, Lee MJ, et al. Anatomical variations of the vertebral artery segment in the lower cervical spine: analysis by three-dimensional computed tomography angiography. Spine (Phila Pa 1976) 2008;33(22):2422–6.

32. Lunardini DJ, Eskander MS, Even JL, et al. Vertebral artery injuries in cervical spine surgery. Spine J 2014;14(8):1520–5.
33. Farey ID, Nadkarni S, Smith N. Modified Gallie technique versus transarticular screw fixation in C1-C2 fusion. Clin Orthop Relat Res 1999;(359): 126–35.
34. Wright NM, Lauryssen C. Vertebral artery injury in C1-2 transarticular screw fixation: results of a survey of the AANS/CNS section on disorders of the spine and peripheral nerves. American Association of Neurological Surgeons/Congress of Neurological Surgeons. J Neurosurg 1998;88(4):634–40.
35. Peng CW, Chou BT, Bendo JA, et al. Vertebral artery injury in cervical spine surgery: anatomical considerations, management, and preventive measures. Spine J 2009;9(1):70–6.
36. Cole T, Veeravagu A, Zhang M, et al. Anterior versus posterior approach for multilevel degenerative cervical disease: a retrospective propensity score-matched study of the MarketScan database. Spine 2015;40(13):1033–8.
37. Hsu WK, Kannan A, Mai HT, et al. Epidemiology and outcomes of vertebral artery injury in 16 582 cervical spine surgery patients: an AOSpine North America Multicenter Study. Global Spine J 2017;7(1 Suppl): 21S–7S.
38. Theologis AA, Burch S. Safety and efficacy of reconstruction of complex cervical spine pathology using pedicle screws inserted with stealth navigation and 3D image-guided (O-Arm) technology. Spine 2015; 40(18):1397–406.
39. Sugawara T, Higashiyama N, Kaneyama S, et al. Accurate and simple screw insertion procedure with patient-specific screw guide templates for posterior C1-C2 fixation. Spine 2017;42(6):E340–6.
40. Hartl R, Alimi M, Abdelatif Boukebir M, et al. Carotid artery injury in anterior cervical spine surgery: multicenter cohort study and literature review. Global Spine J 2017;7(1 Suppl):71S–5S.
41. Chozick BS, Watson P, Greenblatt SH. Internal carotid artery thrombosis after cervical corpectomy. Spine 1994;19(19):2230–2.
42. Yeh YC, Sun WZ, Lin CP, et al. Prolonged retraction on the normal common carotid artery induced lethal stroke after cervical spine surgery. Spine 2004; 29(19):E431–4.
43. Loret JE, Francois P, Papagiannaki C, et al. Internal carotid artery dissection after anterior cervical disc replacement: first case report and literature review of vascular complications of the approach. Eur J Orthop Surg Traumatol 2013;23(Suppl 1): S107–10.
44. Lesoin F, Bouasakao N, Clarisse J, et al. Results of surgical treatment of radiculomyelopathy caused by cervical arthrosis based on 1000 operations. Surg Neurol 1985;23(4):350–5.
45. Radhakrishnan M, Bansal S, Srihari GS, et al. Perioperative stroke following anterior cervical discectomy. Br J Neurosurg 2010;24(5):592–4.
46. Pollard ME, Little PW. Changes in carotid artery blood flow during anterior cervical spine surgery. Spine 2002;27(2):152–5.
47. Yanagisawa T, Mizoi K, Sugawara T, et al. Direct repair of a blisterlike aneurysm on the internal carotid artery with vascular closure staple clips. Technical note. J Neurosurg 2004;100(1):146–9.
48. Shintani A, Zervas NT. Consequence of ligation of the vertebral artery. J Neurosurg 1972;36(4): 447–50.
49. Katsaridis V, Papagiannaki C, Violaris C. Treatment of an iatrogenic vertebral artery laceration with the Symbiot self expandable covered stent. Clin Neurol Neurosurg 2007;109(6):512–5.
50. Gandhoke G, Wu JC, Rowland NC, et al. Anterior corpectomy versus posterior laminoplasty: is the risk of postoperative C-5 palsy different? Neurosurg Focus 2011;31(4):E12.
51. Hashimoto M, Mochizuki M, Aiba A, et al. C5 palsy following anterior decompression and spinal fusion for cervical degenerative diseases. Eur Spine J 2010;19(10):1702–10.
52. Sakaura H, Hosono N, Mukai Y, et al. C5 palsy after decompression surgery for cervical myelopathy: review of the literature. Spine (Phila Pa 1976) 2003; 28(21):2447–51.
53. Thompson SE, Smith ZA, Hsu WK, et al. C5 palsy after cervical spine surgery: a multicenter retrospective review of 59 cases. Global Spine J 2017;7(1 Suppl):64S–70S.
54. Sugawara T. Anterior cervical spine surgery for degenerative disease: a review. Neurol Med Chir (Tokyo) 2015;55(7):540–6.
55. Kalisvaart M, Nassr A, Eck J. C5 palsy after cervical decompression procedures. Neurosurg Q 2009;19: 276–82.
56. Nassr A, Eck JC, Ponnappan RK, et al. The incidence of C5 palsy after multilevel cervical decompression procedures: a review of 750 consecutive cases. Spine (Phila Pa 1976) 2012;37(3):174–8.
57. Wu FL, Sun Y, Pan SF, et al. Risk factors associated with upper extremity palsy after expansive open-door laminoplasty for cervical myelopathy. Spine J 2014;14(6):909–15.
58. Bydon M, Macki M, Kaloostian P, et al. Incidence and prognostic factors of c5 palsy: a clinical study of 1001 cases and review of the literature. Neurosurgery 2014;74(6):595–604 [discussion: 604–5].
59. Liu T, Zou W, Han Y, et al. Correlative study of nerve root palsy and cervical posterior decompression laminectomy and internal fixation. Orthopedics 2010;33(8).
60. Takemitsu M, Cheung KM, Wong YW, et al. C5 nerve root palsy after cervical laminoplasty and posterior

fusion with instrumentation. J Spinal Disord Tech 2008;21(4):267–72.
61. Chen Y, Guo Y, Lu X, et al. Surgical strategy for multilevel severe ossification of posterior longitudinal ligament in the cervical spine. J Spinal Disord Tech 2011;24(1):24–30.
62. Beutler WJ, Sweeney CA, Connolly PJ. Recurrent laryngeal nerve injury with anterior cervical spine surgery risk with laterality of surgical approach. Spine 2001;26(12):1337–42.
63. Netterville JL, Koriwchak MJ, Winkle M, et al. Vocal fold paralysis following the anterior approach to the cervical spine. Ann Otol Rhinol Laryngol 1996; 105(2):85–91.
64. Kilburg C, Sullivan HG, Mathiason MA. Effect of approach side during anterior cervical discectomy and fusion on the incidence of recurrent laryngeal nerve injury. J Neurosurg Spine 2006; 4(4):273–7.
65. Jung A, Schramm J, Lehnerdt K, et al. Recurrent laryngeal nerve palsy during anterior cervical spine surgery: a prospective study. J Neurosurg Spine 2005;2(2):123–7.
66. Kriskovich MD, Apfelbaum RI, Haller JR. Vocal fold paralysis after anterior cervical spine surgery: incidence, mechanism, and prevention of injury. Laryngoscope 2000;110(9):1467–73.
67. Apfelbaum RI, Kriskovich MD, Haller JR. On the incidence, cause, and prevention of recurrent laryngeal nerve palsies during anterior cervical spine surgery. Spine 2000;25(22):2906–12.
68. Dimopoulos VG, Chung I, Lee GP, et al. Quantitative estimation of the recurrent laryngeal nerve irritation by employing spontaneous intraoperative electromyographic monitoring during anterior cervical discectomy and fusion. J Spinal Disord Tech 2009; 22(1):1–7.
69. Gokaslan ZL, Bydon M, De la Garza-Ramos R, et al. Recurrent laryngeal nerve palsy after cervical spine surgery: a multicenter AOSpine clinical research network study. Global Spine J 2017;7(1 Suppl): 53S–7S.
70. Orestes MI, Chhetri DK. Superior laryngeal nerve injury: effects, clinical findings, prognosis, and management options. Curr Opin Otolaryngol Head Neck Surg 2014;22(6):439–43.
71. Tempel ZJ, Smith JS, Shaffrey C, et al. A multicenter review of superior laryngeal nerve injury following anterior cervical spine surgery. Global Spine J 2017;7(1 Suppl):7S–11S.
72. Bulger RF, Rejowski JE, Beatty RA. Vocal cord paralysis associated with anterior cervical fusion: considerations for prevention and treatment. J Neurosurg 1985;62(5):657–61.
73. Dursun G, Sataloff RT, Spiegel JR, et al. Superior laryngeal nerve paresis and paralysis. J Voice 1996;10(2):206–11.
74. Ames CP, Clark AJ, Kanter AS, et al. Hypoglossal nerve palsy after cervical spine surgery. Global Spine J 2017;7(1 Suppl):37S–9S.
75. Haller JM, Iwanik M, Shen FH. Clinically relevant anatomy of high anterior cervical approach. Spine 2011;36(25):2116–21.
76. Grob D, Jeanneret B, Aebi M, et al. Atlanto-axial fusion with transarticular screw fixation. J Bone Joint Surg Br 1991;73(6):972–6.
77. Kang JH, Kim DM, Kim SW. Tapia syndrome after cervical spine surgery. Korean J Spine 2013;10(4): 249–51.
78. Park CK, Lee DC, Park CJ, et al. Tapia's syndrome after posterior cervical spine surgery under general anesthesia. J Korean Neurosurg Soc 2013;54(5): 423–5.
79. Lu J, Ebraheim NA, Nadim Y, et al. Anterior approach to the cervical spine: surgical anatomy. Orthopedics 2000;23(8):841–5.
80. Ebraheim NA, Lu J, Yang H, et al. Vulnerability of the sympathetic trunk during the anterior approach to the lower cervical spine. Spine 2000;25(13): 1603–6.
81. Kiray A, Arman C, Naderi S, et al. Surgical anatomy of the cervical sympathetic trunk. Clin Anat 2005; 18(3):179–85.
82. Saylam CY, Ozgiray E, Orhan M, et al. Neuroanatomy of cervical sympathetic trunk: a cadaveric study. Clin Anat 2009;22(3):324–30.
83. Fountas KN, Kapsalaki EZ, Nikolakakos LG, et al. Anterior cervical discectomy and fusion associated complications. Spine 2007;32(21):2310–7.
84. Nanda A, Sharma M, Sonig A, et al. Surgical complications of anterior cervical diskectomy and fusion for cervical degenerative disk disease: a single surgeon's experience of 1,576 patients. World Neurosurg 2014;82(6):1380–7.
85. Traynelis VC, Malone HR, Smith ZA, et al. Rare complications of cervical spine surgery: Horner's syndrome. Global Spine J 2017;7(1 Suppl): 103S–8S.
86. Traynelis VC, Arnold PM, Fourney DR, et al. Alternative procedures for the treatment of cervical spondylotic myelopathy: arthroplasty, oblique corpectomy, skip laminectomy: evaluation of comparative effectiveness and safety. Spine 2013;38(22 Suppl 1): S210–31.
87. Chacko AG, Turel MK, Sarkar S, et al. Clinical and radiological outcomes in 153 patients undergoing oblique corpectomy for cervical spondylotic myelopathy. Br J Neurosurg 2014;28(1):49–55.
88. Chacko AG, Joseph M, Turel MK, et al. Multilevel oblique corpectomy for cervical spondylotic myelopathy preserves segmental motion. Eur Spine J 2012;21(7):1360–7.
89. Chibbaro S, Mirone G, Makiese O, et al. Multilevel oblique corpectomy without fusion in managing

cervical myelopathy: long-term outcome and stability evaluation in 268 patients. J Neurosurg Spine 2009;10(5):458–65.
90. Kiris T, Kilincer C. Cervical spondylotic myelopathy treated by oblique corpectomy: a prospective study. Neurosurgery 2008;62(3):674–82 [discussion: 674–82].
91. Rocchi G, Caroli E, Salvati M, et al. Multilevel oblique corpectomy without fusion: our experience in 48 patients. Spine (Phila Pa 1976) 2005;30(17):1963–9.
92. Gokcen HB, Erdogan S, Kara K, et al. Bilateral diaphragm paralysis due to phrenic nerve palsy after two-level cervical corpectomy. Spine J 2016;16(7):e431–2.

Options of Management of the Patient with Mild Degenerative Cervical Myelopathy

Izumi Koyanagi, MD

KEYWORDS

• Cervical spondylotic myelopathy • Ossification of the posterior longitudinal ligament
• Degenerative cervical myelopathy • Surgical treatment • Mild myelopathy

KEY POINTS

- Degenerative process of the cervical spine with age causes various pathologic conditions such as disc protrusions, bony spur formation, malalignment of the spinal column, and hypertrophied or ossified spinal ligaments.
- These degenerative changes result in cervical disc hernia, cervical spondylosis, or ossification of the longitudinal ligament (OPLL) according to the affected areas.
- Indication for surgical treatment is controversial because the clinical course often shows spontaneous recovery and patients' needs are different by general and social conditions.
- To understand surgical management of degenerative cervical myelopathy in the actual clinical practice, a personal series of subjects with cervical spondylotic myelopathy or OPLL who underwent surgical treatment were reviewed.

INTRODUCTION

Degenerative process of the cervical spine with age causes various pathologic conditions such as disc protrusions, bony spur formation, malalignment of the spinal column, and hypertrophied or ossified spinal ligaments. These degenerative changes result in cervical disc hernia, cervical spondylosis, or ossification of the longitudinal ligament (OPLL) according to the affected areas. They are the most popular spinal disorders for cervical myelopathy. Indication for surgical treatment is controversial because the clinical course often shows spontaneous recovery and patients' needs are different by general and social conditions. In this study, clinical features and surgical treatment of the degenerative cervical spine disorders, especially the mild form of myelopathy, are reviewed and discussed. To understand surgical management of degenerative cervical myelopathy (DCM) in the actual clinical practice, personal series of the subjects with cervical spondylotic myelopathy (CSM) or OPLL who underwent surgical treatment were reviewed.

CLINICAL FEATURES OF DCM

In the past 5 years, 84 subjects with CSM (50 subjects, 59.5%) or OPLL (34 subjects, 40.5%) were surgically treated. The subjects with reoperation, significant comorbidities, radiculopathy, soft disc herniation, and atlantoaxial lesions were excluded. There were 53 men and 31 women, ages 41 to 90 years (mean 68.9, median 70). Preoperatively,

Disclosures: The author has no potential conflicts of interest.
Department of Neurosurgery, Hokkaido Neurosurgical Memorial Hospital, 1-20, Hachiken 9-jo, Higashi 5-chome, Nishi-ku, Sapporo 063-0869, Japan
E-mail address: koyanagi@hnsmhp.or.jp

Neurosurg Clin N Am 29 (2018) 139–144
https://doi.org/10.1016/j.nec.2017.09.009
1042-3680/18/© 2017 Elsevier Inc. All rights reserved.

44 subjects (52.4%) presented with walking difficulty. Eleven (13.1%) showed severe gait disturbance and needed a wheel chair. Anterior decompression and fusion was performed in 30 subjects (35.7%). Threaded titanium cage was used for discectomy, osteophytectomy, and fusion in 15 subjects, whereas 15 subjects underwent corpectomy and fusion with a titanium mesh cage. Fifty-two subjects (61.9%) underwent posterior decompression by bilateral open-door laminoplasty. The other 2 subjects were treated with laminectomy alone or laminectomy with posterior fusion.

The preoperative neurologic state was evaluated by Neurosurgical Cervical Spine Scale (NCSS) (**Table 1**).[1] This scoring system evaluates motor functions of the lower and upper extremities on a scale of 1 to 5 and sensory function and/or pain from 1 to 4. In total, the neurologic state is scored from 3 to 14 (total disability to normal). The mean of the total NCSS score, lower extremity motor function, upper extremity motor function, and sensory function of 84 subjects were 8.8 (range: 5–11), 3.3 (1–5), 3.1 (2–4), and 2.4 (1–4), respectively.

MILD DCM

In this study, mild myelopathy was defined as 11 or more of the total score of NCSS. Nine (10.7%) out of the 84 subjects met the criteria (**Table 2**). There were 7 men and 2 women, ages 50 to 79 years (mean 62.7, median 62.0). Three subjects were associated with OPLL. Numbness of upper extremities was the most common symptoms at onset (6 subjects). Three had neck pain (**Fig. 1**) or headache (**Fig. 2**). In 1 subject, neck pain was the only symptom (**Fig. 3**). Two subjects presented with motor weakness of upper extremities or 4 extremities. Duration from onset of symptoms to surgery ranged from 1 month to 3 years (mean 11.7 months). Preoperative total NCSS score was 11 in all subjects, with the mean of lower extremity motor function 4.3, upper extremity motor function 3.8, and sensory function 2.9. Preoperative MRI revealed spinal cord compression of various degrees in all subjects. Five subjects showed intramedullary hyperintensity on T2-weighted MRI at the compressed segment. Despite the intramedullary signal changes due to spinal cord compression, these subjects

Table 1
Neurosurgical Cervical Spine Scale for degenerative cervical spine diseases. Total score is 3 to 14, indicating total disability to normal

Score	Lower Extremity Motor Function
1	Total disability: chair-bound or bedridden
2	Severe disability: needs support in walking on flat, and unable to ascend or descend stairways
3	Moderate disability: difficulty in walking on flat, and needs support in ascending or descending stairways
4	Mild disability: no difficulty in walking on flat, but mild difficulty in ascending or descending stairways
5	Normal: normal walking, with or without abnormal reflexes
Score	**Upper Extremity Motor Function**
1	Total disability: totally unable to perform daily activities
2	Severe disability: severe difficulty in daily activities with motor weakness
3	Moderate disability: moderate difficulty in daily activities with hand and/or finger clumsiness
4	Mild disability: no difficulty in daily activities, but mild hand and/or finger clumsiness
5	Normal: normal daily activities, with or without abnormal reflexes
Score	**Sensory Function and/or Pain**
1	Severe disturbance: severe difficulty in daily activities with incapacitating sensory disturbance and/or pain
2	Moderate disturbance: moderate difficulty in daily activities with sensory disturbance and/or pain
3	Mild disturbance: normal daily activities, but mild sensory disturbance and/or pain
4	Normal: neither sensory disturbance nor pain

Table 2
Summary of 9 subjects with mild degenerative myelopathy who underwent surgical treatment

		Preoperative NCSS					
Age & Sex	Disease	L	U	S	Total	IMH	Surgery
56 F	CSM	4	4	3	11	C5-6 (+)	C5-6 anterior fusion
70 M	CSM	4	4	3	11	C7-Th1 (+)	C5-7 laminoplasty
63 M	CSM	5	3	3	11	C3-4 (+)	C3-4 anterior fusion
79 M	CSM	4	3	4	11	(−)	C3-7 laminoplasty
58 M	CSM	4	4	3	11	(−)	C3-5 laminoplasty
68 M	CSM	5	4	2	11	(−)	C5-6,C6-7 anterior fusion
58 F	OPLL	4	4	3	11	C5-6 (+)	C5-6 anterior fusion
50 M	OPLL	5	4	2	11	C3-4 (+)	C2-5 laminoplasty
62 M	OPLL	4	4	3	11	(−)	C4-6 anterior fusion

Abbreviations: F, female; IMH, intramedullary hyperintensity on T2-weighted MRI; L, lower extremity motor function; M, male; S, sensory function and/or pain; U, upper extremity motor function.

presented with only slight or mild long tract symptoms.

All subjects had received conservative treatment such as administration of analgesics or muscle relaxants for their symptoms before the decision of surgical treatment. Five subjects underwent anterior decompression and fusion using titanium cages (see **Figs. 1 and 2**). Bilateral

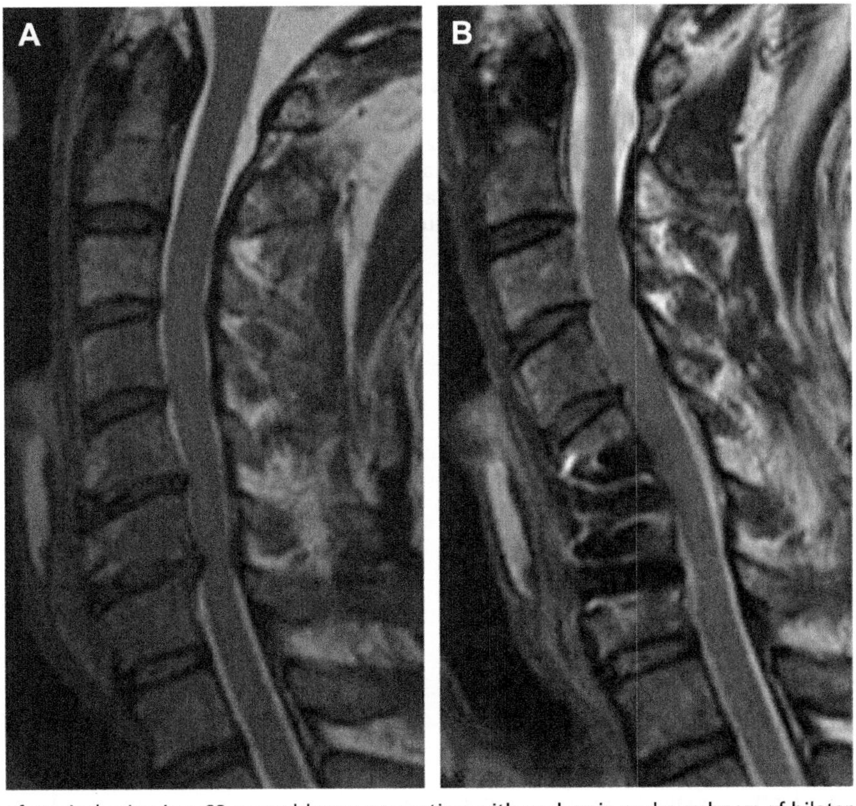

Fig. 1. MRI of cervical spine in a 68-year-old man presenting with neck pain and numbness of bilateral hands for 9 months. (*A*) Preoperative T2-weighted sagittal image showing spinal cord compression at C5-6 and C6-7. (*B*) T2-weighted sagittal image 3 years after anterior fusion at C5-6 and C6-7 using threaded titanium cages showing decompression of the spinal cord.

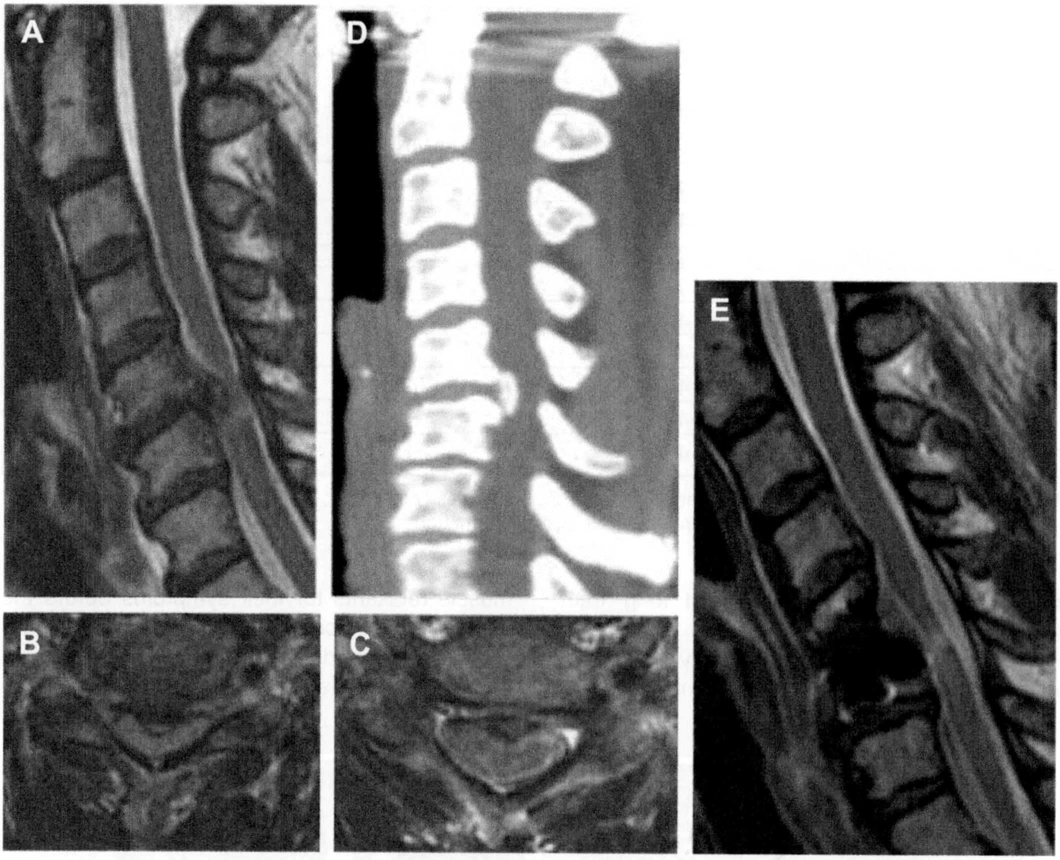

Fig. 2. MRI and CT of the cervical spine in a 58-year-old woman presenting with headache, numbness of bilateral hands, and slight dizziness for 6 months. Preoperative T2-weighted sagittal image (*A*) and axial (*B*, *C*) images at C5-6 showing spinal cord compression with intramedullary hyperintensity. (*D*) Preoperative sagittal reconstruction of CT revealing marked spur formation and OPLL at C5-6. (*E*) T2-weighted sagittal image 3 months after C5-6 anterior decompression and fusion using a titanium mesh cage showing decompression of spinal cord with persistent intramedullary hyperintensity.

open-door laminoplasty was performed in the other 4 subjects (see **Fig. 3**). One subject had a temporary gastrointestinal problem of unknown cause after surgery. There were no postoperative unfavorable events in the other 8 subjects. All subjects showed improved symptoms after surgery, although one subject complained of a persistent headache.

INDICATIONS FOR SURGERY

In this series of mild DCM subjects, 7 subjects (77.8%) complained of numbness of the upper extremities or pain. Persistent pain and/or numbness of upper extremities significantly influenced their quality of life although the motor functions were preserved or slightly impaired. Five subjects (55.6%) were associated with intramedullary signal change on MRI. Such MRI findings promoted the decision to use surgical treatment.

The surgical indication for mild DCM is controversial. According to a randomized study by Kadaěka and colleagues[2] of 64 subjects with the mild or moderate form of CSM, there was no significant difference in clinical outcome evaluated by a mJOA (modified Japanese Orthopedic Association score) scoring system between the conservative and surgical treatment groups. Oshima and colleagues[3] reviewed 45 CSM subjects with mild motor deficits and intramedullary hyperintensity on T2-weighted MRI who were conservatively managed. Their analysis revealed that 56% of these subjects did not deteriorate or did not receive surgery at 10 years. Sumi and colleagues[4] reported on 60 subjects of mild CSM (13 or higher on JOA scoring system) who were conservatively treated. During mean follow-up of 94.3 months, they found that 25.5% showed deterioration of myelopathy, whereas 74.5% maintained mild form of CSM. They also concluded that the mild

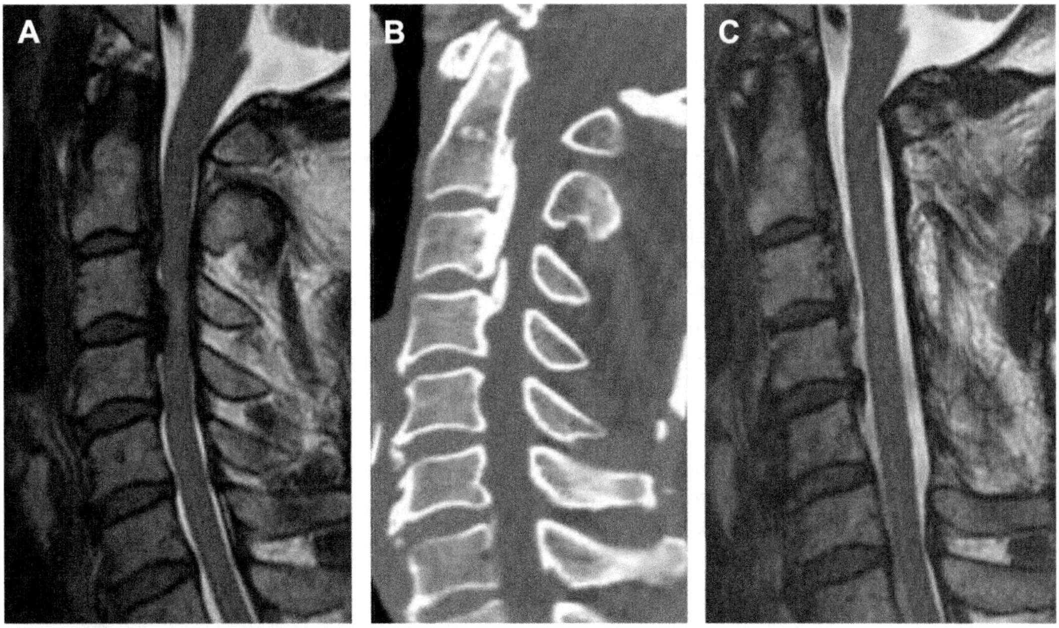

Fig. 3. MRI and CT of the cervical spine in a 50-year-old man presenting with neck pain. (*A*) Preoperative T2-weighted sagittal image showing spinal cord compression from C2 to C5 with intramedullary hyperintensity at C3-4. (*B*) Preoperative sagittal reconstruction of CT demonstrating OPLL from C2 to C4. (*C*) T2-weighted sagittal image 3 years after bilateral open-door laminoplasty from C2 to C5 showing decompression of the spinal cord without intramedullary signal change.

CSM subjects who showed angular-edged deformity of the spinal cord on axial MRI should be considered as candidates for surgical treatment. There have been no reports on the mild form of myelopathy in cervical OPLL. According to Matsunaga and colleagues,[5] 22% of 167 OPLL subjects who were conservatively treated developed aggravated myelopathy with a mean follow-up of 11 years and 2 months. Their analysis indicated that a residual sagittal diameter of the spinal canal less than 6 mm was a definite factor for developing myelopathy, whereas a dynamic factor of the cervical spine influenced myelopathy for the subjects with the residual sagittal diameter of 6 to 14 mm. A study by Koyanagi and colleagues[6] on spinal canal diameter as measured by bone window CT in 64 cervical OPLL subjects showed that a residual sagittal diameter of 8 mm was critical for developing lower extremity motor dysfunction and almost all subjects with residual sagittal diameter of less than 5 mm showed gait disturbance.

INTRAMEDULLARY SIGNAL CHANGE ON MRI

Intramedullary abnormal signal on MRI indicates reversible or irreversible parenchymal changes of the spinal cord. Clinical significance of intramedullary signal changes on MRI has not been fully established, especially in the mild form of DCM. Intramedullary hyperintensity on T2-weighted MRI typically represented cystic degeneration of the gray matter with a snake-eye appearance.[7] Extensive and reversible intramedullary hyperintensity was also reported in CSM patients.[8] Such hyperintensity was observed in 3% of CSM patients and was considered to represent increased interstitial fluid caused by disturbed local venous circulation due to compression.[8] Patients with intramedullary hyperintensity tended to show more severe myelopathy than those without hyperintensity.[7,9,10] Because intramedullary hypointensity on T1-weighted MRI indicated definite cystic change in the spinal cord, patients with signal changes on both on T1-weighted and T2-weighted images were associated with worse postoperative results than those with signal change only in the T2-weighted image in CSM.[11–13] According to Mastronardi and colleagues,[12] reduced areas of intramedullary hyperintensity on a T2-weighted image after surgery was associated with better prognosis.

In the present series, 55.6% of the mild DCM subjects had intramedullary hyperintensity. Postoperative MRI revealed reduced or diminished intramedullary hyperintensity in 3 subjects (see **Fig. 3**).

OPTIONS FOR MANAGEMENT

Treatment of patients with DCM should be determined individually. Patients with mild myelopathy often show preserved quality of life. Conservative treatment, such as use of a cervical collar or medications of muscle relaxant and/or analgesics, should be applied to these cases. Associated pain is an important factor for decision-making if conservative treatment fails to alleviate symptoms. Intramedullary signal change on MRI is another important factor that favors consideration of surgical treatment. To understand the underlying pathologic features of DCM, both MRI and CT scans of the cervical spine should be carefully examined (see **Fig. 2**). From the author's experience, patients with OPLL sometimes show significant spinal cord deformity on MRI with only mild myelopathy. Difficulty of surgery is different in CSM and OPLL patients. Extensive OPLL is often associated with dural ossification.[14] For anterior surgery of extensive OPLL, special surgical techniques, such as careful drilling of OPLL to paper-thin or repair of the dura mater using fibrin glue or fascia tissue, are needed. Management of patients with mild DCM should be decided by considering the benefits and risks of long-term conservative treatments and surgery. The reader is also referred to recent AOSpine-CSRS guidelines on the management of DCM, which provide additional guidance on this topic (available at: http://journals.sagepub.com/toc/gsja/7/3_suppl).

REFERENCES

1. Kadoya S. Grading and scoring system for neurological function in degenerative cervical spine disease–Neurosurgical Cervical Spine Scale. Neurol Med Chir (Tokyo) 1992;32:40–1.
2. Kadaěka Z, Bednařík J, Novotný O, et al. Cervical spondylotic myelopathy: conservative versus surgical treatment after 10 years. Eur Spine J 2011;20:1533–58.
3. Oshima Y, Seichi A, Takeshita K, et al. Natural course and prognostic factors in patients with mild cervical spondylotic myelopathy with increased signal intensity on T2-weighted magnetic resonance imaging. Spine 2012;37:1909–13.
4. Sumi M, Miyamoto H, Suzuki T, et al. Prospective cohort study of mild cervical spondylotic myelopathy without surgical treatment. J Neurosurg Spine 2012;16:8–14.
5. Matsunaga S, Kukita M, Hayashi K, et al. Pathogenesis of myelopathy in patients with ossification of the posterior longitudinal ligament. J Neurosurg 2002;96(2 Suppl):168–72.
6. Koyanagi I, Imamura H, Fujimoto S, et al. Spinal canal size in ossification of the posterior longitudinal ligament of the cervical spine. Surg Neurol 2004;62:286–91.
7. Mizuno J, Nakagawa H, Inoue T, et al. Clinicopathological study of "snake-eye appearance" in compressive myelopathy of the cervical spinal cord. J Neurosurg 2003;99(2 Suppl):162–8.
8. Lee JB, Koyanagi I, Hida K, et al. Spinal cord edema: unusual MR findings in cervical spondylosis. J Neurosurg 2003;99(1 Suppl):8–13.
9. Choi BW, Hum TW. Significance of intramedullary high signal intensity on magnetic resonance imaging in patients with cervical ossification of the posterior longitudinal ligament. Clin Orthop Surg 2015;7:465–9.
10. Koyanagi I, Iwasaki Y, Hida K, et al. Magnetic resonance imaging findings in ossification of the posterior longitudinal ligament of the cervical spine. J Neurosurg 1998;88:247–54.
11. Alafifi T, Kern R, Fehlings M. Clinical and MRI predictors of outcome after surgical intervention for cervical spondylotic myelopathy. J Neuroimaging 2007;17:315–22.
12. Mastronardi L, Elsawaf A, Roperto R, et al. Prognostic relevance of the postoperative evolution of intramedullary spinal cord changes in signal intensity on magnetic resonance imaging after anterior decompression for cervical spondylotic myelopathy. J Neurosurg Spine 2007;7:615–22.
13. Yagi M, Ninomiya K, Kihara M, et al. Long-term surgical outcome and risk factors in patients with cervical myelopathy and a change in signal intensity of intramedullary spinal cord on Magnetic Resonance imaging. J Neurosurg Spine 2010;12:59–65.
14. Hida K, Iwasaki Y, Koyanagi I, et al. Bone window computed tomography for detection of dural defect associated with cervical ossified posterior longitudinal ligament. Neurol Med Chir (Tokyo) 1997;37:173–6.

Management of the Patient with Cervical Cord Compression but no Evidence of Myelopathy

What Should We do?

Kentaro Naito, MD[a], Toru Yamagata, MD[b], Kenji Ohata, MD[a], Toshihiro Takami, MD[a,*]

KEYWORDS

- Aging spine • Cervical spondylotic myelopathy • Degenerative cervical myelopathy
- Degenerative disk disease • Ossification of the posterior longitudinal ligament

KEY POINTS

- Cervical spondylosis, disk herniation, and ossification of the posterior longitudinal ligament are common age-related disorders, collectively referred to as degenerative cervical myelopathy (DCM), that eventually affects not only activities of daily living but also quality of life.
- DCM is usually a gradually progressive, sometimes irreversible, disease of the cervical spinal cord, although there is always a risk of acute deterioration caused by minor trauma.
- There is still not enough evidence regarding the prognosis of mild or moderate DCM without surgical treatment, and conservative treatment seems fairly successful and has an acceptable tolerance rate in the literature.
- Surgeons need to understand the importance of decision making in the surgical management of mild DCM, and they must carefully consider that patients' symptoms of pain or gait disturbance may seriously affect their activities of daily living and overall mental health.
- Careful imaging using not only conventional MRI but also the latest 3T-diffusion tensor imaging technology may help surgeons determine surgical indications in patients with mild DCM.

INTRODUCTION

Cervical spondylosis, disk herniation, and ossification of the posterior longitudinal ligament are common age-related disorders. Cervical spondylosis may result in compression of the spinal cord causing gait disturbance, clumsy hands, and/or sensory disturbance and may eventually affect a patient's quality of life. Collectively, such functional disturbance, accompanied by characteristic

Disclosure Statement: The authors report no conflicts of interest concerning the materials or methods used in this study or the findings specified in this article. All authors who are members of the Japan Neurosurgical Society (JNS) have completed on-line self-reported conflict-of-interest disclosure statement forms through the Web site for JNS members.

[a] Department of Neurosurgery, Osaka City University Graduate School of Medicine, 1-4-3 Asahi-machi, Abeno-ku, Osaka 545-8585, Japan; [b] Department of Neurosurgery, Osaka City General Hospital, 2-13-22 Miyakojima-hondori, Miyakojima-ku, Osaka 531-0021, Japan

* Corresponding author. Department of Neurosurgery, Osaka City University Graduate School of Medicine, 1-4-3 Asahi-machi, Abeno-ku, Osaka 545-8585, Japan.

E-mail address: ttakami@med.osaka-cu.ac.jp

Neurosurg Clin N Am 29 (2018) 145–152
https://doi.org/10.1016/j.nec.2017.09.010
1042-3680/18/© 2017 Elsevier Inc. All rights reserved.

findings on physical examination and concordant imaging abnormalities, is called degenerative cervical myelopathy (DCM).[1–4] DCM is usually a gradually progressive, sometimes irreversible, condition of the cervical spinal cord, although there is always a risk of acute deterioration with minor trauma. Patients with DCM who demonstrate significant neurologic symptoms are excellent candidates for decompressive surgery.[5] Surgical outcomes are usually favorable, although there are sometimes surgery-related complications. It may be acceptable and recommended for patients with moderate or severe neurologic symptoms to have spinal decompression or fusion surgery early after imaging confirmation of cervical cord compression with clear evidence of myelopathy. There is no definite agreement, however, on the surgical indications for patients who have cervical cord compression but no evidence of myelopathy (**Fig. 1**).

This article discusses the clinical issue of how to manage patients who have cervical cord compression but no evidence of myelopathy. Attention is focused on the prognosis for mild DCM without surgical treatment, the indications for prophylactic surgery for mild DCM, and finally the latest imaging technology using 3T–diffusion tensor (DT) MRI parameters to assess the condition of the cervical spinal cord.

PROGNOSIS FOR MILD OR MODERATE DEGENERATIVE CERVICAL MYELOPATHY WITHOUT SURGICAL TREATMENT

Not enough evidence regarding the prognosis for mild DCM without surgical treatment currently exists. A recent literature review suggests its benign or acceptable course without significant deterioration of neurologic conditions (**Table 1**).[6–12] This literature review is also supplemented by recent systematic reviews and guidelines, which have been jointly developed by Fehlings and colleagues with the support of AOSpine and the Cervical Spine Research Society (see http://journals.sagepub.com/toc/gsja/7/3_suppl). These guidelines recommend surgical treatment of patients with moderate or severe DCM and either a structured course of rehabilitation with careful clinical follow-up or operative intervention for patients with mild DCM. For patients with cord compression but myelopathic features, careful clinical follow-up is recommended. Surgery is an option, however, for those individuals with cord compression and symptoms or signs of nerve root compromise.

Matsumoto and colleagues[6] retrospectively investigated whether increased signal intensity on T2-weighted MRI can predict the outcome of DCM with conservative treatment. A satisfactory outcome was recognized in 78% of patients

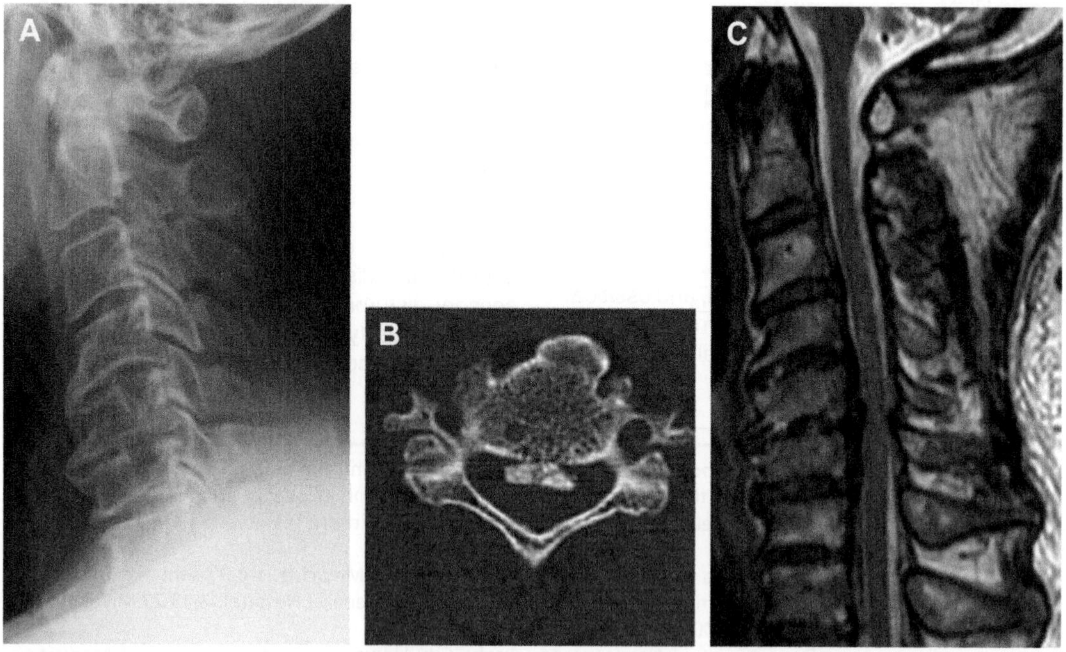

Fig. 1. Mild DCM. (*A*) Plain lateral radiograph of 68-year-old man with mild neck stiffness and JOA score of 16. (*B*) His cervical spine demonstrated a straight spine with ossification of the posterior longitudinal ligament at the C5-6 level that was more evident on CT scan. (*C*) MRI demonstrated moderate compression of the spinal cord at the C5-6 level with faint signal change of the spinal cord on T2-weighted images.

Table 1
Recent literature review of clinical studies focusing on conservative treatment of mild or moderate degenerative cervical myelopathy

Authors, Year	Study Design	No. of Patients	Inclusion Criteria	Duration of Follow-up	Clinical Course (%)		
					Improved	Steady	Deteriorated
Matsumoto et al,[6] 2000	Retrospective	52	JOA $\geq$10	3 y	69		31
Yoshimatsu et al,[7] 2001	Retrospective	69	JOA $\geq$13	29 mo	23	15	62
Kadaňka et al,[8] 2002	Prospective	35	JOA $\geq$12, Age <75 y	3 y	1.9	70.8	27.3
Bednarik et al,[9] 2004	Prospective	66	Without myelopathy With radiculopathy or axial pain	4 y	80.3		19.7
Shimomura et al,[10] 2007	Prospective	56	JOA $\geq$13	35.6 mo	80.4		19.6
Oshima et al,[11] 2012	Retrospective	45	Motor of JOA $\geq$3 (both arms and legs)	78 mo	60.0		40.0
Sumi et al,[12] 2012	Prospective	55	JOA $\geq$13	33.6 mo (deteriorated) 94.3 mo (steady)	74.5		25.5

without increased signal intensity, in 63% of those with focal increased signal intensity, and in 70% of those with multisegmental increased signal intensity. They concluded that increased signal intensity on MRI was not related to the outcome of DCM with conservative treatment. Yoshimatsu and colleagues[7] investigated the results of conservative treatment of cervical spondylotic myelopathy (CSM) in 69 patients. Multivariate analysis indicated a significant correlation between clinical outcome and the disease duration or the presence of rigorous conservative treatment. They suggested the importance of timely surgical intervention when the symptoms do not change or are exacerbated with conservative treatment. Kadaňka and colleagues[8] conducted a 3-year prospective randomized study to compare conservative and surgical treatment of mild, moderate, nonprogressive, and slowly progressive types of DCM. They randomly divided the patients into 2 groups: conservative treatment and surgical treatment. Their 3-year follow-up study did not show that surgical treatment is superior to conservative treatment of mild or moderate DCM. Bednarik and colleagues[9] conducted a cohort study of clinically asymptomatic patients with DCM. A total of 66 patients with MRI signs of spondylotic cervical cord compression but without clear clinical signs of myelopathy was followed prospectively for at least 2 years. The tolerance rate in their study was 80.3%. They suggested that electrophysiological abnormalities with clinical signs of cervical radiculopathy could predict clinical manifestations of preclinical spondylotic cervical cord compression. Shimomura and colleagues[10] conducted a prospective clinical study for mild DCM. Nonsurgical treatment was selected for 56 patients with mild DCM (Japanese Orthopedic Association [JOA] score $\geq$13 points). The tolerance rate in their study was 80.4%. They suggested that the most important prognostic factor for mild DCM was circumferential spinal cord compression in the maximally compressed segment on axial MRI. Oshima and colleagues[11] conducted a retrospective comparative study to investigate the natural course and prognostic factors in patients with mild DCM, focusing on intramedullary increased signal intensity on T2-weighted MRI. A total of 45 patients were enrolled in their study. Twenty of 45 patients (60%) were stable during a mean follow-up period of 78 months. They suggested that a large range of motion, segmental kyphosis, and instability at the narrowest canal were adverse prognostic factors. Sumi and colleagues[12] analyzed the prognosis of mild CSM without surgical intervention by evaluation of clinical symptoms and MRI findings. They classified patients into 2 study groups: ovoid deformity and angular-edge deformity based on the spinal cord shape seen on axial slices on T1-weighted MRI. They suggested that the overall tolerance rate for mild CSM was 70%, although the tolerance rate for patients with angular-edged deformity was 58%. They concluded that surgical treatment of mild CSM should be considered when patients with mild CSM have an angular-edge deformity on MRI.

The prognosis for mild DCM without surgical treatment seems fairly successful, with an acceptable tolerance rate in the literature. Surgeons need to be aware of the role of nonsurgical intervention for mild DCM, although there is always a risk of acute deterioration after minor trauma or with poor response to conservative treatment. Careful follow-up helps surgeons determine the indications for and timing of surgical intervention.

INDICATIONS FOR PROPHYLACTIC SURGERY FOR MILD DEGENERATIVE CERVICAL MYELOPATHY

There is no clear agreement on the surgical indications for mild DCM, and various reports in the literature have suggested the superiority or inferiority of surgery versus conservative treatment.[13–15] Some patients with mild or moderate DCM present with gradual or slowly progressive symptoms, and others present with acute deterioration after minor trauma. It is still difficult, however, to predict possible clinical outcomes without surgical treatment. There may be general agreement on predictive factors affecting surgical outcomes, such as age or duration of symptoms, although MRI or physiologic studies cannot accurately differentiate patients who will benefit from surgery from those who will not. Surgical treatment, such as laminectomy or laminoplasty, may improve neurologic dysfunction in some patients with DCM and prevent worsening in others but is associated with significant surgery-related risks. These risks should be carefully considered when determining the indications for prophylactic surgery in patients with mild or moderate DCM.

Tracy and Bartleson[16] proposed that neurologists should be familiar with this very common condition and suggested that surgical decompression from an anterior or posterior approach should be considered in patients with progressive and moderate-to-severe neurologic deficits. Neo and colleagues[17] suggested that decompression surgery can rescue well-informed and deliberately selected patients with only slight myelopathy because it can improve their symptoms and free them from persistent anxiety. Stoffman and colleagues[18] surveyed a cohort of

89 patients with CSM during 1 year. They demonstrated that 29% of the cohort had a depressed mood and 38% had an anxious mood, and higher depression scores were associated worse myelopathy, compared with arm scale, sphincter scale, or sensory scale. They concluded that ambulatory dysfunction may cause or exacerbate the symptoms of depression and anxiety in patients with CSM. Recent analysis of the AOSpine North America prospective multicenter study indicated that cervical decompression not only arrested progression but also improved neurologic outcomes, functional status, and quality of life in patients regardless of the degree of myelopathy.[19] Although indications and careful consideration of selection for anterior or posterior cervical spine surgery need to be discussed, there may be no significant differences in functional and quality-of-life outcomes between patients treated with anterior surgery and those treated with posterior surgery for DCM. There is no absolute indication to determine the association between surgical approach and postoperative outcome or surgery-related complications. Another analysis of the prospective AOSpine international and North America multicenter study focusing on comparison of clinical outcomes in patients with and without preexisting depression or bipolar disorder undergoing surgery for DCM demonstrated that patients with depression or bipolar disorder have fewer functional and quality-of-life improvements after surgery compared with patients without psychiatric comorbidities.[20]

Although there is no clear agreement on the surgical indications for mild DCM, symptoms of pain or gait disturbance may be the key factors suggesting the need for surgical intervention because they may considerably affect not only the activities of daily living but also overall mental health in patients with mild or moderate DCM. Surgeons need to carefully consider the indications for surgery using both evidence-based medicine and narrative-based medicine.

Illustrative Case 1

A 37-year-old man presented with mild neck stiffness. He had a transient episode of acute neck pain after physical exercise. Careful assessment revealed his activities of daily living using the JOA score to be 16. Plain lateral radiograph of his cervical spine demonstrated a mildly kyphotic spine at C5-6. MRI demonstrated the existence of a disk herniation at C5-6 with moderate compression of the spinal cord (**Fig. 2**A). The

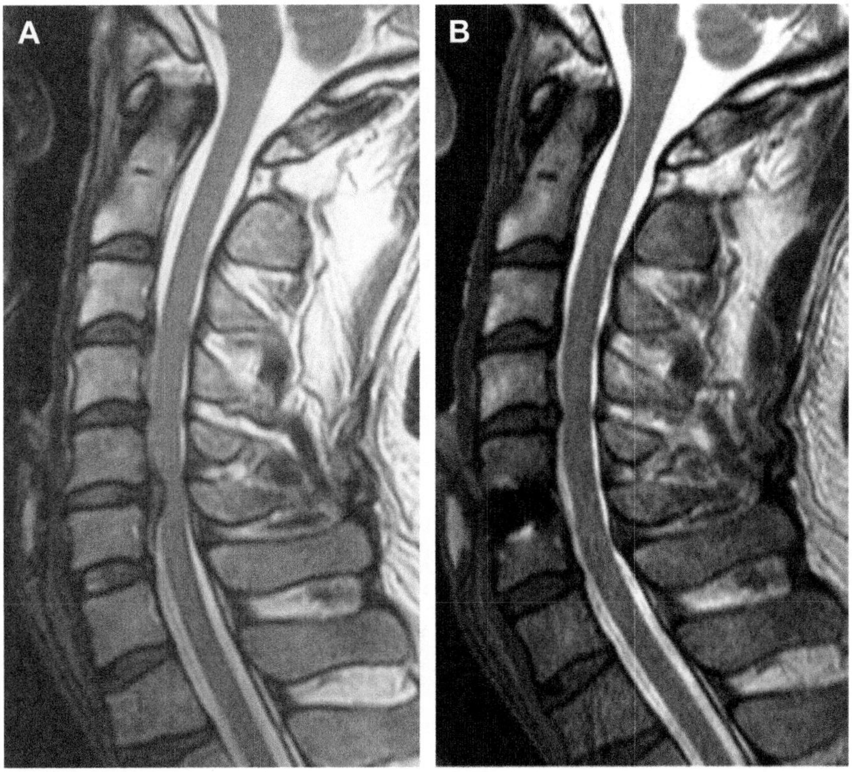

Fig. 2. Illustrative case 1 — before and after surgery. (*A*) Before surgery; (*B*) 13 years after anterior cervical discectomy and fusion at C5-6 using a rectangular titanium stand-alone cage.

patient demonstrated a significantly anxious mood and decreased ability to participate in strenuous work. He underwent anterior cervical discectomy and fusion at C5-6 using a rectangular titanium stand-alone cage. His postoperative course was uneventful. Thirteen years after surgery, he is without significant symptoms or limitations and is actively working as a surgeon (**Fig. 2**B).

Illustrative Case 2

A 68-year-old woman presented with dysesthesia and limb apraxia of her hands as well as mild gait disturbance. Careful assessment revealed her JOA score to be 14. Plain lateral radiograph of the cervical spine demonstrated a straight spine. MRI demonstrated the existence of multisegment stenosis of the spinal cord without increased signal intensity on T2-weighted imaging (**Fig. 3**A). Conservative treatment eventually failed to improve her symptoms. She underwent posterior cervical decompression with selective laminectomy. Her postoperative course was uneventful. Postoperative MRI demonstrated good decompression of the spinal cord (**Fig. 3**B).

3T–DIFFUSION TENSOR MRI PARAMETERS

Diagnostic imaging using CT or MRI is available for spinal structural diagnosis. These modalities can suggest the presence of myelopathy to some degree in cases of DCM, but there have been some exceptions reported of patients without myelopathy despite anatomic cord compression. Intramedullary T2-weighted magnetic resonance (MR) signals are most commonly applied to clarify the spinal cord condition, for example, to suggest myelomalacia.[21] The degree of intramedullary T2-weighted MR signals, however, does not necessarily correlate with neurologic function. The assessment for diseases of the spinal cord is not always straightforward, even with these diagnostic studies. To examine for the existence or degree of DCM, subjective neurologic scoring or grading systems are still widely used. Motor function can be examined to some degree by assessing muscle strength, but objective sensory or autonomic nervous system examination can be easily affected by mood or psychological conditions. Somatosensory evoked magnetic field dipole measurements by magnetoencephalography may be somewhat helpful for the objective assessment of sensory function.[22]

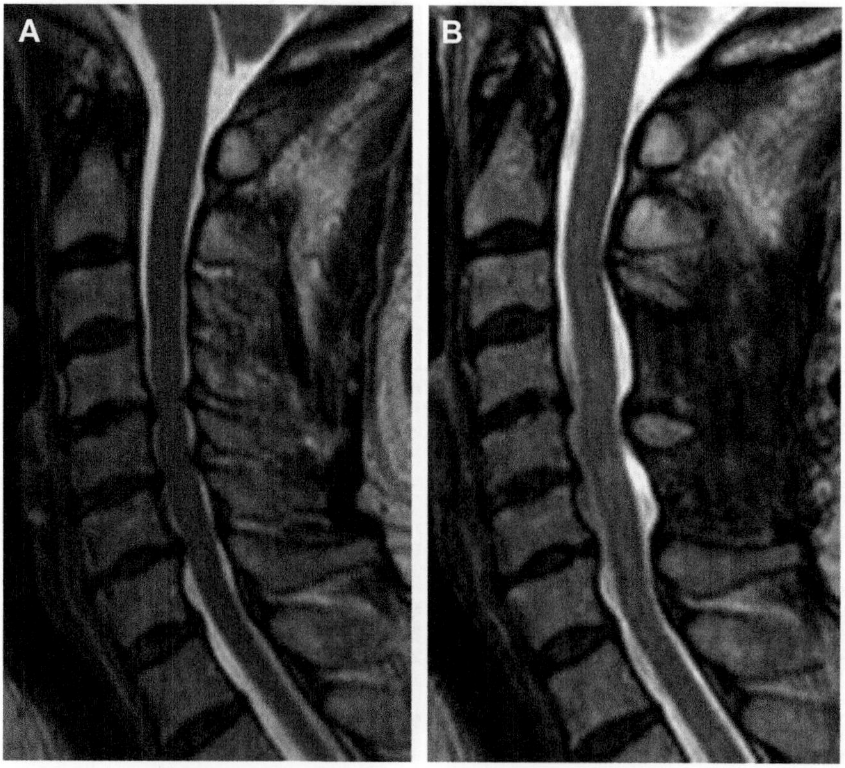

Fig. 3. Illustrative case 2 — before and after surgery. (*A*) Before surgery; (*B*) 1 year after posterior cervical decompression with selective laminectomy.

Magnetoencephalography is available, however, only at a few institutions and is not in widespread use. Therefore, more accurate and objective diagnostic modalities for the assessment of conditions of the spinal cord are truly necessary to determine the surgical indications in patients with DCM.

DT imaging is an MRI-based technology and is becoming popular in its use.[23–25] It can provide not only fiber tracking images but also quantitative diffusion parameters. Mean diffusivity (MD) and fractional anisotropy (FA) are commonly used as quantitative DT parameters. MD represents the degree of diffusional motion of water molecules (regardless of direction) and can be measured in units of square millimeters per second (mm^2/s). FA represents a rotationally invariant parameter ranging from 0 to 1; 0 represents completely isotropic diffusion, and 1 represents extremely limited diffusion in only 1 direction. These DT parameters are promising modalities for quantitative evaluation of the condition of the spinal cord and may be more sensitive for the assessment of early-stage DCM than conventional diagnostic imaging.[26–33] Quantitative analysis using DT parameters is a well-established technique for the detection of pathologic changes that are not evident in conventional MRI, even at a very early stage. Application of DT imaging to the spinal cord has been limited because of anatomic disadvantages that include the relatively small size of the spinal cord and surrounding structures (such as the cerebrospinal fluid, vertebrae, and air in the trachea). These disadvantages tend to produce susceptibility artifacts. More recently, technical advancements have made it possible to acquire good-quality DT images of the cervical spinal cord. For clinical applications, there have been several studies evaluating demyelination and degenerative spinal cord diseases with DT parameters. Increased MD and/or decreased FA at lesion sites seem to reflect tissue condition. These changes have been attributed to a chronically poor blood supply and histopathologic changes (including gliosis, microcystic degeneration, venous congestion, and extracellular edema) that lead to increased water mobility and decrease anisotropy. DT parameters can provide information regarding structural damage of the cervical spinal cord that may be closely related to the extent of neurologic dysfunction. In symptomatic patients with DCM, DT parameters could potentially suggest the neurologic condition or the prognosis, even after surgery.

SUMMARY

The surgical outcomes for DCM are usually favorable, although there are surgery-related complications in limited cases. There may be agreement on the surgical indications for moderate or severe DCM, but there is still no definite agreement on the surgical indications for mild or moderate or DCM. The prognosis for mild or moderate DCM without surgical treatment seems fairly successful, with an acceptable tolerance rate in the literature. Surgeons need to understand the importance of decision making in the surgical management of mild or moderate DCM, and they must carefully consider that patients' symptoms of pain or gait disturbance may seriously affect their activities of daily living and overall mental health. Careful imaging analysis using conventional MRI as well as the latest 3T-DT imaging technology may help surgeons to determine the surgical indications in patients with mild or moderate DCM.

REFERENCES

1. Kalsi-Ryan S, Karadimas SK, Fehlings MG. Cervical spondylotic myelopathy: the clinical phenomenon and the current pathobiology of an increasingly prevalent and devastating disorder. Neuroscientist 2013;19(4):409–21.
2. Fehlings MG, Tetreault LA, Wilson JR, et al. Cervical spondylotic myelopathy: current state of the art and future directions. Spine (Phila Pa 1976) 2013;38(22 Suppl 1):S1–8.
3. Nouri A, Tetreault L, Singh A, et al. Degenerative cervical myelopathy: epidemiology, genetics, and pathogenesis. Spine (Phila Pa 1976) 2015;40(12): E675–93.
4. Tetreault L, Goldstein CL, Arnold P, et al. Degenerative cervical myelopathy: a spectrum of related disorders affecting the aging spine. Neurosurgery 2015;77(Suppl 4):S51–67.
5. Lawrence BD, Shamji MF, Traynelis VC, et al. Surgical management of degenerative cervical myelopathy: a consensus statement. Spine (Phila Pa 1976) 2013;38(22 Suppl 1):S171–2.
6. Matsumoto M, Toyama Y, Ishikawa M, et al. Increased signal intensity of the spinal cord on magnetic resonance images in cervical compressive myelopathy. Does it predict the outcome of conservative treatment? Spine (Phila Pa 1976) 2000;25(6): 677–82.
7. Yoshimatsu H, Nagata K, Goto H, et al. Conservative treatment for cervical spondylotic myelopathy. prediction of treatment effects by multivariate analysis. Spine J 2001;1(4):269–73.
8. Kadaňka Z, Mares M, Bednaník J, et al. Approaches to spondylotic cervical myelopathy: conservative versus surgical results in a 3-year follow-up study. Spine (Phila Pa 1976) 2002; 27(20):2205–11.

9. Bednarik J, Kadanka Z, Dusek L, et al. Presymptomatic spondylotic cervical cord compression. Spine (Phila Pa 1976) 2004;29(20):2260–9.
10. Shimomura T, Sumi M, Nishida K, et al. Prognostic factors for deterioration of patients with cervical spondylotic myelopathy after nonsurgical treatment. Spine (Phila Pa 1976) 2007;32(22):2474–9.
11. Oshima Y, Seichi A, Takeshita K, et al. Natural course and prognostic factors in patients with mild cervical spondylotic myelopathy with increased signal intensity on T2-weighted magnetic resonance imaging. Spine (Phila Pa 1976) 2012;37(22):1909–13.
12. Sumi M, Miyamoto H, Suzuki T, et al. Prospective cohort study of mild cervical spondylotic myelopathy without surgical treatment. J Neurosurg Spine 2012;16(1):8–14.
13. Sampath P, Bendebba M, Davis JD, et al. Outcome of patients treated for cervical myelopathy. A prospective, multicenter study with independent clinical review. Spine (Phila Pa 1976) 2000;25(6):670–6.
14. Kadaňka Z, Bednařík J, Novotný O, et al. Cervical spondylotic myelopathy: conservative versus surgical treatment after 10 years. Eur Spine J 2011; 20(9):1533–8.
15. Li FN, Li ZH, Huang X, et al. The treatment of mild cervical spondylotic myelopathy with increased signal intensity on T2-weighted magnetic resonance imaging. Spinal Cord 2014;52(5):348–53.
16. Tracy JA, Bartleson JD. Cervical spondylotic myelopathy. Neurologist 2010;16(3):176–87.
17. Neo M, Fujibayashi S, Takemoto M, et al. Clinical results of and patient satisfaction with cervical laminoplasty for considerable cord compression with only slight myelopathy. Eur Spine J 2012;21(2):340–6.
18. Stoffman MR, Roberts MS, King JT Jr. Cervical spondylotic myelopathy, depression, and anxiety: a cohort analysis of 89 patients. Neurosurgery 2005; 57(2):307–13.
19. Fehlings MG, Wilson JR, Kopjar B, et al. Efficacy and safety of surgical decompression in patients with cervical spondylotic myelopathy: results of the AOSpine North America prospective multi-center study. J Bone Joint Surg Am 2013;95(18):1651–8.
20. Tetreault L, Nagoshi N, Nakashima H, et al. Impact of depression and bipolar disorders on functional and quality of life outcomes in patients undergoing surgery for degenerative cervical myelopathy: analysis of a combined prospective dataset. Spine (Phila Pa 1976) 2017;42(6):372–8.
21. Wada E, Ohmura M, Yonenobu K. Intramedullary changes of the spinal cord in cervical spondylotic myelopathy. Spine (Phila Pa 1976) 1995;20(20): 2226–32.
22. Goto T, Tsuyuguchi N, Ohata K, et al. Usefulness of somatosensory evoked magnetic field dipole measurements by magnetoencephalography for assessing spinal cord function. J Neurosurg 2002;96(1 Suppl):62–7.
23. Ries M, Jones RA, Dousset V, et al. Diffusion tensor MRI of the spinal cord. Magn Reson Med 2000; 44(6):884–92.
24. Le Bihan D, Mangin JF, Poupon C, et al. Diffusion tensor imaging: concepts and applications. J Magn Reson Imaging 2001;13(4):534–46.
25. Wheeler-Kingshott CA, Hickman SJ, Parker GJ, et al. Investigating cervical spinal cord structure using axial diffusion tensor imaging. Neuroimage 2002; 16(1):93–102.
26. Facon D, Ozanne A, Fillard P, et al. MR diffusion tensor imaging and fiber tracking in spinal cord compression. AJNR Am J Neuroradiol 2005;26(6): 1587–94.
27. Mamata H, Jolesz FA, Maier SE. Apparent diffusion coefficient and fractional anisotropy in spinal cord: age and cervical spondylosis-related changes. J Magn Reson Imaging 2005;22(1):38–43.
28. Hori M, Okubo T, Aoki S, et al. Line scan diffusion tensor MRI at low magnetic field strength: feasibility study of cervical spondylotic myelopathy in an early clinical stage. J Magn Reson Imaging 2006;23(2): 183–8.
29. Agosta F, Lagana M, Valsasina P, et al. Evidence for cervical cord tissue disorganisation with aging by diffusion tensor MRI. Neuroimage 2007;36(3): 728–35.
30. Ellingson BM, Ulmer JL, Kurpad SN, et al. Diffusion tensor MR imaging in chronic spinal cord injury. AJNR Am J Neuroradiol 2008;29(10):1976–82.
31. Uda T, Takami T, Sakamoto S, et al. Normal variation of diffusion tensor parameters of the spinal cord in healthy subjects at 3.0-Tesla. J Craniovertebr Junction Spine 2011;2(2):77–81.
32. Uda T, Takami T, Tsuyuguchi N, et al. Assessment of cervical spondylotic myelopathy using diffusion tensor magnetic resonance imaging parameter at 3.0 tesla. Spine (Phila Pa 1976) 2013;38(5): 407–14.
33. Arima H, Sakamoto S, Naito K, et al. Prediction of the efficacy of surgical intervention in patients with cervical myelopathy by using diffusion tensor 3T-magnetic resonance imaging parameters. J Craniovertebr Junction Spine 2015;6(3):120–4.

Clinical Characteristics and Management of C3-4 Degenerative Cervical Myelopathy

Masato Tomii, MD*, Junichi Mizuno, MD, PhD

KEYWORDS

- C3-4 level • Cervical spondylotic myelopathy • Degenerative cervical myelopathy
- Anterior cervical discectomy and fusion • Instability

KEY POINTS

- C3-4 myelopathy cases show that the patients were elderly.
- Cervical motion was dependent on the C3-4 segment.
- A dynamic factor (instability) at C3-4 level contributed more to the major causes of myelopathy than the static factors.

INTRODUCTION

Cervical spondylosis (CS) at the C3-4 level (segment) usually presents with cervical spondylotic myelopathy (CSM), which is the most common subtype of degenerative cervical myelopathy (DCM). A variety of symptoms are characteristic, such as hand clumsiness and cerebellar signs, and the incidence is 5 times higher in older than younger patients.[1–4] On the other hand, lower cervical level anterior cervical discectomy and fusion (ACDF) is commonly performed in relatively young patients compared with C3-4 ACDF patients. The morphologic features of patients with CSM caused by C3-4 level spondylosis were studied to understand this unique phenomenon.

MATERIALS AND METHODS

Between February 2003 and January 2013, 713 patients were surgically treated by ACDF in the Department of Neurosurgery, Southern TOHOKU General Hospital, and Department of Neurosurgery, Southern TOHOKU Research Institute for Neuroscience, Southern TOHOKU General Hospital. Single-level ACDF at C3-4 was performed in 53 CSM patients (38 men and 15 women) (group I). Clinical outcomes were assessed according to the Japanese Orthopedic Association (JOA) score, the Neurosurgical Cervical Spine Scale (NCSS), and the Nurick scale. The evaluation system for CSM proposed by the JOA score (maximum score = 17 points) was used to evaluate the severity of myelopathy.[5] The recovery rate of the JOA score (%) was calculated using the following formula: (postoperative JOA score − preoperative JOA score)/(17 − preoperative JOA score) × 100. The neurologic state of the patient was evaluated using the NCSS (maximum score = 14 points), a method of scoring motor function of the upper and lower extremities and sensory deficits.[6] The recovery rate of the NCSS (%) was calculated using the following formula: (postoperative

Conflicts of Interest Disclosure: The authors declare that they have no conflict of interest.
Department of Neurosurgery, Southern TOHOKU General Hospital, Iwanuma, Miyagi, Japan
* Corresponding author. Department of Neurosurgery, Southern TOHOKU General Hospital, 1-2-5 Satonomori Iwanuma, Iwanuma, Miyagi 989-2483, Japan.
E-mail address: masatotomii@ybb.ne.jp

Neurosurg Clin N Am 29 (2018) 153–158
https://doi.org/10.1016/j.nec.2017.09.011
1042-3680/18/© 2017 Elsevier Inc. All rights reserved.

NCSS − preoperative NCSS)/(14 − preoperative NCSS) ×100. Changes of disability in walking were rated according to the Nurick scale.[7] Patients were examined, and the data were recorded preoperatively and at the latest postoperative follow-up. The mean duration of follow-up was 67.2 months (range, 21–114 months). Next, the following radiological parameters were recorded: (1) anteroposterior (AP) spinal canal diameter at the center level of the C3 vertebral body; (2) C2-7 lordosis (alignment); (3) C3-4 range of intervertebral motion (ROM); (4) C2-7 ROM; and (5) %ROM at C3-4. (1) and (2) were assessed by measuring preoperative lateral cervical spine radiographs in the neutral position. Lateral cervical spine radiographs were taken with a distance of 1.5 m between the x-ray tube and the film in all subjects, and the films were correctly placed along a gravity plumb line. Spinal canal diameter at the center level of the C3 vertebral body was measured by Boijsen method.[8] C2-7 lordosis was measured by the Jackson physiologic stress lines method for measuring cervical curvature.[9] The method requires drawing 2 lines, both parallel to the posterior surface of the C7 and C2 vertebral bodies and measuring the angle between them. A positive value means lordosis. C3-4 ROM and C2-7 ROM were assessed by measuring cervical spine radiographs that were taken with the neck in maximum flexion and extension positions. Percent segmental mobility at C3-4 (%ROM) was calculated by (C3-4 ROM/C2-7 ROM) × 100 (%). In addition, to compare the pathogenesis of CS of the non–C3-4 ACDF patients, a randomly sampled group of 53 non–C3-4 ACDF patients (40 men and 13 women), including 32 with CSM and 21 with radiculopathy, was also studied (group II). Each patient was examined, and the data were recorded preoperatively and at the latest postoperative follow-up. Clinical outcomes were then assessed. The mean duration of follow-up was 60.8 months (range, 36–121 months). The radiological findings for numbers (2) to (5) were evaluated in group II as in group I. All images were transferred to the computer as Digital Imaging and Communications in Medicine data. Each parameter was measured by 2 experienced neurosurgeons (M.T. and J.M.) using imaging software (GE Medical Systems [Milwaukee, Wisconsin], Centricity Enterprise Web V 3.0.10). Average value was taken as the final measurement value to minimize intraobserver error.

Statistical Analysis

Continuous variables are presented as means ± SD with ranges. The Mann-Whitney U-test was used for evaluating intergroup differences. Differences were considered significant at a probability level of 95% ($P \leq .05$). All statistical analyses were performed with a commercially available software program (IBM SPSS Statistics for Windows, Version 19.0. Armonk, NY: IBM Corp., USA).

RESULTS

The mean age at the time of operation was 72.3 years ± 10.1 years (range, 34–89 years) in group I and 59.4 years ± 13.2 years (range, 35–83 years) in group II; the difference was significant ($P<.001$). The mean duration of preoperative symptoms was 6.0 months ± 8.4 months in group I and 6.4 months ± 7.0 months in group II, with no significant difference between the 2 groups ($P = .1126$).

As for clinical outcome, in group I, the JOA score ranged from 11.4 ± 2.7 preoperatively to 14.7 ± 1.9 at the final follow-up. The NCSS ranged from 9.2 ± 2.0 preoperatively to 12.1 ± 1.5 at the final follow-up. The Nurick score ranged from 2.1 ± 1.2 preoperatively to 1.2 ± 0.9 at the final follow-up. All 3 scores were significantly improved after surgery ($P<.001$ for the JOA score and NCSS, $P = .0004$ for the Nurick score). Meanwhile in group II, the JOA score ranged from 12.1 ± 1.6 preoperatively to 14.9 ± 1.7 at the final follow-up. The NCSS ranged from 9.3 ± 1.7 preoperatively to 12.1 ± 1.3 at the final follow-up. The Nurick score ranged from 0.6 ± 0.8 preoperatively to 0.3 ± 0.5 at the final follow-up. The JOA score and NCSS were significantly improved after surgery ($P<.001$ for the JOA score and NCSS), but there was no difference in the Nurick score between before and after surgery ($P = .1599$).

The recovery rates of the JOA score and the NCSS in group I were 62.5% ± 23.0% and 62.1% ± 23.6%, respectively. The recovery rates of the JOA score and NCSS in group II were 61.3% ± 20.9% and 61.1% ± 23.2%, respectively. There were no significant differences between the 2 groups in both scores ($P = .9500$ for the JOA score and 0.7792 for the NCSS).

The AP canal diameter of group I was 11.3 mm ± 2.3 mm. For standing sagittal alignment, C2-7 lordosis was 18.3 ± 11.6° in group I and 9.5 ± 6.5° in group II; there was a significant difference between the 2 groups ($P<.001$). C2-7 ROM was 37.5 ± 15.4° in group I and 39.1 ± 12.5° in group II; there was no significant difference between the 2 groups ($P = .3318$). C3-4 ROM was 13.3 ± 5.8° in group I and 6.5 ± 3.9° in group II, however, and C3-4 %ROM was 39.8 ± 23.0% in group I and 16.9% ± 10.3% in group II. There were significant differences between the 2 groups

($P<.001$ for C3-4 ROM and C3-4 %ROM). Group I showed greater C3-4 ROM than group II (**Table 1**).

ILLUSTRATIVE CASE

An 84-year-old woman presented with a 6-month history of numbness and pain in both hands and legs. Neurologic examination showed spastic tetraparesis, and fine finger movement was severely impaired. Her gait was spastic; she could not walk without assist. Radiological examination revealed severe cervical canal stenosis with instability at C3-4 (C2-7 lordosis 9°, C2-7 ROM 34.6°, C3-4 ROM 16.8°, and C3-4 %ROM 48.6%) (**Fig. 1**). Preoperative JOA score, NCSS, and Nurick score were 9, 7, and 4, respectively. We proceeded ACDF at C3-C4 with two m-cages (porous 6 mm) (Ammtec, Suginami, Tokyo, Japan) (**Fig. 2**). Postoperatively, the patient experienced improved numbness and left-hand pain, and she was able to walk with a cane as of the 4-year follow-up. Postoperative JOA score, NCSS, and Nurick score at the latest postoperative follow-up (4 years after surgery) were 12, 10, and 3, respectively. The recovery rates of the JOA score and the NCSS were both 42.9%. Postoperative radiography demonstrated no instability of the operated site. Postoperative MRI after 1 month after surgery showed decompression of the spinal cord (**Fig. 3**).

DISCUSSION

This study is mainly a radiological study but also a clinical study of single-level ACDF patients at C3-4. Static factors, such as a degenerative disk, posterior longitudinal ligament, yellow ligament, and osteophytes are pathologic factors of canal stenosis (CSM). The authors' study shows that the patients were elderly with CSM. In these cases, a dynamic factor (instability) at C3-4 level contributed more to the major causes of CSM than the static factors.

In general, degenerative changes develop in the cervical spine and its surrounding tissues as manifestations of the aging process. The level most loaded during cervical movement is the C5-6 level.[10] As a result, at the first step of spondylosis, degenerative changes of disks and ligaments may develop at lower cervical levels in the younger group (less than 65 years), followed by osteophytes. As a consequence, the middle and/or lower cervical spine is already less mobile in the elderly group (65 years or older). Thus, this condition causes overloading at the upper cervical level during cervical movement,[10] leading to the development of degenerative spondylolisthesis[2] and comparatively greater mobility at this level.[1] Hypermobility at the C3-4 segment, which still maintains mobility, compensates for decreased mobility at the lower segments. Cervical movement is dependent on the motion of the C3-4 segment, which accounted for 39.8% of C2-7 total motion in the present cases. Hayashi and colleagues[1] reported that posterior osteophytes at the C5-6 and C6-7 segments and retrolisthesis at the C3-4 or C4-5 segment were the major causes of dynamic canal stenosis. In the present cases, C3-4 ACDF patients presented with significant lordosis compared with other level ACDF patients due to increased ROM at the C3-4 level, as previously reported.[3,6,11] To conclude greater segmental angulation and hypermobility at the C3-4 segment were identified as potential contributors to the high incidence of pathology at the C3-4 segment in elderly patients with CSM,[2,3] and not only static factors but also dynamic factors may contribute to the development of CSM.

Most C3-4 ACDF patients were elderly. This may be due to the following reason. People develop lower cervical level spondylotic changes when young, and C3-4 ACDF patients were asymptomatic with these changes. Lower cervical level ACDF patients, however, were symptomatic

Table 1
Comparison of C3-C4 ACDF and non C3-C4 ACDF patients

	C3/4 ACDF Patients (Group I)	Non C3/4 ACDF Patients (Group II)	*P* Value
C2-C7 lordosis (°)	18.3 ± 11.6	9.5 ± 6.5	$P<.001$
C2-C7 ROM (°)	37.5 ± 15.4	39.1 ± 12.5	$P=.3318$
C3-C4 ROM (°)	13.3 ± 5.8	6.5 ± 3.9	$P<.001$
C3-C4%ROM (%)	39.8 ± 23.0	16.9 ± 10.3	$P<.001$

Values are mean ± SD.
Abbreviation: ACDF, anterior cervical discectomy and fusion.

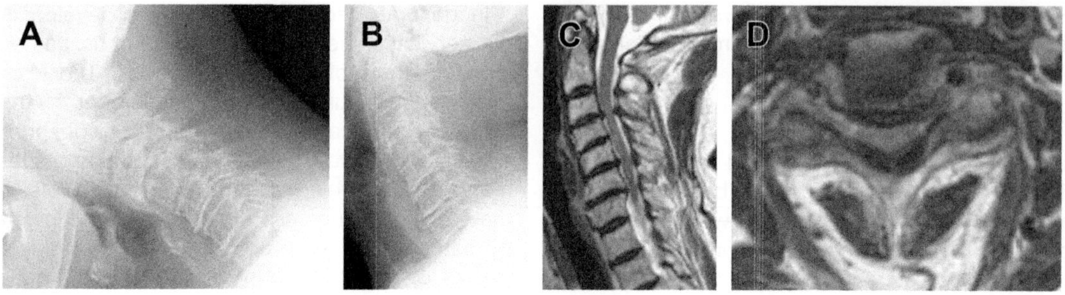

Fig. 1. Lateral radiograph of the cervical spine with the neck in flexion (*A*) and in extension (*B*), showing distinct instability at C3-4 segment. Sagittal (*C*) and axial (*D*) T2-weighted MRI, showing severe cervical canal stenosis with high signal intensity at C3-4 segment.

and presented with CS. As discussed previously, C3-4 spondylotic changes develop gradually for several decades after lower cervical level spondylotic changes develop. Thus, C3-4 ACDF patients presented with myelopathy when older. This raises another question about the difference between being symptomatic with lower cervical level ACDF patients and asymptomatic with C3-4 ACDF patients when younger with lower cervical level spondylotic changes. The difference between the 2 groups may be attributable mainly to the difference in the initial size of the cervical spinal canal. Cervical spinal canal diameter is a good indicator for detecting myelopathy.[11] It has been reported that patients with a sagittal cervical spinal canal diameter of less than 10 mm had myelopathy, and that those with a diameter of 10 mm to 13 mm had premyelopathic changes.[12] In the present C3-4 ACDF patients, the mean AP canal diameter was 11.3 mm. This is a critical canal diameter for myelopathy. Meanwhile, the original cervical canal diameters at lower cervical levels of C3-4 ACDF patients might be wider than those of other patients, so that C3-4 ACDF patients may have escaped CS due to lower cervical spondylotic changes when young. Okamoto and colleagues[13] reported an investigation of surgical CSM cases and found that the old patients were more than 70 year old and had a sagittal diameter of the cervical canal that was stenotic but wider than that of patients in their 50s and 60s, supporting the authors' hypothesis. In C3-4 ACDF patients, lower cervical level spondylotic changes might have been asymptomatic when they were young, but they presented with CSM in their old age in conjunction with hypermobility at the C3-4 level.

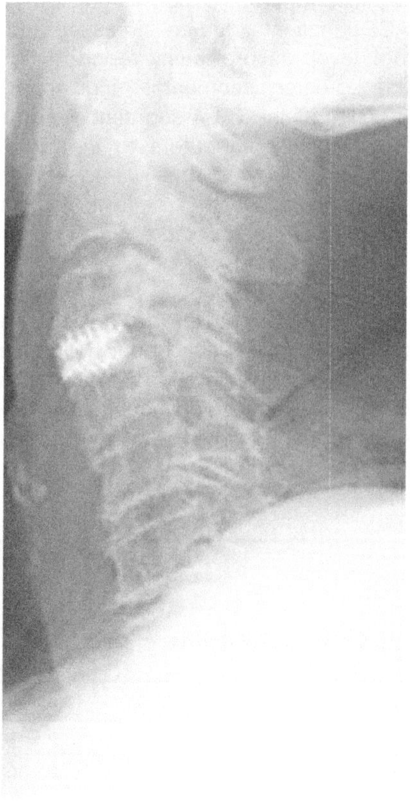

Fig. 2. Lateral radiograph of the cervical spine with the neck in neutral position after surgery, showing C3-4 segment was fixed with titanium cages.

CLINICAL SYMPTOMS AND OUTCOMES OF OPERATION

The symptoms of C3-4 ACDF patients were varied, and these symptoms may have suggested cerebellar and other disorders, causing confusion and delaying treatment. These symptoms are suspected to be caused by a disorder of the propriospinal neurons in the gray matter of the cervical cord at the C3 and C4 levels.[14] It has been reported that half of aged patients (more than 65 years of age) with CSM had serious falls within

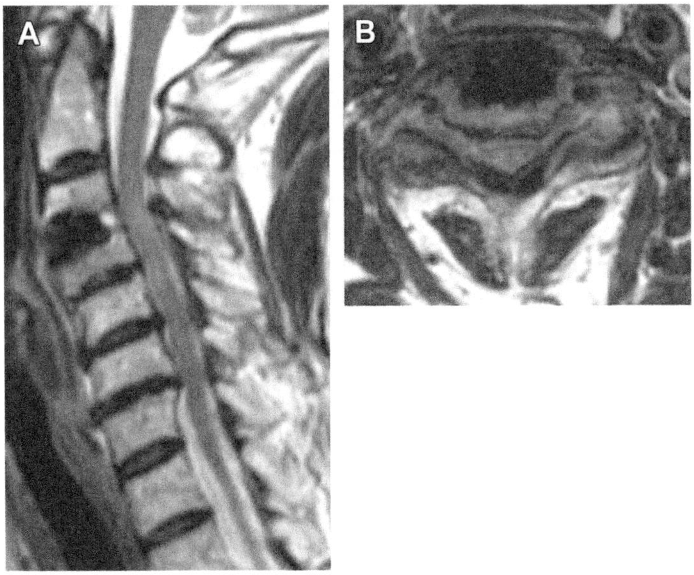

Fig. 3. Sagittal (*A*) and axial (*B*) T2-weighted MRI 1 month after surgery, showing decompression of the spinal cord at C3-4 segment.

6 months, and their preoperative conditions were worse than those of younger patients.[3] In the present cases, the mean duration of preoperative symptoms was 6.0 months, and the symptoms of C3-4 ACDF patients tended to be caused by multisegmental lesions and large segmental mobility at the C3-4 level. These features made the etiology of C3-4 ACDF patients complicated, and the clinical signs were often confused, making it difficult to distinguish their symptoms from those of intracranial disorders. In the present cases, the outcome of C3-4 ACDF patients was generally good but slightly worse than that of the non–C3-4 ACDF patients. One of the reasons could be the difference in the preoperative clinical conditions of each group. Basically, C3-4 ACDF patients all presented with CSM, whereas among non–C3-4 patients, 60% presented with CSM, and 40% presented with radiculopathy. Another reason could be the difference in the preoperative clinical scores of each group. Preoperative clinical scores of C3-4 ACDF patients were slightly worse than that of the non–C3-4 ACDF patients. This may be the reason that the elderly generally have a low activities of daily living; thus, a slight disturbance does not affect the activities. They have a tendency to visit a hospital after CSM has considerably developed. In the present study, however, there was no difference in outcomes between the C3-4 ACDF patients and non–C3-4 patients. Outcome of surgery may depend on age, duration of the disease, severity of the preoperative deficit and spinal cord plasticity, and so forth. There is a point at which irreversible damage is done to the cord. But surgery is sometimes carried out to arrest the progression of myelopathy despite the length of the clinical disability.[15] Early diagnosis and treatment lead to improvement of the outcomes of C3-4 CSM patients.

SUMMARY

This clinical study of single-level ACDF at C3-4 shows that the patients were elderly with CSM. In these cases, a dynamic factor (instability) at C3-4 level contributed more to the major causes of CSM than the static factors.

REFERENCES

1. Hayashi H, Okada K, Hashimoto J, et al. Cervical Spondylotic myelopathy in the aged patient. A radiographic evaluation of the aging changes in the cervical spine and etiologic factors of myelopathy. Spine 1988;13:618–25.
2. Kawasaki M, Tani T, Ushida T, et al. Anterolisthesis and retrolisthesis of the cervical spine in cervical spondylotic myelopathy in the elderly. J Orthop Sci 2007;12:207–13.
3. Mihara H, Ohnari K, Hachiya M, et al. Cervical myelopathy caused by C3-C4 spondylosis in elderly patiens. Spine 2000;25:796–800.
4. Tsunoda K, Morikawa M, Nagata I. Clinical study of C3-4 level cervical spondylotic myelopathy. Spinal Surg 2009;23:24–8 [in Japanese].
5. Japanese Orthopaedic Association. Japanese orthopaedic association score for spondylotic myelopathy. J Jpn Orthop Assoc 1975;99. prefatory note.
6. Kadoya S. Grading and scoring system for neurological function in degenerative cervical spine

disease-neurosurgical cervical spine scale. Neurol Med Chir (Tokyo) 1992;32:40–1.
7. Nurick S. The pathogenesis of the spinal cord disorder associated with cervical spondylosis. Brain 1972;95:87–100.
8. Boijsen E. The cervical spinal canal in intraspinal expansive process. Acta Radiol 1954;42:101–15.
9. Jacson R. The cervical syndrome. 2nd edition. Springfield, IL: Charles C. Thomas; 1958.
10. Nishizawa S, Yokoyama T, Kaneko M. High cervical disc lesions in elderly patients-presentation and surgical approach. Acta Neurochir (Wien) 1999;141:119–26.
11. Yukawa Y, Kato F, Suda K. Age-related changes in osseous anatomy, alignment, and range of motion of the cervical spine. Part I: radiographic data from over 1200 asymptomatic subjects. Eur Spine J 2012;21:1492–8.
12. Morishita Y, Naito M, Hymanson H, et al. The relationship between the cervical spinal canal diameter and the pathological changes in the cervical spine. Eur Spine J 2009;18:877–83.
13. Okamoto A, Shinomiya K, Matuoka T, et al. Surgical treatment for aged patients with cervical spondylotic myelopathy. East Jpn Clin Orthopedics 1990;2:229–31 [in Japanese].
14. Ikegami H, Tanaka T, Endo K, et al. The clinical study of C3-C4 level cervical spondylosis with unusual clinical signs. Surg Tech Spine Spinal Nerves 2004;6:103–6 [in Japanese].
15. Soo MY, Tran-Dinh HD, Dorsch NWC, et al. Cervical spine degenerative diseases: An evaluation of clinical and imaging features in surgical decisions. Aust Radiol 1997;41:351–6.

Intraoperative Neurophysiologic Monitoring for Degenerative Cervical Myelopathy

Masaaki Takeda, MD, PhD*, Satoshi Yamaguchi, MD, PhD,
Takafumi Mitsuhara, MD, PhD, Masaru Abiko, MD,
Kaoru Kurisu, MD, PhD

KEYWORDS

• Degenerative cervical myelopathy • Intraoperative neurophysiologic monitoring
• Somatosensory evoked potential • Motor evoked potential

KEY POINTS

- Multimodal intraoperative neurophysiologic monitoring is a reliable tool for detecting intraoperative spine injury and is recommended during surgery for degenerative cervical myopathy (DCM).
- Somatosensory evoked potential (SEP) can be used to monitor spine and peripheral nerve injury during positioning in surgery for DCM.
- Compensation technique for transcranial evoked muscle action potentials (tcMEPs) should be adopted in intraoperative monitoring during surgery for DCM.
- Free-running electromyography is a useful real-time monitoring add-on modality in addition to SEP and tcMEP.

INTRODUCTION

In the past, a wake-up test was considered a gold standard for detection of spinal cord injury during spinal corrective surgery.[1] Because spinal cord injury occurs during surgical maneuver, such as corrective instrumentation, however, wake-up tests can easily lead to false-negative findings.[2] In the 1970s, somatosensory evoked potential (SEP) had been applied in scoliosis corrective surgery as intraoperative sensory tract monitoring.[3] In 1980, Merton and Morton[4] reported a breakthrough method called transcranial evoked muscle action potentials (tcMEPs) for monitoring motor tracts. With the widespread use of total intravenous anesthesia (TIVA) using propofol and opioids, intraoperative monitoring with tcMEPs has become popular in spine surgery.[5,6] Each method has characteristic advantages and disadvantages; therefore, a combination of multiple methods has been developed and accepted for intraoperative neurophysiologic monitoring (IONM) during spine surgery.[7] IONM is established as an effective method to predict an increased risk of the adverse outcome of paralysis after spine surgery.[8] IONM in spine surgery has become a standard during resection of spinal tumors and surgical correction for scoliosis. A large retrospective study reported that the incidence of major spinal cord injuries in cervical spine was 3 per 1000.[9] Although the likelihood of complication is low, IONM during

Disclosure Statement: The authors have nothing to disclose regarding this article.
Department of Neurosurgery, Hiroshima University Graduate School of Biomedical and Health Sciences, Hiroshima City, Hiroshima, Japan
* Corresponding author. 1-2-3, Kasumi, Minami-ku, Hiroshima City, Hiroshima 7348551, Japan.
E-mail address: tkdmsk@hiroshima-u.ac.jp

Neurosurg Clin N Am 29 (2018) 159–167
https://doi.org/10.1016/j.nec.2017.09.012
1042-3680/18/© 2017 Elsevier Inc. All rights reserved.

decompressive surgery of degenerative cervical myelopathy (DCM) should be adopted.

SOMATOSENSORY EVOKED POTENTIAL

As IONM for spine surgery, SEP was first reported and suggested as having great potential for improving outcome of spine surgery. SEP, as an IONM tool, has been used in spine surgery for more than 40 years.[10] SEP is the most widely popularized technique among different modalities of IONM. In cervical decompression surgery, SEP is used not only to assess the function of somatosensory pathways but also to avoid injury to the spinal cord or the peripheral nerves during positioning.[11]

Surgery for cervical myelopathy requires monitoring of the 4 nerves of the extremities.[12] SEPs for IONM are typically elicited by stimulating the median nerve and the posterior tibial nerve in the upper and lower extremities, respectively.[13] Various electrodes can be used for stimulation of target nerves, such as bar electrodes, electroencephalographic metal disc electrodes, surface electrodes, and subdermal needle electrodes. Each electrode has characteristic advantages and disadvantages. For IONM, the most suitable stimulating electrodes are surface electrodes. The cortical potentials of SEP are recorded from CP3 and CP4 in the upper extremities and CPz in the lower extremities (depending on the 10–20 international electrode system).[14]

Evoked potentials of SEP are very low in amplitude and require averaging several times. Therefore, reducing or diminishing the noise of operating theater is necessary and requires a few minutes to evaluate the change in waveform. A warning signal is generally issued when there is a 50% decrease in amplitude or 10% increase in latency compared with baseline values.[14] SEP signal changes, however, are not always related to a postoperative neurologic deficit. The specificity of SEP during IONM was reported as 27%, whereas the sensitivity was 99%.[11] Low specificity of intraoperative SEP affects the utility of SEP alone for IONM. Waveform of SEP is influenced by many factors, such as blood pressure, body temperature, partial pressure of alveolar carbon dioxide, and anesthetic drugs, in addition to spinal interference.[15] Deletis and Sala[16] pointed out that the isolated use of SEP monitoring for IONM is inappropriate. The lack of specificity of SEP has favored the use of muscle evoked potential (MEP) for IONM during cervical decompression surgery.[16]

In addition, cases of degenerative cervical myelopathy have a potential risk of spinal cord compression or peripheral nerve injury during positioning.[11,17,18] Recording prepositioning and postpositioning SEP for spine surgery in skeletal dysplasia was reported by Ofiram and colleagues.[19] Only a few studies have reported the application of neurophysiologic monitoring for the position-related spinal cord dysfunction during anterior cervical discectomy and fusion (ACDF).[20] Chen and colleagues[21] reported postoperative neurologic deficits due to positioning by unrecognized coexisting cervical disk herniation during lumbar laminectomy. Although recording of MEP at the same time is ideal, it is often difficult because of the muscle relaxants used during intubation. It is the authors' practice to monitor prepositioning and postpositioning SEP as described in **Fig. 1**. Detection of postpositioning SEP changes can contribute to prevention of neurologic deficits.

SEP can also detect and prevent peripheral nerve injury during cervical spine surgery.[22] Peripheral nerve injury occurs in patients who are malpositioned during surgery.[23] Both prone and supine positions have a possibility of peripheral nerve injury and SEP can detect arm position-related waveform changes. The rate of reversible SEP changes with tucked arms were 1.8% in supine and 2.1% in prone positions.[24] IONM of SEP, including positioning-related changes, are of value in identifying and preventing spine and peripheral nerve injury during cervical spine surgery.

TRANSCRANIAL MOTOR EVOKED POTENTIALS

MEPs derived from transcranial stimulation for IONM have been used for more than 20 years and rapidly became popular in spine surgery.[25] Usefulness of tcMEP has been reported during spine surgery.[26–29] tcMEP is recognized as the most sensitive technique compared with other techniques, such as SEP or spinal cord evoked potential.[30] Some investigators argue that surgical decompression for symptomatic cervical spine may be safely done without IONM.[31] Contrarily, other reports conclude that intraoperative MEP monitoring during surgery for degenerative cervical spondylotic myelopathy may have prevented occurrence of permanent postoperative neurologic injury.[32] Although the requirement of IONM for DCM is controversial and literature specific to DCM is sparse, articles supporting the usefulness of IONM are increasing in recent years. tcMEP could detect acute-type postoperative C5 palsy after cervical laminoplasty for DCM.[33] A large study of multichannel tcMEP suggested its benefit

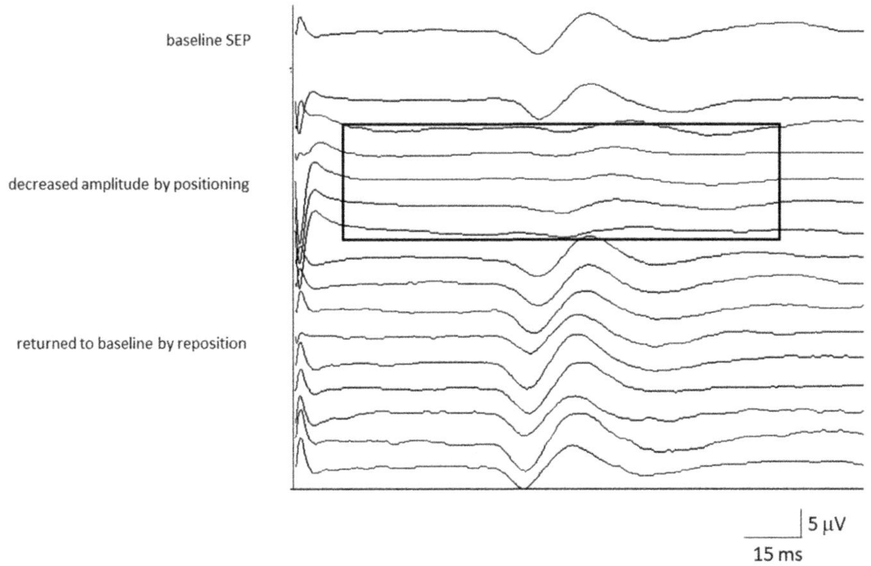

Fig. 1. Posterior tibial nerve cortical SEP demonstrated disappearance of waveform due to spinal cord compression on positioning. After repositioning neck to neutral position, waveform recovered to baseline.

for the detection of spinal injury during ACDF surgery.[34] Guidelines and reviews declare the usefulness of tcMEP for spine surgery, including surgery for DCM.[8,35–37]

To depolarize the corticospinal system to elicit MEP waveform, needle or corkscrew electrodes for transcranial electrical stimulation are placed on the scalp over motor cortex in general. The stimulating electrodes are positioned at C3, C4, C1, C2, and a point 6 cm in front of C2. The stimulation parameters of a train of 5 to 7 pulses (0–200 mA or 0–800 V) with a pulse duration of 0.5 ms and an interstimulus interval of 4 ms is commonly used. tcMEPs are recorded by a pair of needle or surface electrodes inserted in or installed on target muscles (typically abductor pollicis brevis [APB] and tibialis anterior muscle).[14,38–40] Reliable 4-extremity monitoring is necessary during surgery for DCM but an optimal stimulating point for lower extremity has not been established. Murata and colleagues[41] accomplished lower extremity MEP recording during brain surgery using monopolar direct cortical stimulation with subdural electrodes. Direct cortical stimulation during surgery for DCM is highly invasive; therefore, Szelényi and colleagues[38] recommended stimulating montage of Cz/Cz+6 cm for lower extremity (tibialis anterior muscle) tcMEP monitoring.

FREE-RUNNING ELECTROMYOGRAPHY

SEP and tcMEP are intermittent recording modalities; therefore, detecting the exact moment of spine injury during surgical procedure is difficult. To complement those situations, free-running electromyography (EMG) has recently been used as a real-time monitoring modality. Free-running EMG records intermittent burst activity generated by traction of spinal nerve root or compression of spinal cord. Santiago-Pérez and colleagues[42] reported free-running EMG recording as a simple technique and provided continuous information about functional integrity of lumbosacral spinal roots throughout surgery. Intraoperative free-running EMG contributed to reducing the incidence of postoperative C5 palsy after cervical decompression surgery.[43] Fotakopoulos and colleagues[44] reported effectiveness of free-running EMG during ACDF. During the operation, free-running EMG monitoring prompted a surgical alert of imminent damage to the neural structures.[44] Sutter and colleagues[45] reported that IONM with free-running EMG reduced postoperative complications and improved long-term results.

Triggered EMG elicited by electrical stimulation of pedicle screw has been applied to posterior lumbar fusion to detect malposition of pedicle screw.[14,46] Few reports have been published about electrical stimulation of lateral mass and pedicle screws. Djurasovic and colleagues[47] concluded that electrical screw stimulation provided a 99% predictive value for suitable position of screws in cervical pedicle or lateral mass. Multimodality neuromonitoring using free-running EMG and the pedicle screw stimulation technique was considered a practical option in a position statement by the American Society of Neurophysiological Monitoring.[48]

D-WAVE

D-waves are recorded directly from spinal cord with electrical stimulation from the cranial side of the lesion, including transcranial stimulation.[49] D-waves are one of the most reliable methods to monitor motor function. A decrease in D-wave amplitude more than 50% correlates with postoperative motor deficits.[50] D-waves are resistant to inhalation anesthetics and neuromuscular blockage, thereby favoring their utility as primary monitoring modality in spinal tumor surgery.[51,52] To record D-waves, installation of epidural electrode is necessary. During operations for diseases that require exposure of spine, electrode installation is easy; however, for routine surgery of DCM, percutaneous insertion is required. Percutaneous insertion of epidural electrode has a possibility of nerve root or spinal cord injury, infection, and epidural hematoma.[53] Although D-wave monitoring has major advantages and is important during cervical tumor surgery, it is not usually applied during routine decompressive surgery for DCM.

MULTIMODAL INTRAOPERATIVE NEUROPHYSIOLOGIC MONITORING DURING SURGERY FOR DEGENERATIVE CERVICAL MYOPATHY

Multiple modalities exist for IONM during surgery for DCM, such as SEP, tcMEP, D-wave, and free-running EMG. Each modality has limitations in identifying postoperative neurologic deficits during operation by isolated application. Therefore, utilization of multimodal IONM has been routine in several institutes.[54] Many investigators have reported effectiveness of SEP and MEP as IONM for detecting intraoperative neurologic deficits. May and colleagues[11] reported SEP monitoring in cervical surgery with sensitivity and specificity of 99% and 27%, respectively, for predicting a new deficit. On the contrary, Dennis and colleagues[55] concluded that median nerve SEP during cervical spine surgery was not specific for detecting intraoperative neurologic deficits. Smith and colleagues[56] reported postoperative central cord syndrome after ACDF without SEP deterioration. As described previously, IONM of SEP alone is less reliable for cervical spine surgery.

Bose and colleagues[57] reported superiority of tcMEP during surgery for DCM compared with SEP. In this study, 1 of 119 patients undergoing ACDF developed a new deficit with waveform change only on tcMEP but not on SEP.[57] Hilibrand and colleagues[58] also reported postoperative new neurologic deficit without changes on SEP. They reported 25% sensitivity and 100% specificity of SEP in contrast to 100% sensitivity and specificity of tcMEP. These results suggest that tcMEP is more sensitive for detecting neurologic deficits than SEP during surgery for DCM. Clark and colleagues[32] reported usefulness of IONM of MEP in patients undergoing surgery for DCM. The sensitivity and specificity of SEP and MEP during cervical spine surgery were reported as 43% to 71% and 94% to 99.2%, respectively.[32,59,60] Lee and colleagues[61] reported that application of multimodal IONM during posterior cervical operations may be useful to detect intraoperative neurologic injury. Their overall sensitivity of IONM was 50% and the specificity was 100%. The effectiveness of multimodal IONM for spinal tumor has been clearly shown.[62] Guidelines published by the American Academy of Neurology established the utility of multimodal IONM in spine surgeries, including surgery for cervical lesion.[8] Despite few studies, the usefulness of IONM during surgery for DCM has been reported and effort should be made to use these techniques to ensure better postoperative outcome. **Fig. 2** presents a representative screen shot of multimodal IONM.

CORRESPONDENCE WITH SIGNIFICANT CHANGES OF INTRAOPERATIVE NEUROPHYSIOLOGIC MONITORING

In brain surgery, a greater than 50% reduction criterion is advocated for brain, brainstem, and facial nerve MEP monitoring as a warning criterion.[63–65] In contrast, only a few articles report the alarm criteria of MEP or SEP for DCM. As discussed previously, alert criteria for SEP of 50% decrease in amplitude and 10% increase in latency have been advocated in spine surgery.[14] Many alert criteria for tcMEP have been reported, including 50% decrease to total loss of amplitude. An amplitude decrease of 50% to 80% is commonly used in spine surgery, including DCM and scoliosis correction.[66–69]

If an IONM technologist detects significant changes in waveforms, causes other than surgical technique should be ruled out before warning. The representative points to be checked are disconnection of the recording or stimulating electrodes, unexpected administration of anesthetic agents such as muscle relaxants, or changes in general condition such as body temperature or blood

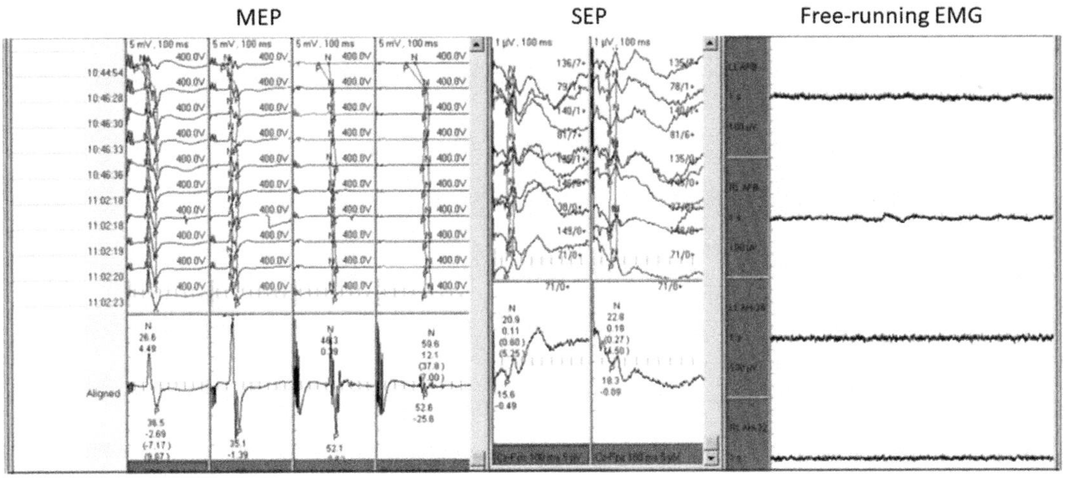

Fig. 2. Multimodal IONM during surgery for DCM.

pressure. If no clear explanation is found, surgeons should suspect the possibility of iatrogenic spinal cord injury. If waveform change does not recover or neurotonic EMG does not disappear even after waiting, removal of instruments, additional decompression, or administration of methylprednisolone should be opted.[70] Additional foraminotomy to prevent postoperative C5 palsy based on IONM during laminectomy for DCM has been reported.[71] Some investigators advocate the effectiveness of immediate administration of intravenous bolus methylprednisolone.[70,72] There is no absolute approach, however, for significant IONM changes during DCM surgery.

ANESTHESIA FOR INTRAOPERATIVE NEUROPHYSIOLOGIC MONITORING

General Features of Anesthesia

tcMEP is the most sensitive IONM modality for detecting intraoperative nerve injuries during cervical spine surgery.58 tcMEP waveforms, however, are known to be strongly influenced by various anesthetic agents, especially neuromuscular blocking agents. Selection of the appropriate anesthetic regimen is necessary to acquire stable recording of IONM. Furthermore, inhalational agents affect evoked potentials, such as SEP, more than intravenous agents.[13] Among halogenated agents, nitrous oxide has a limited influence on SEP. When selecting nitrous oxide as anesthetic agent during IONM, a nitrous-narcotic technique is preferred. The modern version of nitrous-narcotic technique consists of a high-dose remifentanil infusion (0.2–0.5 μg/kg/min) with 60% to 70% inhaled fraction of NO.[73] Neuromuscular blocking agents strongly suppress MEP; therefore, anesthetic technique without neuromuscular blockage is necessary to obtain stable MEP. Recently, TIVA based on continuous propofol infusion and supplementation with intravenous opioid has been preferred for IONM. Propofol and fentanyl or remifentanil anesthesia is most suitable for IONM during spine surgery. Use of neuromuscular blockage is recommended only for intubation.[36,39,74]

Compensation of Anesthetic Effect

As described previously, tcMEP is strongly influenced by anesthetic agents, especially muscle relaxants. To compensate for this effect, a technique using compound muscle action potentials (CMAPs) of muscles evoked by peripheral nerve stimulation has recently been reported. Even if neuromuscular blockage is used only for intubation, remnant agents may reduce the amplitude of MEP at the beginning of the operation. As a reference waveform of tcMEP during neurosurgical surgery, CMAP of the APB obtained by median nerve stimulation has been reported (**Fig. 3**).[75] In DCM cases of severe myelopathy causing amyotrophy of the upper extremities, a reference waveform of APB-CMAP might be unstable.[76] An alternative proposal of facial CMAP, as a reference waveform, derived from transcranial electrical stimulation has recently been reported.[77] The investigators speculated that transcranially evoked facial CMAP is not influenced by cervical myelopathy, making it more suitable as a reference waveform contrary to previous methods. Besides TIVA with opioid, compensatory technique should be considered along with IONM, including MEP during surgery for DCM.

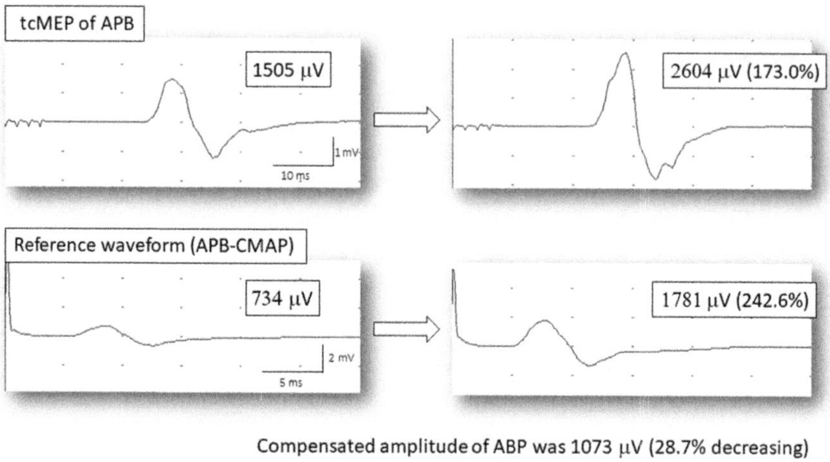

Fig. 3. Amplitude changes of target muscle and reference waveforms. Amplitude of tcMEP of APB increased after fading of the effect of neuromuscular blocking agent, administered at oral intubation (*upper*). At the same time, the amplitude of APB-CMAP as reference waveforms elicited from median nerve stimulation also increased in similar fashion. Compensated amplitude of tcMEP of APB demonstrated 28.7% decrease compared with the baseline value (*lower*). Although the amplitude of tcMEP of APB demonstrated apparent increment, compensated amplitude was decreased.

SUMMARY

Postoperative neurologic complications must be avoided after surgery for DCM. Advances in IONM have helped reduce morbidity in spine surgery. Despite development of newer modalities, SEP plays an important role in IONM. tcMEP is one of the most reassuring modalities for assessing motor function in IONM. For real-time monitoring of functional integrity of spine, free-running EMG is most effective and is frequently used. Each monitoring technique has advantages and disadvantages. IONM is merely a technique for detecting change in spinal function and does not give a definite answer. Despite limitations, it is desirable to use IONM during surgery for DCM, understanding the meaning of each modalities.

REFERENCES

1. Vauzelle C, Stagnara PJP. Functional monitoring of spinal cord activity during spinal surgery. Clin Orthop Relat Res 1973;93:173–8.
2. Diaz JH, Lockhart CH. Postoperative quadriplegia after spinal fusion for scoliosis with intraoperative awakening. Anesth Analg 1987;66(10):1039–42.
3. Engler GL, Spielholz NJ, Bernhard WN, et al. Somatosensory evoked potentials during Harrington instrumentation for scoliosis. J Bone Joint Surg Am 1978;60(4):528–32.
4. Merton PA, Morton HB. Stimulation of the cerebral cortex in the intact human subject. Nature 1980; 285(5762):227.
5. Kalkman CJ, Drummond JC, Ribberink AA, et al. Effects of propofol, etomidate, midazolam, and fentanyl on motor evoked responses to transcranial electrical or magnetic stimulation in humans. Anesthesiology 1992;76(4):502–9.
6. Pechstein U, Cedzich C, Nadstawek J, et al. Transcranial high-frequency repetitive electrical stimulation for recording myogenic motor evoked potentials with the patient under general anesthesia. Neurosurgery 1996;39(2):335–44.
7. Magit DP, Hilibrand AS, Kirk J, et al. Questionnaire study of neuromonitoring availability and usage for spine surgery. J Spinal Disord Tech 2007;20(4): 282–9.
8. Nuwer MR, Emerson RG, Galloway G, et al. Evidence-based guideline update: intraoperative spinal monitoring with somatosensory and transcranial electrical motor evoked potentials*. J Clin Neurophysiol 2012;29(1):101–8.
9. Cramer DE, Maher PC, Pettigrew DB, et al. Major neurologic deficit immediately after adult spinal surgery: incidence and etiology over 10 years at a single training institution. J Spinal Disord Tech 2009; 22(8):565–70.
10. Nash CL, Lorig RA, Schatzinger LA, et al. Spinal cord monitoring during operative treatment of the spine. Clin Orthop Relat Res 1977;(126):100–5.
11. May DM, Jones SJ, Crockard HA. Somatosensory evoked potential monitoring in cervical surgery: identification of pre- and intraoperative risk factors associated with neurological deterioration. J Neurosurg 1996;85(4):566–73.
12. Baumann SB, Welch WC, Bloom MJ. Intraoperative SSEP detection of ulnar nerve compression or

ischemia in an obese patient: a unique complication associated with a specialized spinal retraction system. Arch Phys Med Rehabil 2000;81(1):130–2.
13. Toleikis JR. Intraoperative monitoring using somatosensory evoked potentials. J Clin Monit Comput 2005;19(3):241–58.
14. Simon Mirela V. Neurophysiologic tests in the operating room. In: Deletis V, Shils JL, editors. Intraoperative neurophysiology a comprehensive guide to monitoring and mapping. New York: Demos Medical Publishing; 2010. p. 1–44.
15. Cui H, Luk KDK, Hu Y. Effects of physiological parameters on intraoperative somatosensory-evoked potential monitoring: results of a multifactor analysis. Med Sci Monit 2009;15(5):CR226–30.
16. Deletis V, Sala F. Intraoperative neurophysiological monitoring of the spinal cord during spinal cord and spine surgery: a review focus on the corticospinal tracts. Clin Neurophysiol 2008;119(2):248–64.
17. Kamel I. Positioning patients for spine surgery: Avoiding uncommon position-related complications. World J Orthop 2014;5(4):425.
18. Than KD, Mummaneni PV, Smith ZA, et al. Brachial plexopathy after cervical spine surgery. Global Spine J 2017;7(1_suppl):17S–20S.
19. Ofiram E, Lonstein JE, Skinner S, et al. "The disappearing evoked potentials": a special problem of positioning patients with skeletal dysplasia: case report. Spine (Phila Pa 1976) 2006;31(14):E464–70.
20. Schwartz DM, Sestokas AK, Hilibrand AS, et al. Neurophysiological identification of position-induced neurologic injury during anterior cervical spine surgery. J Clin Monit Comput 2006;20(6): 437–44.
21. Chen S-H, Hui Y-L, Yu C-M, et al. Paraplegia by acute cervical disc protrusion after lumbar spine surgery. Chang Gung Med J 2005;28(4):254–7.
22. Jones SC, Fernau R, Woeltjen BL. Use of somatosensory evoked potentials to detect peripheral ischemia and potential injury resulting injury resulting from positioning of the surgical patient: case reports and discussion. Spine J 2004;4(3):360–2.
23. Uribe JS, Kolla J, Omar H, et al. Brachial plexus injury following spinal surgery. J Neurosurg Spine 2010;13(4):552–8.
24. Kamel IR, Drum ET, Koch SA, et al. The use of somatosensory evoked potentials to determine the relationship between patient positioning and impending upper extremity nerve injury during spine surgery: a retrospective analysis. Anesth Analg 2006;102(5):1538–42.
25. Burke D, Hicks R, Stephen J, et al. Assessment of corticospinal and somatosensoty conduction simultaneously during scoliosis surgery. Electroencephalogr Clin Neurophysiol 1992;85(6):388–96.
26. Langeloo DD, Journée HL, de Kleuver M, et al. Criteria for transcranial electrical motor evoked potential monitoring during spinal deformity surgery. A review and discussion of the literature. Neurophysiol Clin 2007;37(6):431–9.
27. Bartley K, Woodforth IJ, Stephen JP, et al. Corticospinal volleys and compound muscle action potentials produced by repetitive transcranial stimulation during spinal surgery. Clin Neurophysiol 2002; 113(1):78–90.
28. Langeloo DD, Lelivelt A, Louis Journée H, et al. Transcranial electrical motor-evoked potential monitoring during surgery for spinal deformity: a study of 145 patients. Spine (Phila Pa 1976) 2003;28(10): 1043–50.
29. Lang EW, Chesnut RM, Beutler AS, et al. The utility of motor-evoked potential monitoring during intramedullary surgery. Anesth Analg 1996;83(6): 1337–41.
30. Sala F, Palandri G, Basso E, et al. Motor evoked potential monitoring improves outcome after surgery for intramedullary spinal cord tumors: a historical control study. Neurosurgery 2006;58(6):1129–41.
31. Traynelis VC, Abode-Iyamah KO, Leick KM, et al. Cervical decompression and reconstruction without intraoperative neurophysiological monitoring. J Neurosurg Spine 2012;16(2):107–13.
32. Clark AJ, Safaee M, Chou D, et al. Comparative sensitivity of intraoperative motor evoked potential monitoring in predicting postoperative neurologic deficits: nondegenerative versus degenerative myelopathy. Global Spine J 2016;6(5):452–8.
33. Fujiwara Y, Manabe H, Izumi B, et al. The efficacy of intraoperative neurophysiological monitoring using transcranial electrically stimulated muscle-evoked potentials (TcE-MsEPs) for predicting postoperative segmental upper extremity motor paresis after cervical laminoplasty. Clin Spine Surg 2016;29(4): E188–95.
34. Kim D-G, Jo S-R, Park Y-S, et al. Multi-channel motor evoked potential monitoring during anterior cervical discectomy and fusion. Clin Neurophysiol Pract 2017;2:48–53.
35. Fehlings MG, Brodke DS, Norvell DC, et al. The evidence for intraoperative neurophysiological monitoring in spine surgery: does it make a difference? Spine (Phila Pa 1976) 2010;35(9 Suppl):S37–46.
36. Stecker M. A review of intraoperative monitoring for spinal surgery. Surg Neurol Int 2012;3(4):174.
37. Gavaret M, Jouve JL, Péréon Y, et al. Intraoperative neurophysiologic monitoring in spine surgery. Developments and state of the art in France in 2011. Orthop Traumatol Surg Res 2013; 99(6 SUPPL):S319–27.
38. Szelényi A, Kothbauer KF, Deletis V. Transcranial electric stimulation for intraoperative motor evoked potential monitoring: stimulation parameters and electrode montages. Clin Neurophysiol 2007; 118(7):1586–95.

39. Kothbauer KF. Intraoperative neurophysiologic monitoring for intramedullary spinal-cord tumor surgery. Neurophysiol Clin 2007;37(6):407–14.
40. Clark AJ, Ziewacz JE, Safaee M, et al. Intraoperative neuromonitoring with MEPs and prediction of postoperative neurological deficits in patients undergoing surgery for cervical and cervicothoracic myelopathy. Neurosurg Focus 2013;35(1):E7.
41. Maruta Y, Fujii M, Imoto H, et al. Intra-operative monitoring of lower extremity motor-evoked potentials by direct cortical stimulation. Clin Neurophysiol 2012;123(6):1248–54.
42. Santiago-Pérez S, Nevado-Estévez R, Aguirre-Arribas J, et al. Neurophysiological monitoring of lumbosacral spinal roots during spinal surgery: continuous intraoperative electromyography (EMG). Electromyogr Clin Neurophysiol 2007;47(7–8):361–7.
43. Jimenez JC, Sani S, Braverman B, et al. Palsies of the fifth cervical nerve root after cervical decompression: prevention using continuous intraoperative electromyography monitoring. J Neurosurg Spine 2005;3(2):92–7.
44. Fotakopoulos G, Alexiou GA, Pachatouridis D, et al. The value of transcranial motor-evoked potentials and free-running electromyography in surgery for cervical disc herniation. J Clin Neurosci 2013; 20(2):263–6.
45. Sutter M, Deletis V, Dvorak J, et al. Current opinions and recommendations on multimodal intraoperative monitoring during spine surgeries. Eur Spine J 2007;16(SUPPL. 2):232–7.
46. Toleikis JR, Skelly JP, Carlvin AO, et al. The usefulness of electrical stimulation for assessing pedicle screw placements. J Spinal Disord 2000;13(4):283–9.
47. Djurasovic M, Dimar JR 2nd, Glassman SD, et al. A prospective analysis of intraoperative electromyographic monitoring of posterior cervical screw fixation. J Spinal Disord Tech 2005;18(6):515–8.
48. Leppanen RE. Intraoperative monitoring of segmental spinal nerve root function with free-run and electrically-triggered electromyography and spinal cord function with reflexes and F-responses. J Clin Monit Comput 2005;19(6):437–61.
49. Patton H, Amassian VD. Single and multiple-unit analysis of cortical stage of pyramidal tract activation. J Neurophysiol 1954;17(4):345–63.
50. Morota N, Deletis V, Constantini S, et al. The role of motor evoked potentials during surgery for intramedullary spinal cord tumors. Neurosurgery 1997; 41(6):1327–36.
51. Deletis V. Intraoperative neurophysiology and methodologies used to monitor the functional integrity of the motor system. In: Deletis V, Shils JL, editors. Neurophysiology in neurosurgery: a modern intraoperative approach. London: Academic Press; 2002. p. 25–51.
52. Scheufler KM, Reinacher PC, Blumrich W, et al. The modifying effects of stimulation pattern and propofol plasma concentration on motor-evoked potentials. Anesth Analg 2005;100(2):440–7.
53. Yamada T, Tucker M, Husain AM. Spinal cord surgery. In: Husain AM, editor. A practical approach to neurophysiologic intraoperative monitoring. Second edition. New York: Demos Medical Publishing; 2015. p. 106–26.
54. Sutter MA, Eggspuehler A, Grob D, et al. Multimodal intraoperative monitoring (MIOM) during 409 lumbosacral surgical procedures in 409 patients. Eur Spine J 2007;16(SUPPL. 2):S221–8.
55. Dennis GC, Dehkordi O, Millis RM, et al. Monitoring of median nerve somatosensory evoked potentials during cervical spinal cord decompression. J Clin Neurophysiol 1996;13(1):51–9.
56. Smith PN, Balzer JR, Khan MH, et al. Intraoperative somatosensory evoked potential monitoring during anterior cervical discectomy and fusion in nonmyelopathic patients-a review of 1,039 cases. Spine J 2007;7(1):83–7.
57. Bose B, Sestokas AK, Schwartz DM. Neurophysiological monitoring of spinal cord function during instrumented anterior cervical fusion. Spine J 2004; 4(2):202–7.
58. Hilibrand AS, Schwartz DM, Sethuraman V, et al. Comparison of transcranial electric motor and somatosensory evoked potential monitoring during cervical spine surgery. J Bone Joint Surg Am 2004;86-A:1248–53.
59. Eggspuehler A, Sutter MA, Grob D, et al. Multimodal intraoperative monitoring (MIOM) during cervical spine surgical procedures in 246 patients. Eur Spine J 2007;16(SUPPL. 2):S209–15.
60. Xu R, Ritzl EK, Sait M, et al. A role for motor and somatosensory evoked potentials during anterior cervical discectomy and fusion for patients without myelopathy: Analysis of 57 consecutive cases. Surg Neurol Int 2011;2:133.
61. Lee HJ, Kim IS, Sung JH, et al. Significance of multimodal intraoperative monitoring for the posterior cervical spine surgery. Clin Neurol Neurosurg 2016; 143:9–14.
62. Sutter M, Eggspuehler A, Grob D, et al. The validity of multimodal intraoperative monitoring (MIOM) in surgery of 109 spine and spinal cord tumors. Eur Spine J 2007;16(SUPPL. 2):S197–208.
63. Neuloh G, Pechstein U, Cedzich C, et al. Motor evoked potential monitoring with supratentorial surgery. Neurosurgery 2004;54(5):1061–70.
64. Dong CCJ, Macdonald DB, Akagami R, et al. Intraoperative facial motor evoked potential monitoring with transcranial electrical stimulation during skull base surgery. Clin Neurophysiol 2005;116(3):588–96.
65. Szelényi A, Hattingen E, Weidauer S, et al. Intraoperative motor evoked potential alteration in intracranial tumor surgery and its relation to signal alteration in postoperative magnetic resonance imaging. Neurosurgery 2010;67(2):302–13.

66. Schwartz DM, Sestokas AK, Dormans JP, et al. Transcranial electric motor evoked potential monitoring during spine surgery: is it safe? Spine (Phila Pa 1976) 2011;36(13):1046–9.
67. Pastorelli F, Plasmati R, Michelucci R, et al. P496: Multimodality monitoring of somatosensory (SSEPs) and transcranial electric motor evoked potentials (tce-MEPs) during surgical correction of neuromuscular scoliosis in patients with central or peripheral nervous system diseases. Abstr 30th Int Congr Clin Neurophysiol IFCN March 20–23, 2014, Berlin (German). 2014;125(1):S182.
68. Bhagat S, Durst A, Grover H, et al. An evaluation of multimodal spinal cord monitoring in scoliosis surgery: a single centre experience of 354 operations. Eur Spine J 2015;24:1399–407.
69. Thirumala PD, Muralidharan A, Loke YK, et al. Value of intraoperative neurophysiological monitoring to reduce neurological complications in patients undergoing anterior cervical spine procedures for cervical spondylotic myelopathy. J Clin Neurosci 2016;25:27–35.
70. Simon MV. Decompressive surgery of the spine. In: Intraoperative neurophysiology a comprehensive guide to monitoring and mapping. New York: Demos Medical Publishing; 2010. p. 209–21.
71. Fan D, Schwartz DM, Vaccaro AR, et al. Intraoperative neurophysiologic detection of iatrogenic C5 nerve root injury during laminectomy for cervical compression myelopathy. Spine (Phila Pa 1976) 2002;27(22):2499–502.
72. Bracken MB. Steroids for acute spinal cord injury. In: Bracken MB, editor. Cochrane database of systematic reviews. Chichester (United Kingdom): John Wiley & Sons, Ltd; 2012.
73. Khan SA, James ML. Anesthetic consideration. In: Husain AM, editor. A practical approach to neurophysiologic intraoperative monitoring. New York: Demos Medical Publishing; 2015. p. 76–84.
74. Haghighi SS, Blaskiewicz DJ, Ramirez B, et al. Can intraoperative neurophysiologic monitoring during cervical spine decompression predict post-operative segmental C5 palsy? J Spine Surg 2016; 2(3):167–72.
75. Tanaka S, Kobayashi I, Sagiuchi T, et al. Compensation of intraoperative transcranial motor-evoked potential monitoring by compound muscle action potential after peripheral nerve stimulation. J Clin Neurophysiol 2005;22(4):271–4.
76. Moldovan M, Alvarez S, Krarup C. Motor axon excitability during Wallerian degeneration. Brain 2009; 132(2):511–23.
77. Morishige M. Application of compound action potential of facial muscles evoked by transcranial stimulation as a reference waveform of motor-evoked potential in spinal surgery. Hiroshima J Med Sci 2017;66(1):1–5.

Health Economics and the Management of Degenerative Cervical Myelopathy

Christopher D. Witiw, MD, MS[a], Fabrice Smieliauskas, PhD[b], Michael G. Fehlings, MD, PhD, FRCSC[c,*]

KEYWORDS

• Degenerative cervical myelopathy • Health economics • Cervical spine • Surgery
• Cost-effectiveness • Value • Health related quality of life

KEY POINTS

- In the current era of value-based medicine, cost as well as effectiveness must be included when evaluating a medical intervention, particularly for management of degenerative cervical myelopathy where surgery is costly and the demand for interventions is likely to increase with aging demographics.
- The growing body of literature pertaining to the health economics of surgery for degenerative cervical myelopathy supports that surgery is very cost effective compared with nonoperative management.
- Further study is needed to determine which patient subgroups derive the greatest value from surgical intervention and which surgical approaches are the most appropriate from cost and health-related quality-of-life perspectives.

INTRODUCTION

Degenerative cervical myelopathy (DCM) is recognized as the leading cause of spinal cord impairment worldwide.[1] The chronic compressive forces on the cervical spinal cord, which result from osteoarthritic degeneration and/or ligamentous aberrations, lead to neurologic symptoms, functional impairment, and reduced quality of life.[2] The natural history of DCM is variable, but recent multicenter, prospective studies suggest that surgical intervention is associated with improved neurologic symptoms and reduced functional impairment, regardless of disease severity.[3,4] This has, in part, led to a shift in perspective. Within the past 5 years, surgery has been increasingly viewed as a means to improve health-related quality of life (HRQOL) rather than simply to halt disease progression.

Although demonstrably effective for DCM, spine surgery is costly; the interventions rank among some of the most costly surgical procedures.[5] Concerns regarding health care sustainability have driven the need to optimize resource

Disclosure Statement: The authors have no personal, financial or institutional interest in any of the drugs, materials or devices described in this article. Dr M.G. Fehlings wishes to declare consulting agreements with Pfizer, Zimmer Biomet and InVivo Therapeutics.

[a] Division of Neurosurgery, Department of Surgery, University of Toronto, Toronto Western Hospital, 4WW, Toronto, Ontario M5T 2S8, Canada; [b] Health Services Research, The University of Chicago, 5841 South Maryland Avenue, MC 2000, Room W249, Chicago, IL 60637-1447, USA; [c] Department of Surgery, University of Toronto, Toronto Western Hospital, 399 Bathurst Street, 4WW-449, Toronto, Ontario M5T 2S8, Canada
* Corresponding author.
E-mail address: Michael.Fehlings@uhn.ca

Neurosurg Clin N Am 29 (2018) 169–176
https://doi.org/10.1016/j.nec.2017.09.013
1042-3680/18/© 2017 Elsevier Inc. All rights reserved.

allocation and have brought quality and value assessments to the forefront of health policy making. In response, a body of research has emerged on the health economics of surgery for DCM.

It is imperative that spine surgeons remain appraised of value considerations when evaluating commonly performed interventions. This review aims to provide a focused overview of key concepts of health economics pertaining to DCM. This is followed by discussion of research available to guide clinicians and health policy decision makers on the value of surgery for DCM and concludes with comments on important questions that remain to be answered.

KEY HEALTH ECONOMIC CONCEPTS RELATED TO DEGENERATIVE CERVICAL MYELOPATHY

This section provides a brief review of the primary considerations in assessing value, to help frame the subsequent survey of health economic literature on the management of DCM. Specifically, the focus is on defining costs, estimating metrics for HRQOL, and combining cost and HRQOL to estimate value and evaluate cost-effectiveness using willingness-to-pay (WTP) thresholds.

Defining Costs

Costs in health economic evaluations can be classified as either health care costs or non–health care costs.[6] Health care costs include all resources consumed resulting from an intervention. With respect to spinal surgery, these may include the cost of the hospital stay, surgical devices, surgeon remuneration, diagnostic tests, and other costs. At times, microlevel costs from case-costing databases can be challenging to obtain because hospitals often do not publically release these data. As alternatives, investigators may choose to use payment data from public or private insurance plans or else hospital discharge data. Charge amounts from hospital discharge data can serve as proxy measures for health care costs; however, it should be recognized that charges are not synonymous with costs, and cost-to-charge ratios (CCRs) should be applied to provide more accurate estimates.[7,8] Costs outside the health care sector also result from medical interventions, including lost productivity, time costs, child care for patients while undergoing treatment, and others. These non–health care costs are often more difficult to estimate but methods, including the human capital-cost approach and the friction-cost approach, are typically used.[9]

The perspective chosen for an economic analysis determines which costs are included in an analysis. Generally, health economic evaluations in spine surgery can be performed from 1 of 3 perspectives: hospital, payer, or society.[10] The societal perspective is the most inclusive and incorporates all health care and non–health care costs. This perspective is recommended by cost-effectiveness methodological guidelines; however, in many instances the scope of data required is not available.[6] The hospital and payer perspectives are narrower in scope but are the perspectives more commonly used in practice.

A final important cost-related consideration pertains to the timeframe over which the economic evaluation is performed. Typically, in the surgical management of degenerative spinal conditions, the upfront costs are high but subsequent costs are much lower—and may be lower than under medical management. Health outcomes from the intervention are often durable over prolonged periods of time. Thus, it is best to evaluate the intervention over a long time horizon, ideally over a lifetime. This provides the most comprehensive estimation of the relative cost of surgery. Extending the timeframe of evaluation has been noted to substantially change findings regarding cost-effectiveness in the spinal literature.[11]

Evaluating Health-related Quality of Life

HRQOL can be defined using a multitude of metrics. Within the domain of health economics in spinal surgery, HRQOL is often measured as health utility. Health utility ranges from 0 to 1 and reflects a person's health status valuation. These can be measured with direct methods, such as time tradeoff, standard gamble, or magnitude estimation.[12,13] It is more common, however, to use preference-based measures, such as the Short Form (SF)-6D and the EuroQol-5D (EQ-5D). EQ-5D is a 5-dimension instrument that includes mobility, self-care, usual activities, pain/discomfort, and depression/anxiety.[14] The SF-6D is a health utility index derived from the SF-36 health questionnaires.[15] A total of 8 dimensions are covered, including physical function, bodily pain, role limitations due to physical health problems, role limitations due to personal or emotional problems, emotional well-being, social functioning, energy/fatigue, and general health perceptions.[16]

Determining Value

Once the cost and health outcomes of an intervention are known, there are 2 common methods of determining value: (1) cost-minimization analysis and (2) cost-effectiveness analysis (CEA) (**Table 1**). A cost minimization analysis is the simpler of the 2 methods; however, it relies on an assumption that the intervention assessed is equivalent in health

Table 1
Common methods for determining the value of a health care intervention

Classification	Methodology	Units for Value Comparison
Cost minimization analysis	Direct cost comparison between 2 interventions Relies on the assumption of equivalent clinical efficacy	Cost difference
Cost-effectiveness analysis	Direct comparison of cost and effectiveness No equivalency in outcomes assumed	ICER (difference in cost divided over difference in outcome)
Cost utility analysis	Subgroup of Cost-effectiveness analysis Direct comparison of cost and effectiveness, with effectiveness measured in QALYs	ICUR (difference in cost divided over difference QALYs)

outcomes to the standard on which it is compared. With the assumption of equivalency, the costs are compared directly and the one of greater value is the one of lesser cost. Unfortunately, this approach is often not applicable. It is uncommon for 2 different interventions to provide precisely equivalent outcomes and without this the approach loses its relevance.

A CEA is more generally applicable because it does not require equivalency in health outcomes. In this method, the difference in cost and in health between the new intervention and the standard is determined concurrently. Once both parameters are known, the ratio of the difference between the 2 is calculated. This gives a value referred to as an incremental cost-effectiveness ratio (ICER) for the intervention in question (Equation 1). This ICER may then be assessed based on where it falls on a cost-effectiveness plane (**Fig. 1**). In a CEA, HRQOL measures other than health utilities may be used. For example, change in the modified Japanese Orthopedic Association (mJOA) score could be used as a HRQOL measure in a CEA of 2 treatment approaches for DCM. Thus, the results of such a comparison would be reported as a dollar value per unit of mJOA gained. This is somewhat difficult to interpret because there is no well-accepted dollar value per mJOA unit gained.

To overcome this, a cost-utility analysis, which is a type of CEA, incorporates the standardized quality-adjusted life year (QALY) as the measure of quality. A QALY is equal to 1 year of life in perfect health. QALYs gained are determined by estimating the improvement in HRQOL using a health utility measure, such as the SF-6D or EQ-5D, and multiplying that by years of life lived during the time horizon of the study, using appropriate discounting. The ratio of the difference in cost and the difference in QALYs gives an incremental cost-utility ratio (ICUR) value for the treatment in question (Equation 2). This ICUR may then be treated in a similar manner to the ICER using a cost-effectiveness plane to determine the relative value of the intervention. Those interventions that have ICURs, which fall in the northeast quadrant of the plane may be compared with standard WTP thresholds, which are described in the following section, to determine if the intervention should be adopted.

$$ICUR = \frac{Cost_{new} - Cost_{standard}}{QALY_{new} - QALY_{standard}} \quad (2)$$

Willingness to Pay

In health economics, the WTP threshold is the monetary amount that decision makers (such as payers or policymakers) are willing to forego to receive one additional QALY.[17] Any intervention with an ICUR under this threshold value is deemed cost effective (**Fig. 2**). The precise threshold level used in making this determination, however, is generally not fixed or absolute. It is influenced by a multitude of factors, including a nation's economic state and standard of living, the nature and burden of a specific disease, among others.[18] In the United Kingdom, the National Institute for Health and Care Excellence defined treatments that range from \$40,000 to \$60,000 per QALY gained as cost effective.[19] Studies performed in

$$ICER = \frac{Cost_{new} - Cost_{standard}}{Health\ Outcome_{new} - Health\ Outcome_{standard}} \quad (1)$$

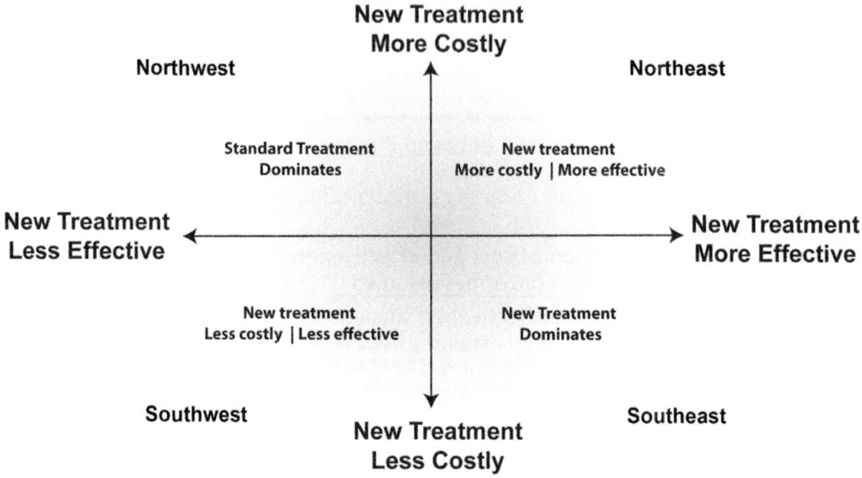

Fig. 1. Four-quadrant cost-effectiveness plane. If the ICER falls in the northwest quadrant, the new treatment is less effective and costlier; thus, the standard treatment dominates and the new treatment should not be adopted. The southeast quadrant represents the opposite, where the new treatment is more effective and less costly and thereby dominates the standard treatment. If the ICER falls in the southwest quadrant, the new treatment provides a cost saving but is less effective. Generally, treatments that are less effective than the standard are not well accepted. The northeast quadrant provides the greatest challenge to health economists. Here, the new treatment is costlier but also more effective. The decision regarding adaptation depends on the WTP threshold. See **Fig. 2** for further details.

the United States most commonly use a $50,000 or a $100,000 threshold.[20] The World Health Organization (WHO) has established a more generalizable definition. An intervention with an ICUR falling below the threshold set at the level of a given country's gross domestic product (GDP) per capita is considered "very cost effective," those that are between 1 and 3 times the GDP of the country are "cost effective," and those that exceed 3 times the GDP per capita are "not cost effective."[21]

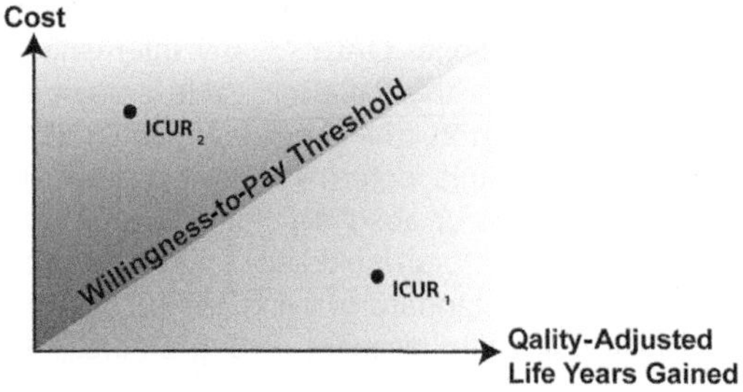

Fig. 2. A WTP in the northeast quadrant of a cost-effectiveness plane. Here any ICUR that falls within the northeast quadrant indicates that a new intervention that is more effective than the standard but also costlier. In a case of the ICUR falling below the WTP, the tradeoff between cost and QALY gained is acceptable and the new intervention should be adopted ($ICUR_1$). In the case of ICUR exceeding WTP, the tradeoff between quality gained and costs is unacceptable and the new intervention should not be adopted ($ICUR_2$).

CURRENT EVIDENCE PERTAINING TO VALUE IN THE MANAGEMENT OF DEGENERATIVE CERVICAL MYELOPATHY

The health economic research on the management of DCM is focused primarily on operative interventions. Nonoperative treatment modalities, such as medication (nonsteroidal anti-inflammatory drugs, and gabapentin), spinal injections, physical therapy, cervical orthoses, and traction therapy, have been described but not evaluated using formal health economic methods.[22] Using the concepts described in the preceding section as a framework, this section serves to provide an up-to-date synopsis of the current health economic literature available relating to the value of surgical intervention for DCM.

Value of Surgery Versus Nonoperative Management

There have been 2 health economic evaluations aimed at estimating the ICUR of surgery to conservative management. The first study was published in 2012 and included outcome data from all 278 subjects enrolled in the AOSpine North America Cervical Spondylotic Myelopathy study.[23] Utility of surgical intervention was determined using the SF-6D. Costs were calculated from a hospital perspective applied to 70 patients enrolled at a single Canadian tertiary care center specializing in the surgical management of complex spinal pathology. The direct costs of medical treatment were just over $21,000 and the ICUR was estimated to be $32,916 (Canadian dollars [CAD])/QALY gained. This was the first evidence that surgery for DCM is cost effective from a payer perspective. There are, however, some notable limitations with this investigation. Namely, a method for determining uncertainty in the estimate was not provided, an estimation of the counterfactual outcome of nonoperative management was not provided for this single arm study, and the horizon over which the ICUR was calculated was set at 10 years, which may underestimate the benefit of this intervention for a chronic degenerative process.

The second study was published in 2016 and set out to address some of these limitations.[24] This updated study included SF-6D health utility data from both the AOSpine North America and AOSpine International studies. A total of 171 subjects were included from the same Canadian tertiary care center. The primary differences between this study and the preceding investigation were methodological. The study was conducted in accordance with the Consolidated Health Economic Evaluation Reporting Standards statement.[25] The ICUR was estimated using a Markov state transition model whereby a counterfactual nonoperative treatment arm was included with outcomes based on the best data available on the natural history of DCM.[26] Furthermore, multiple 1-way deterministic and Monte Carlo probabilistic sensitivity analyses were included in the model to account for parameter uncertainty. Using this model, the estimated lifetime ICUR of surgical intervention for DCM was estimated to be $11,496.02/QALY gained over a lifetime horizon; 97.9% of the estimates obtained in the sensitivity analyses would be considered very cost effective under the WHO WTP threshold, discussed previously (**Fig. 3**). This ICUR is notably lower than in the prior investigation, owing principally to the Markov state transition model approach, which allowed for estimation of the HRQOL outcomes of nonoperative management as well as the lifetime horizon over which the comparison was conducted.

Overall, these results are strongly suggestive that surgical intervention for DCM is very cost effective. One limitation to these studies, however, is that costs from a hospital budgetary perspective were used rather than society's perspective. Another limitation is the inability to observe the counterfactual nonoperative outcomes and the consequent need to project these outcomes using natural history data and Markov modeling. These limitations and the potential to address them are discussed later.

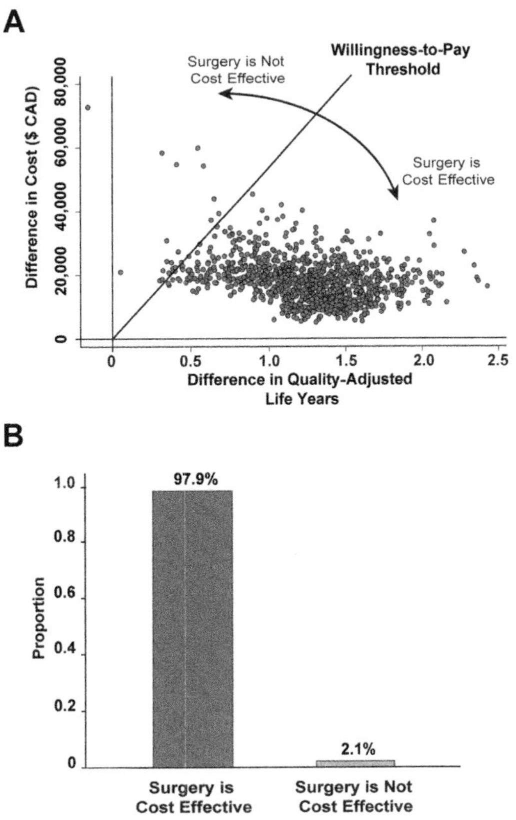

Fig. 3. Markov state transition model with Monte Carlo probabilistic sensitivity analysis for lifetime estimates of ICUR of surgical intervention for DCM. (*A*) Cost-effectiveness plane (partial northwest and northeast quadrants) demonstrating that a majority of estimates fall below WTP threshold set by the WHO to define an intervention as very cost effective. (*B*) Proportion of ICUR estimates (97.9%) that fall within the WHO WTP threshold. (*Adapted from* Witiw CD, Tetreault LA, Smieliauskas F, et al. Surgery for degenerative cervical myelopathy: a patient-centered quality of life and health economic evaluation. Spine J 2017;17(1):23; with permission.)

Anterior Versus Posterior Surgical Approach

Although surgical intervention in general seems cost effective, when compared with nonoperative management it must be recognized that surgery for DCM may be approached using a variety of interventions. These include posterior laminectomy, posterior laminectomy and fusion, posterior laminoplasty, anterior cervical discectomy and fusion, and anterior cervical corpectomy and fusion, to name the most common. Broadly, the health economic literature pertaining to the choice of surgical procedure is limited to comparisons of anterior versus posterior approaches, as described in this section.

An analysis of American hospital administrative data conducted by Shamji and colleagues[27] used National Inpatient Sample data from 2002 to 2005 to study patients with DCM undergoing cervical decompression and fusion of 2 or more levels. Patients undergoing surgery from a posterior approach had a significantly higher rate of immediate postoperative complications and resource utilization (increased length of stay and inflation-adjusted cost) than patients from an anterior approach. This was echoed in a more recent article. Tanenbaum and colleagues[28] included data from the National Inpatient Sample from 1998 to 2011 and used propensity score matching methods to balance groups on observed covariates. They found that patients undergoing a posterior surgical approach for cervical decompression had substantially greater costs and longer hospital stays and were less likely to be discharged home under self-care than those undergoing an anterior approach. Although both studies provide compelling evidence of cost savings from anterior approaches, neither investigation was able to incorporate HRQOL data as a measure of outcome, and both studies were limited by restrictions inherent with administrative databases.[29,30] Although proxy measures, such as length of stay, discharge disposition, and adverse outcomes, are helpful, none provides valid quantification of the impact of surgical intervention on HRQOL. Thus, these studies are in effect cost-minimization analyses; however, to draw meaningful conclusions, matched HRQOL is needed.

Two small studies from a multicenter database of patients undergoing surgical decompression for DCM have sought to compare surgical approaches using both cost and HRQOL data. The first, published in 2011, was a nonrandomized prospective comparative study that included 50 subjects.[31] The investigators found that HRQOL, as measured by the EQ-5D, was significantly improved at 12-month follow-up in both groups but did not find the between group difference to be statistically different. They did find, however, that costs were significantly lower for the anterior group (\$19,245 vs \$29,465; $P = .005$). The investigators refrained from drawing strong conclusions regarding the health economics of anterior versus posterior surgery for DCM but indicated that the pilot study results justified conducting a larger randomized control trial of effectiveness and cost-effectiveness.

In a follow-up study published in 2012, using the same methodology but with an expanded patient cohort that included 85 patients, the average costs after adjustment using Medicare CCR methods were still significantly less for anterior approaches (\$21,563 vs \$27,942; $P = .02$), and the between-group difference in the improvement in EQ-5D scores at 12-month follow-up was again not significantly different (0.13 vs 0.16; $P = .56$).[32] These estimates were then used to determine the ICUR of anterior versus posterior surgery for DCM, concluding that anterior approaches dominate posterior ones because both costs and HRQOL favor anterior procedures. These results are novel and interesting; however, caution in interpreting the findings is warranted. The investigators appropriately highlighted that costing methods may have a substantial impact on the results. They found that anterior surgery was only less costly when using Medicare CCR methods; when using Medicare payment rates, anterior surgeries had higher costs than posterior procedures. Moreover, the groups were not randomly assigned treatment nor were between-group baseline and surgical differences accounted for when comparing outcomes using methods, such as regression adjustment or propensity score matching. Uncertainty in the estimates was also not provided using standard deterministic or probabilistic methods.

In sum, these studies provide novel and helpful information comparing surgical approaches from a health economic perspective, but the methodological and data limitations preclude definitive conclusions regarding the optimal surgical approach from a value perspective.

FUTURE DIRECTIONS

Much remains to be learned about the health economics of the surgical management of DCM. Existing research on the cost-utility of surgery over nonoperative management strongly suggests that surgery is very cost effective over a lifetime horizon.[23,24] These data, however, are derived from a heterogeneous group of individuals participating in the AOSpine studies. Surgery may not be equally effective in improving HRQOL in every type of patient. A larger patient sample permits research to estimate cost-effectiveness in various patient subgroups. These may include younger patients with substantial life-expectancy and earning potential or those with focal compression who only require short segment decompressions with short hospital stays and minimal costs. Moreover, these studies used a hospital budgetary perspective in a single-payer health system. External generalizability to multipayer systems, such as the United States, remains a limitation, as does a lack of information on costs outside the health care system, which would permit using a societal perspective when comparing surgery with nonoperative management. Although it is reasonable to postulate that because operative intervention provides a significant improvement in functionality, costs, such as caregiver burden and lost productivity, could be reduced by surgery, this remains to be shown empirically.

Estimating the magnitude of potential societal impact of surgery for DCM has also remained a challenge. This stems from a limited understanding of the epidemiology of DCM; in particular, accurate estimates of prevalence. DCM encompasses a spectrum of degenerative spinal pathologic conditions, all of which present in a similar manner, thereby making specific epidemiologic classification difficult.[1,2] There is no specific diagnostic classification code within the *International Classification of Diseases, Ninth Revision*, or *Tenth Revision*, to identify DCM to assist with identification in large population based databases. The best data suggest a conservative North American prevalence of 605 per million population; however, these are derived from literature on nontraumatic spinal cord injury and may not include those with mild disability and thus underestimate the prevalence.[1]

Other factors, such as the cost of injury avoidance, have also yet to be factored into health economic considerations when assessing the management of DCM. It has been suggested that individuals with cervical spinal stenosis are at a greater risk of traumatic quadriplegia or quadraparesis from a minor traumatic event to the cervical spine compared with controls without stenosis.[33,34] Drawing from the literature on traumatic spinal injury, the health care costs in the first year for an individual with tetraplegia from a cervical spinal cord injury has been estimated at between $770,264 and $1,065,980 in the United States,[35] and total costs are thought to exceed $1.7 billion in 2009.[36] The economics pertaining to the avoidance of 1 cervical spinal cord injury with decompressive surgery remains to be demonstrated empirically, but this may represent an additional source of value from surgical intervention.

Finally, the question regarding the relative value of anterior versus posterior approaches remains unanswered. Most of the existing literature suggests posterior approaches are costlier. These findings are largely limited, however, by the inherent difficulties in balancing the groups on observable covariates, such as extent of cervical cord compression, sagittal cervical spinal deformity, and specifics regarding presurgical impairment. It is likely that future studies aiming to compare the 2 approaches using randomized treatment allocation and rigorous inclusion/exclusion criteria with concurrent, careful collection of cost data will help answer these questions.[37]

SUMMARY

A growing body of literature supports the cost-effectiveness of surgery for DCM when compared with nonoperative treatment. Further investigation is needed to determine the specific patient subgroups and surgical approaches that result in the most value from surgical intervention. Addressing these questions will be helpful for clinicians and policymakers alike in the face of shifting population demographics and increasing pressures on already strained health care resources.

REFERENCES

1. Nouri A, Tetreault L, Singh A, et al. Degenerative cervical myelopathy: epidemiology, genetics, and pathogenesis. Spine (Phila Pa 1976) 2015;40(12): E675–93.
2. Witiw CD, Fehlings MG. Degenerative cervical myelopathy. CMAJ 2017;189(3):E116.
3. Tetreault LA, Kopjar B, Vaccaro A, et al. A clinical prediction model to determine outcomes in patients with cervical spondylotic myelopathy undergoing surgical treatment: data from the prospective, multi-center AOSpine North America study. J Bone Joint Surg Am 2013;95(18):1659–66.
4. Witwer BP, Trost GR. Cervical spondylosis: ventral or dorsal surgery. Neurosurgery 2007;60(1 Supp1 1): S130–6.
5. Weiss AJ, Elixhauser A, Andrews RM. Characteristics of operating room procedures in U.S. hospitals, 2011: statistical brief #170. Healthcare Cost and Utilization Project (HCUP) Statistical Briefs. Rockville (MD): Agency for Healthcare Research and Quality; 2014.
6. Neumann PJ, Sanders GD, Russell LB, et al. Cost-effectiveness in health and medicine. 2nd edition. New York: Oxford University Press; 2017.
7. Healthcare Cost and Utilization Project (HCUP). Cost-to-charge Ratio Files. 2016. Available at: https://www.hcup-us.ahrq.gov/db/state/costtocharge.jsp. Accessed May 20, 2017.
8. Tumeh JW, Moore SG, Shapiro R, et al. Practical approach for using Medicare data to estimate costs for cost-effectiveness analysis. Expert Rev Pharmacoecon Outcomes Res 2005;5(2):153–62.
9. Liljas B. How to calculate indirect costs in economic evaluations. PharmacoEconomics 1998;13(1 Pt 1): 1–7.

10. Alvin MD, Miller JA, Lubelski D, et al. Variations in cost calculations in spine surgery cost-effectiveness research. Neurosurg Focus 2014;36(6):E1.
11. Tosteson AN, Tosteson TD, Lurie JD, et al. Comparative effectiveness evidence from the spine patient outcomes research trial: surgical versus nonoperative care for spinal stenosis, degenerative spondylolisthesis, and intervertebral disc herniation. Spine (Phila Pa 1976) 2011;36(24):2061–8.
12. Froberg DG, Kane RL. Methodology for measuring health-state preferences–II: Scaling methods. J Clin Epidemiol 1989;42(5):459–71.
13. Brazier J, Deverill M, Green C. A review of the use of health status measures in economic evaluation. J Health Serv Res Policy 1999;4(3):174–84.
14. Rabin R, de Charro F. EQ-5D: a measure of health status from the EuroQol Group. Ann Med 2001; 33(5):337–43.
15. Brazier J, Roberts J, Deverill M. The estimation of a preference-based measure of health from the SF-36. J Health Econ 2002;21(2):271–92.
16. Ware JE Jr. SF-36 health survey update. Spine (Phila Pa 1976) 2000;25(24):3130–9.
17. Claxton K, Briggs A, Buxton MJ, et al. Value based pricing for NHS drugs: an opportunity not to be missed? BMJ 2008;336(7638):251–4.
18. King JT Jr, Tsevat J, Lave JR, et al. Willingness to pay for a quality-adjusted life year: implications for societal health care resource allocation. Med Decis Making 2005;25(6):667–77.
19. McCabe C, Claxton K, Culyer AJ. The NICE cost-effectiveness threshold: what it is and what that means. Pharmacoeconomics 2008;26(9):733–44.
20. Neumann PJ, Cohen JT, Weinstein MC. Updating cost-effectiveness–the curious resilience of the $50,000-per-QALY threshold. N Engl J Med 2014; 371(9):796–7.
21. Cost effectiveness and strategic planning (WHO-CHOICE), Cost-effectiveness levels. Available at: http://www.who.int/choice/costs/CER_levels/en/. Accessed May 19, 2017.
22. Rhee JM, Shamji MF, Erwin WM, et al. Nonoperative management of cervical myelopathy: a systematic review. Spine (Phila Pa 1976) 2013;38(22 Suppl 1): S55–67.
23. Fehlings MG, Jha NK, Hewson SM, et al. Is surgery for cervical spondylotic myelopathy cost-effective? A cost-utility analysis based on data from the AO-Spine North America prospective CSM study. J Neurosurg Spine 2012;17(1 Suppl):89–93.
24. Witiw CD, Tetreault LA, Smieliauskas F, et al. Surgery for degenerative cervical myelopathy: a patient-centered quality of life and health economic evaluation. Spine J 2017;17(1):15–25.
25. Husereau D, Drummond M, Petrou S, et al. Consolidated health economic evaluation reporting standards (CHEERS) statement. BMJ 2013;346:f1049.
26. Karadimas SK, Erwin WM, Ely CG, et al. The pathophysiology and natural history of cervical spondylotic myelopathy. Spine 2013;38(22S):521–36.
27. Shamji MF, Cook C, Pietrobon R, et al. Impact of surgical approach on complications and resource utilization of cervical spine fusion: a nationwide perspective to the surgical treatment of diffuse cervical spondylosis. Spine J 2009;9(1):31–8.
28. Tanenbaum JE, Lubelski D, Rosenbaum BP, et al. Propensity-matched analysis of outcomes and hospital charges for anterior versus posterior cervical fusion for cervical spondylotic myelopathy. Clin Spine Surg 2016. [Epub ahead of print].
29. Wolff N, Helminiak TW. Nonsampling measurement error in administrative data: implications for economic evaluations. Health Econ 1996;5(6):501–12.
30. Peabody JW, Luck J, Jain S, et al. Assessing the accuracy of administrative data in health information systems. Med Care 2004;42(11):1066–72.
31. Ghogawala Z, Martin B, Benzel EC, et al. Comparative effectiveness of ventral vs dorsal surgery for cervical spondylotic myelopathy. Neurosurgery 2011; 68(3):622–30 [discussion: 630–1].
32. Whitmore RG, Schwartz JS, Simmons S, et al. Performing a cost analysis in spine outcomes research: comparing ventral and dorsal approaches for cervical spondylotic myelopathy. Neurosurgery 2012; 70(4):860–7 [discussion: 867].
33. Ruegg TB, Wicki AG, Aebli N, et al. The diagnostic value of magnetic resonance imaging measurements for assessing cervical spinal canal stenosis. J Neurosurg Spine 2015;22(3):230–6.
34. Chang V, Ellingson BM, Salamon N, et al. The risk of acute spinal cord injury after minor trauma in patients with preexisting cervical stenosis. Neurosurgery 2015;77(4):561–5.
35. National Spinal Cord Injury Statistical Center, Facts and Figures at a Glance. 2016; Available at: https://www.nscisc.uab.edu/Public/Facts 2016.pdf. Accessed May 29, 2017.
36. Mahabaleshwarkar R, Khanna R. National hospitalization burden associated with spinal cord injuries in the United States. Spinal Cord 2014;52(2):139–44.
37. Ghogawala Z, Benzel EC, Heary RF, et al. Cervical spondylotic myelopathy surgical trial: randomized, controlled trial design and rationale. Neurosurgery 2014;75(4):334–46.

Managing the Complex Patient with Degenerative Cervical Myelopathy

How to Handle the Aging Spine, the Obese Patient, and Individuals with Medical Comorbidities

Geoffrey Stricsek, MD[a], John Gillick, MD[b], George Rymarczuk, MD[b], James S. Harrop, MD[c,d,*]

KEYWORDS

- Degenerative cervical myelopathy • Comorbidities • Functional outcome
- Perioperative complication

KEY POINTS

- Surgery is an effective treatment for degenerative cervical myelopathy (DCM).
- Age is correlated with functional outcomes and the risk of perioperative morbidity following surgery for DCM, but it is a nonmodifiable risk factor.
- Cardiovascular comorbidity, diabetes, and obesity are all associated with reduced functional improvement following surgery for DCM.
- Many comorbidities can increase the risk of perioperative complication.

INTRODUCTION

Degenerative cervical myelopathy (DCM) encompasses multiple degenerative conditions including cervical spondylotic myelopathy (CSM), ossification of the posterior longitudinal ligament, ossification of the ligamentum flavum, and degenerative disc disease.[1] Forms of degenerative myelopathy are the most common cause of nontraumatic spinal cord injury in the aging population.[2,3] Although the natural history of DCM is unclear,[4] Fehlings and Arvin[5] documented an important clinical observation that even clinically stable, mild myelopathy can be associated with significant functional limitations.[5] Prospective data from AOSpine North American and International

Disclosure Statement: None of the authors have any relevant disclosures.
[a] Department of Neurological Surgery, Jack and Vickie Farber Institute for Neuroscience, Thomas Jefferson University, 909 Walnut Street, 3rd Floor, Philadelphia, PA 19107, USA; [b] Spine Division, Department of Neurological Surgery, Jack and Vickie Farber Institute for Neuroscience, Thomas Jefferson University, 909 Walnut Street, 3rd Floor, Philadelphia, PA 19107, USA; [c] Division of Spine and Peripheral Nerve Surgery, Department of Neurological Surgery, Jack and Vickie Farber Institute for Neuroscience, Thomas Jefferson University, 909 Walnut Street, 3rd Floor, Philadelphia, PA 19107, USA; [d] Department of Orthopedic Surgery, Thomas Jefferson University Hospital, 909 Walnut Street, 3rd Floor, Philadelphia, PA 19107, USA
* Corresponding author. 909 Walnut Street, 3rd Floor, Philadelphia, PA 19107.
E-mail address: james.harrop@jefferson.edu

Neurosurg Clin N Am 29 (2018) 177–184
https://doi.org/10.1016/j.nec.2017.09.014
1042-3680/18/© 2017 Elsevier Inc. All rights reserved.

cohorts of patients with cervical myelopathy have demonstrated that surgery provides a significant functional benefit, significantly improves quality of life, and is cost-effective.[6–8] Age, medical comorbidities, and smoking status are associated with functional outcomes following surgery.[9–11] Achieving a positive outcome relies on understanding how these factors influence patient selection, surgical decision making, and functional improvement.

AGE

Approximately 90% of patients older than 65 will have some evidence of cervical spondylosis on imaging studies.[12] However, the existence of degenerative changes or spinal cord compression on imaging does not necessarily correlate with symptoms of myelopathy.[13,14] Degenerative changes will continue to progress over time[15] and may result in the development of functional deficits. Bednarik and colleagues[14] prospectively followed asymptomatic patients with cervical spondylosis and observed the development of myelopathy in more than 22% of patients within a median follow-up time of 44 months. Thus, as the average age of the general population and life expectancy both increase, it is likely that the number of people with DCM will also climb.

Prospectively collected data has shown that surgery provides a significant clinical benefit for patients with cervical myelopathy,[6,7,16] but how does age affect outcomes? Data from the international arm of the AOSpine CSM study found preoperative modified Japanese Orthopedic Association (mJOA) scores were significantly lower and preoperative Nurick scores were significantly higher in elderly patients (aged 65 or older) when compared with the younger cohort.[10] Postoperatively, elderly and nonelderly patients were found to have a significant improvement in Nurick and mJOA scores following surgery; however, younger patients still had significantly higher mJOA and lower Nurick scores (**Table 1**).[10] Tetreault and colleagues[17] used combined data from the AOSpine CSM-International and CSM-North American studies to construct prediction models for the minimum clinically important difference (MCID) in mJOA score after surgery for cervical myelopathy; MCID was defined as a 1 point improvement for mild, 2 points for moderate, and 3 points for severe myelopathy. Younger age was found to be a significant predictor of achieving the MCID on postoperative mJOA score; for every 10-year increase in age, a patient was 8% to 9% less likely to achieve the MCID.[9,11] A separate prospective study by Machino and colleagues[16,18] also concluded that patient age of 65 or older was a significant risk factor for lower preoperative and postoperative JOA score and lower JOA recovery rate.

Table 1
Preoperative and 24-month postoperative modified Japanese Orthopedic Association (mJOA) and Nurick scores compared between elderly and nonelderly patients

Outcome Measure	Younger Patients, <65	Elderly Patients, ≥65	*P*
Baseline			
mJOA	12.86	11.41	<.0001
Nurick	3.16	3.75	<.0001
24-mo postoperative			
mJOA	15.45	14.08	<.0001
Nurick	1.64	2.44	<.0001

Data from Nakashima H, Tetreault L, Nagoshi N, et al. Does age affect surgical outcomes in patients with degenerative cervical myelopathy? Results from the prospective multicenter AOSpine International study on 479 patients. J Neurol Neurosurg Psychiatry 2016;87:734–40.

Data from larger retrospective articles[19,20] concur with the findings from the prospective studies by AOSpine and Machino and colleagues.[16,18] A meta-analysis from Madhavan and colleagues[19] looked at more than 2800 patients from 18 different studies, calculated the average age for elderly and nonelderly patients, and compared preoperative and postoperative outcomes. Average age for elderly patients was 74, nonelderly average age was 55, and the investigators concluded that elderly patients had significantly lower preoperative and postoperative JOA scores compared with nonelderly, leading to a significantly lower recovery rate. A systematic review by Tetreault and colleagues[20] identified 36 articles that examined the impact of age on surgical outcome, and then categorized them as "Excellent," "Good," or "Poor" using a modified version of the Scottish Inter-Collegiate Guidelines Network scoring system. Sixteen articles were identified as "Excellent" and collectively suggested that age may be a predictor of outcome using JOA, mJOA, or Nurick scores.[20] However, when "Good" and even "Poor" articles were included in their assessment, age was not found to be a significant predictor of outcome.[20]

In addition to functional outcomes, there are also significant age-related differences in surgical approach. Sixty-five percent of younger patients (age <65) in the AOSpine CSM-International study had anterior surgery, whereas 59% of elderly patients (age ≥65) had posterior surgery.[10] Of the elderly patients treated anteriorly, a significantly higher percentage had a combined discectomy and corpectomy when compared with younger patients (28% vs 13%).[10] Elderly patients also had more levels decompressed than younger patients, most likely a result of the increasing degenerative changes that accumulate with age, thus explaining the bias toward posterior surgery.[10,15] Age-related differences in functional outcomes remained significant after controlling for differences in surgical approach.[10]

Although the evidence supports a significant interaction between age and functional improvement after surgery for DCM, it is also important to consider the impact of age on postoperative recovery and the rate of surgical complication. Older patients have been found to have significantly longer hospital stays,[10,19,21] but similar operative time and less blood loss.[10,18,19] Data regarding the relationship between age and complication rate are mixed. Results from the AOSpine CSM-International study and the cohort of Machino and colleagues did not find any significant difference in perioperative complication rate with regard to age.[10,18,22] The meta-analysis of Madhavan and colleagues[19] made similar conclusions except that older patients had a higher rate of perioperative delirium.[19] However, a retrospective review of more than 54,000 patients from the Nationwide Inpatient Sample (NIS) who underwent surgery for cervical myelopathy found that patients older than 65 had a significantly higher risk for perioperative complications, including cardiac, respiratory, gastrointestinal, and wound healing.[21,23]

Age is a nonmodifiable risk factor; its impact on functional recovery and perioperative complication should be an important part of any preoperative consultation, but it cannot be adjusted. Although age is a fixed predictor, it also has been shown to correlate with the incidence and severity of preoperative comorbidities.[10,18,21] Increasing comorbid score has been shown to be a negative predictor for achieving the MCID in functional scores[9] and the presence of some comorbidities increases the risk of perioperative complication following surgery for cervical myelopathy (**Tables 2** and **3**).[22] Identifying and optimizing modifiable comorbidities should be a priority in the preoperative setting to maximize outcomes.

MEDICAL COMORBIDITIES

Cardiovascular

Cardiovascular comorbidity was the most common comorbidity among enrollees in the combined cohorts of the prospective AOSpine CSM study, occurring in 45% of patients.[9] Specific comorbidities included the following: history of myocardial infarct, congestive heart failure, arrhythmia, hypertension, and peripheral vascular disease.[22] Functional outcomes analysis found cardiovascular comorbidity to be a significant predictor for not obtaining the MCID following surgery.[9,11] Maeno and colleagues[24] retrospectively reviewed their patients with cervical myelopathy who had undergone laminoplasty and also found that patients with hypertension had significantly lower preoperative and postoperative JOA scores, leading to a lower recovery rate.

Table 2
Univariate analysis assessing the relationship between various clinical factors and perioperative complications

Clinical Predictor	Odds Ratio	95% Confidence Interval	*P*
Comorbidities	2.03	1.18–3.47	.01
Number of comorbidities	1.32	1.11–1.56	.002
Comorbidity score	1.19	1.05–1.34	.006
Cardiovascular	1.64	1.01–2.68	.046
Diabetes	2.83	1.54–5.20	<.001
Psychiatric	0.17	0.50–2.76	.72

Data from Tetreault L, Tan G, Kopjar B, et al. Clinical and surgical predictors of complications following surgery for the treatment of cervical spondylotic myelopathy: results from the multicenter, prospective AOSpine International Study of 479 patients. Neurosurgery 2016;79:33–44.

Table 3
Univariate analyses evaluating the association between various clinical predictors and achieving an MCID on the mJOA scale at 2 years following surgery

Clinical Predictor	Relative Risk	95% Confidence Interval	*P*
Age	0.918	0.881–0.955	<.0001
Comorbidities	0.948	0.859–1.046	.285
Comorbidity score	0.966	0.935–0.998	.035
Cardiovascular	0.894	0.808–0.989	.029
Endocrine	0.879	0.760–1.016	.080
Psychiatric	1.058	0.929–1.206	.397

Data from Tetreault L, Tan G, Kopjar B, et al. Clinical and surgical predictors of complications following surgery for the treatment of cervical spondylotic myelopathy: results from the multicenter, prospective AOSpine International Study of 479 patients. Neurosurgery 2016;79:33–44.

A retrospective analysis of patients with symptomatic cervical stenosis looked at the correlation among hypertension, MRI findings, and functional scores.[25] All patients with a diagnosis of hypertension, either controlled or uncontrolled, were significantly more likely to have increased signal intensity (ISI) on sagittal T2-weighted MRI when compared with patients who were not hypertensive, and the ISI surface area was significantly larger in hypertensive patients than nonhypertensive.[25] When looking at controlled versus uncontrolled hypertensive patients, the surface area of ISI in uncontrolled hypertensive patients was significantly larger than those with adequately controlled blood pressure; maximal canal stenosis was equivalent between all groups.[25] The presence of signal changes in the spinal cord were found to correlate with worse mJOA and Nurick scores independent of the surface area of ISI.[25]

Patients with cardiovascular comorbidity in the CSM-International study, in addition to worse functional outcomes, were also significantly more likely to have postoperative complications, with hypertension carrying the greatest risk.[22] Retrospective review of more than 54,000 patients from the NIS database found that congestive heart failure, peripheral vascular disorders, and cardiac valvular disease were also associated with a significantly increased risk of perioperative complication.[23] However, hypertension (grouped as complicated and uncomplicated) had no impact on perioperative morbidity, but was associated with a decreased risk of mortality.[23] The investigators of this review surmised that a known diagnosis of hypertension led to better preoperative optimization of patients, yielding the observed mortality benefit.[23]

Cardiovascular comorbidities have been shown to correlate with perioperative complications and functional outcome following surgery for CSM. Although the interaction between hypertension and perioperative morbidity is unclear, hypertension may significantly compound the neurologic damage caused by cervical spondylosis. The impact of cardiovascular comorbidities on outcomes should be discussed with the patient and optimized before elective surgery to minimize the risk of perioperative complication and maximize the chances for functional improvement.

Diabetes

The rate of diabetes among patients undergoing surgery for DCM is cited at 9% to 36%, making it the second most common comorbidity in this population.[26–30] Although chronic diabetes is known to have neurologic sequelae, data regarding preoperative functional scores in diabetic patients with DCM are mixed: retrospective data from a few small studies suggests that diabetic patients do not have significantly worse preoperative JOA[24,27,28,31] or Nurick scores.[32] However, one prospective study found diabetic patients had a significantly higher preoperative Nurick score, but no difference in mJOA,[26] whereas another study observed significantly lower preoperative JOA scores in diabetic patients compared with nondiabetic patients.[29] Regardless of preoperative differences, diabetic patients appear to have a significant improvement in functional scores after surgery.[26–28] Some studies have found total postoperative JOA, mJOA, and Nurick scores to be significantly worse among diabetic versus nondiabetic patients,[26,29,32] whereas others have found significantly less recovery of only lower extremity motor and sensory function based on JOA score.[27,31] Despite these differences, univariate analysis from the AOSpine CSM studies found that endocrine comorbidities did not significantly impact realization of an MCID on the mJOA scale.[9,11] Although individual diagnoses within the endocrine category were not evaluated, diabetes undoubtedly constituted a significant component.

The impact of diabetes on outcomes following surgery for DCM has also been evaluated based on hemoglobin A1c (HbA1c) and serum blood glucose levels. Preoperative HbA1c levels in diabetic patients with DCM ranged from 6.5% to 8.3%[16,27,31] and were found to negatively correlate with postoperative JOA recovery rate (**Table 4**).[29,31] One retrospective study found higher average perioperative glucose values in diabetic patients negatively correlated with improvement in Nurick score; stratification using an average blood glucose cutoff of 150 mg/dL found significantly improved outcomes for diabetic patients with values less than 150.[32] Although absolute values make it easier to monitor and adjust perioperative care, 2 other studies, 1 prospective and 1 retrospective, observed no correlation between either fasting blood glucose levels or highest perioperative blood glucose level and JOA recovery rate.[16,31] Duration of diabetes also may be important, as one prospective study observed patients who had diabetes for more than 10 years had a lower JOA recovery rate after surgery.[16] Kawaguchi and colleagues[31] did not find a similar association, but their conclusion was based on an average duration of diabetes of 6.7 years.

In addition to functional recovery, it is also important to consider how diabetes impacts the perioperative process. Diabetes is not associated with significantly increased length of surgery or

Table 4
HbA1c levels are correlated with outcomes following surgery for DCM in diabetic patients; poor outcome defined as recovery rate of less than 50%

Variable	Good Outcome	Poor Outcome	*P*
Preoperative			
JOA score	10.6	0.7	.075
HbA1c level, %	6.8	7.2	.0165
Postoperative			
JOA score	15.2	11.2	<.0001
Recovery rate of JOA score	73.8	22.3	<.0001

Abbreviations: DCM, degenerative cervical myelopathy; HbA1C, hemoglobin A1C; JOA, Japanese Orthopedic Association.

Data from Machino M, Yukawa Y, Ito K, et al. Risk factors for poor outcome of cervical laminoplasty for cervical spondylotic myelopathy in patients with diabetes. J Bone Joint Surg Am 2014;96:2049–55.

greater blood loss when compared with nondiabetic patients.[29,31] Although some studies have found no difference in major surgical complication rates between diabetic and nondiabetic patients,[26,27,29,31] larger data sets have suggested that diabetic patients do have a significantly increased risk of perioperative complications including respiratory complications, cardiac and peripheral vascular complications, dysphagia, dysphonia, and an increased transfusion requirement.[22,23,30] Importantly, most studies agree that although diabetic patients may sometimes have delayed superficial wound healing, there was no significant difference in the rate of surgical site infection.[22,30] When comparing well-controlled with poorly controlled diabetic patients, those with poor control were found to have a significantly higher risk of perioperative mortality, cardiac complication, hematoma formation, infection, and nonroutine discharge, but still no difference in the rate of wound complication.[30] The review by Cook and colleagues[30] of the NIS database also found that diabetic patients were more likely to have longer hospital stays and higher hospitalization costs.[30]

Although diabetes does not preclude a patient from gaining meaningful functional recovery following surgery for DCM, it does appear to limit the extent of recovery and is associated with a higher risk of perioperative complication when compared with nondiabetic patients. Patients with a prolonged history of poorly controlled diabetes are the least likely to gain significant functional recovery and the most likely to suffer from perioperative complications. Furthermore, diabetic patients are also more likely to have general cardiovascular comorbidities,[26] including hypertension,[29] and tend to be older than nondiabetic patients.[10,26] Preparing for positive outcomes in the diabetic patient must go beyond controlling HbA1c and blood glucose to identify other conditions that can impact improvement and recovery.

Psychiatric: Depression and Bipolar

Psychiatric comorbidity, including depression and bipolar disorder, is observed in 14% to 25% of patients with DCM.[11,33] Data analyzing the impact of psychiatric comorbidities on the management of patients with CSM are in limited supply. The AOSpine CSM-International study observed that patients with depression or bipolar disorder had significantly worse preoperative neck disability index (NDI) scores compared with those who did not, but mJOA and Nurick scores were not significantly different.[33] Postoperatively, patients had statistically significant improvement in mJOA, Nurick, and NDI scores, and although improvement in mJOA and Nurick scores was similar between patients with depression and those without, changes in NDI were significantly larger in patients without psychiatric disorders.[33] Univariate analysis confirmed that psychiatric comorbidities were not significantly correlated with achieving a postoperative MCID in mJOA score.[11] Zong and colleagues[34] also prospectively looked at the impact of depression in patients with CSM. Whereas the AOSpine study relied on patient-reported and clinical review of medical records to diagnose psychiatric comorbidity, Zong and colleagues[34] obtained Beck Depression Index (BDI) scores for a group of 511 patients; patients with a BDI score of 10 or higher were considered to have depression. They found that patients with depression had significantly less change in mJOA following surgery; however, their final analysis excluded all patients who had recovered from their depression or had subsequently become depressed following surgery.[34]

Evaluation of the impact of psychiatric comorbidity on functional outcomes is limited by the volume and quality of data. Although there does not appear to be an interaction with functional outcome, no study has compared outcomes between well-controlled and poorly controlled patients, or considered the duration of depression in their evaluation. Although data from the AOSpine CSM-International study found that psychiatric comorbidities were not a predictor for increased risk of perioperative complication,[22] they have been shown to correlate with a higher incidence of cardiovascular disease.[33] Thus, preoperative evaluation of the patient with DCM with psychiatric comorbidity should take this into account and include adequate screening and optimization as necessary given the impact of cardiovascular comorbidity as outlined previously.

Body Mass Index

Of the more than 700 patients enrolled in the AOSpine CSM-North American and International studies, 25% were found to be obese (body mass index [BMI] >30 kg/m^2), with an additional 36% classified as overweight (BMI >24.99 kg/m^2).[35] At baseline, elevated BMI was correlated with an increased NDI but not associated with mJOA; similar observations were made 1 year after surgery.[35] Categorization of outcomes based on weight class found postoperative NDI was an average of 4.2 points higher in overweight patients and 7.6 points higher in obese patients when compared with normal-weight patients; only obese patients exhibited a significant difference in NDI.[35] The likelihood of obese patients achieving the MCID for NDI scores at 1 year was also significantly less than for normal-weight patients.[35] A prospective study by Machino and colleagues[16,29] used JOA scores and also observed that patients with a BMI of 25 kg/m^2 or higher did not have a significantly increased risk for poor functional outcome, but they did not separately evaluate the obese population.

Outside of functional improvement, it is also important to consider the impact of body weight on the perioperative process. The average BMI of patients in AOSpine CSM-International study was 25.8, falling into the "overweight" category; univariate analysis of this population found that despite the elevated BMI, there was no increased risk of perioperative complication.[22] Retrospective review of more than 54,000 patients from the NIS database found that obese patients had a significantly higher risk of perioperative complication, although they also had a lower perioperative mortality.[23]

Although BMI may not directly influence functional outcomes, the obese patient's perception of how their daily activities are impacted by DCM is significantly worse than the nonobese patient. Additionally, obesity was shown to significantly increase the risk of perioperative morbidity. Body weight may be a modifiable risk factor that, when optimized, can improve patient-perceived outcomes and reduce perioperative complications.

TOBACCO USE

Data from the combined AOSpine CSM-North American and International studies found that 27% of enrolled patients were smokers.[36] Although smokers tended to be younger than nonsmokers, smokers had significantly less improvement in mJOA and NDI scores 1 year after surgery.[36] A separate, retrospective study observed smokers to have significantly less improvement in Nurick scores and found a significant negative correlation between number of packs smoked per day and postoperative change in Nurick score.[37] Further analysis of the AOSpine cohorts confirmed that smoking status was a significant predictor for achieving an MCID on the mJOA 2 years after surgery and the likelihood of having an MCID decreased by 16% if the patient is a smoker.[9] Tobacco use was not found to be associated with a higher rate of perioperative complication.[22]

Smoking is a modifiable risk factor that can significantly impact patient outcomes. The nonsmoker has a significantly higher chance of gaining significant functional recovery following surgery. Tobacco use was also found to interact with other comorbidities that influence outcomes, including diabetes and older age; in combination, the chance of poor outcomes is further increased.[28] Smoking cessation should be a preoperative priority in the patient with DCM.

SUMMARY

DCM is the most common cause of nontraumatic spinal cord injury in adults.[3] Surgery has been shown to be a safe treatment option that offers significant functional improvement, is cost-effective, and improves patient quality of life.[6–8,18] However, successful outcomes depend on adequate patient counseling and effective management of modifiable risk factors. Although age is a not a modifiable risk factor, older patients are more likely to have medical comorbidities; taking the time to look for cardiovascular, endocrine, and psychiatric conditions in this population can improve functional recovery and limit perioperative complications. Additionally, weight loss in the obese patient and smoking cessation in the tobacco user can also improve outcomes. Surgery is a valuable therapy for the treatment of DCM, but that value relies on proactively identifying obstacles and minimizing their impact.

REFERENCES

1. Nouri A, Tetreault L, Singh A, et al. Degenerative cervical myelopathy: epidemiology, genetics, and pathogenesis. Spine 2015;40(12):E675–93.

2. Moore A, Blumhardt L. A prospective survey of the causes of non-traumatic spastic paraparesis and tetraparesis in 585 patients. Spinal Cord 1997;35:361–7.
3. Kalsi-Ryan S, Karadimas S, Fehlings M. Cervical spondylotic myelopathy: the clinical phenomenon and the current pathobiology of an increasingly prevalent and devastating disorder. Neuroscientist 2013;19:409–21.
4. Matz P, Anderson P, Holly L, et al. The natural history of cervical spondylotic myelopathy. J Neurosurg Spine 2009;11:104–11.
5. Fehlings M, Arvin B. Surgical management of cervical degenerative disease: the evidence related to indications, impact, and outcome. J Neurosurg Spine 2009;11:97–100.
6. Fehlings M, Ibrahim A, Tetreault L, et al. A global perspective on the outcomes of surgical decompression in patients with cervical spondylotic myelopathy. Spine 2015;40:1322–8.
7. Fehlings M, Wilson J, Kopjar B, et al. Efficacy and safety of surgical decompression in patients with cervical spondylotic myelopathy: results of the AO-Spine North America prospective multi-center study. J Bone Joint Surg Am 2013;95:1651–8.
8. Witiw C, Tetreault L, Smieliauskas F, et al. Surgery for degenerative cervical myelopathy: a patient-centered quality of life and health economic evaluation. Spine J 2017;17:15–25.
9. Tetreault L, Wilson J, Kotter M, et al. Predicting the minimum clinically important difference in patients undergoing surgery for the treatment of degenerative cervical myelopathy. Neurosurg Focus 2016;40(6):E14.
10. Nakashima H, Tetreault L, Nagoshi N, et al. Does age affect surgical outcomes in patients with degenerative cervical myelopathy? Results from the prospective multicenter AOSpine International study on 479 patients. J Neurol Neurosurg Psychiatry 2016;87:734–40.
11. Tetreault L, Kopjar B, Cote P, et al. A clinical prediction rule for functional outcomes in patients undergoing surgery for degenerative cervical myelopathy. J Bone Joint Surg Am 2015;97:2038–46.
12. Lawrence J. Disc degeneration. Its frequency and relationship to symptoms. Ann Rheum Dis 1969;28:121–38.
13. Gore D, Sepic S, Gardner G. Roentgenographic findings of the cervical spine in asymptomatic people. Spine (Phila Pa 1976) 1986;11:521–4.
14. Bednarik J, Kadanka Z, Dusek L, et al. Presymptomatic spondylotic cervical myelopathy: an updated predictive model. Eur Spine J 2008;17:421–31.
15. Wilder F, Fahlman L, Donnelly R. Radiographic cervical spine osteoarthritis progression rates: a longitudinal assessment. Rheumatol Int 2011;31:45–8.
16. Machino M, Yukawa Y, Ito K, et al. Risk factors for poor outcome of cervical laminoplasty for cervical spondylotic myelopathy in patients with diabetes. J Bone Joint Surg Am 2014;96:2049–55.
17. Tetreault L, Nouri A, Kopjar B, et al. The minimum clinically important difference of the modified Japanese Orthopaedic Association scale in patients with degenerative cervical myelopathy. Spine 2015;40:1653–9.
18. Machino M, Yukawa Y, Imagama S, et al. Surgical treatment assessment of cervical laminoplasty using quantitative performance evaluation in elderly patients: a prospective comparative study in 505 patients with cervical spondylotic myelopathy. Spine (Phila Pa 1976) 2016;41:757–63.
19. Madhavan K, Chieng L, Foong H, et al. Surgical outcomes of elderly patients with cervical spondylotic myelopathy: a meta-analysis of studies reporting on 2868 patients. Neurosurg Focus 2016;40:E13.
20. Tetreault L, Karpova A, Fehlings M. Predictors of outcome in patients with degenerative cervical spondylotic myelopathy undergoing surgical treatment: results of a systematic review. Eur Spine J 2015;24(Suppl 2):S236–51.
21. Jalai C, Worley N, Marascalchi B, et al. The impact of advanced age on peri-operative outcomes in the surgical treatment of cervical spondylotic myelopathy. Spine 2016;41:E139–47.
22. Tetreault L, Tan G, Kopjar B, et al. Clinical and surgical predictors of complications following surgery for the treatment of cervical spondylotic myelopathy: results from the multicenter, prospective AOSpine International Study of 479 patients. Neurosurgery 2016;79:33–44.
23. Kaye I, Maraschalchi B, Macagno A, et al. Predictors of morbidity and mortality among patients with cervical spondylotic myelopathy treated surgically. Eur Spine J 2015;24:2910–7.
24. Maeno T, Okuda S, Yamashita T, et al. Age-related surgical outcomes of laminopasty for cervical spondylotic myelopathy. Global Spine J 2015;5:118–23.
25. Kalb S, Zaidi H, Ribas-Nijkerk J, et al. Persistent outpatient hypertension is independently associated with spinal cord dysfunction and imaging characteristics of spinal cord damage among patients with cervical spondylosis. World Neurosurg 2015;84:351–7.
26. Arnold P, Fehlings M, Kopjar B, et al. Mild diabetes is not a contraindication for surgical decompression in cervical spondylotic myelopathy: results of the AOSpine North American multicenter prospective study (CSM). Spine J 2014;14:65–72.
27. Dokai T, Nagashima H, Nanjo Y, et al. Surgical outcomes and prognostic factors of cervical spondylotic myelopathy in diabetic patients. Arch Orthop Trauma Surg 2012;132:577–82.

28. Kim H, Moon S, Kim H, et al. Diabetes and smoking as prognostic factors after cervical laminoplasty. J Bone Joint Surg Br 2008;90:1468–72.
29. Machino M, Yukawa Y, Ito K, et al. Impact of diabetes on the outcomes of cervical laminoplasty: a prospective cohort study of more than 500 patients with cervical spondylotic myelopathy. Spine 2014; 39:220–7.
30. Cook C, Tackett S, Shah A, et al. Diabetes and perioperative outcomes following cervical fusion in patients with myelopathy. Spine 2008;33:E254–60.
31. Kawaguchi Y, Matsui H, Ishihara H, et al. Surgical outcome of cervical expansive laminoplasty in patients with diabetes mellitus. Spine 2000;25:551–5.
32. Kusin D, Ahn U, Ahn N. The influence of diabetes on surgical outcomes in cervical myelopathy. Spine 2016;41:1436–40.
33. Tetreault L, Nagoshi N, Nakashmia H, et al. Impact of depression and bipolar disorders on functional and quality of life outcomes in patients undergoing surgery for degenerative cervical myelopathy. Spine 2017;42:372–8.
34. Zong Y, Xue Y, Zhao Y, et al. Depression contributed an unsatisfactory surgery outcome among the posterior decompression of the cervical spondylotic myelopathy patients: a prospective clinical study. Neurol Sci 2014;35:1373–9.
35. WIlson J, Tetreault L, Schroeder G, et al. Impact of elevated body mass index and obesity on long-term surgical outcomes for patients with degenerative cervical myelopathy. Spine 2017;42(3):195–201.
36. Arnold P, Kopjar B, Tetreault L, et al. Tobacco smoking and outcomes of surgical decompression in patients with symptomatic degenerative cervical spondylotic myelopathy. Neurosurgery 2016; 63(Suppl 1):165.
37. Kusin D, Ahn U, Ahn N. The effect of smoking on spinal cord healing following surgical treatment of cervical myelopathy. Spine 2015;40:1391–6.

Future Directions and New Technologies for the Management of Degenerative Cervical Myelopathy

Mario Ganau, MD, PhD[a,*], Langston T. Holly, MD[b],
Junichi Mizuno, MD, PhD[c], Michael G. Fehlings, MD, PhD, FRCSC[a]

KEYWORDS

• Degenerative cervical myelopathy • Nanotechnology • Biomedical engineering • Biomaterials • Osteobiologics • Spinal implants • Neuroprotective drugs • Regenerative strategies

KEY POINTS

- Biomarkers are sought to both detect early structural changes of the spinal cord in degenerative cervical myelopathy (DCM) and to predict the outcome. Clinical studies are testing whether multiparameter analysis of high-Tesla MRI sequences and metabolic images could enhance diagnostic and prognostic information.
- Biomedical engineering is fostering the next generation of spinal implants to correct spinal alignment, increase fusion rate, and preserve range of motion at adjacent levels. To address these needs, engineers are designing hybrid systems, incorporating microelectromechanical and nanoelectromechanical systems, and using functionalized coatings with osteoinducing properties.
- Biomaterials proposed for innovative spinal implants include metals, alloys, and ceramics with nonperiodic nanostructure that enhance the interaction and activity of osteoblasts. Nanoscaffolds, nanoleaves, and nanoneedles are all good examples of this type of nanofabrication.
- Minimally invasive anterior and posterior approaches are already part of the surgical practice; nonetheless, given the refinement of biomaterials and the better understanding of the pathologic processes leading to DCM, their role could potentially become more important in the next years in the setting of a truly personalized medicine.
- Neuroprotective agents (eg, preoperative and postoperative administration of Riluzole, a sodium-channel blocker preserving mitochondrial function and reducing oxidative damage in neurons) and regenerative strategies (eg, application on the decompressed dural layer of Cethrin, a Rho inhibitor promoting axonal sprouting) may soon become common strategies for augmenting the effects of surgical treatment.

INTRODUCTION

Spinal surgery is witnessing a fast-paced evolution in management strategies for degenerative cervical myelopathy (DCM). This metamorphosis has been prompted by the need to address the issue of an expected increase in the prevalence of DCM (due to an aging population prone to

Disclosure: The authors have nothing to disclose.
[a] Department of Neurosurgery, Toronto Western Hospital, University Health Network, 399 Bathurst Street 4WW-449, Toronto, Ontario M5T 258, Canada; [b] Department of Neurosurgery, Ronald Reagan UCLA Medical Center, 1250 16th Street, Santa Monica, CA 90404, USA; [c] Department of Neurological Surgery, Aichi Medical University, 480-1195 Aichi Prefecture, Aichi, Japan
* Corresponding author.
E-mail address: mario.ganau@alumni.harvard.edu

Neurosurg Clin N Am 29 (2018) 185–193
https://doi.org/10.1016/j.nec.2017.09.006
1042-3680/18/© 2017 Elsevier Inc. All rights reserved.

developing the disease), and has been due to the fruitful collaboration with basic scientists.

Progressive compression of the cervical spinal cord due to degeneration and narrowing of the spinal canal is the main pathophysiology underlying DCM. The optimal timing of intervention in DCM is still an area of ongoing debate; however, experimental studies have shown that delays in decompression could increase the extent of ischemia-reperfusion injury and astrogliosis, resulting in poorer neurologic recovery.[1–3] Given the progressive and irreversible nature of DCM, which has an enormous effect on patients' quality of life, early diagnosis and appropriately chosen surgical treatment are the mainstays of current management. For an effective improvement in terms of both clinical outcome and health-economic parameters, it is extremely important to understand the pathologic process as early as possible to intervene in a timely manner and block progression. Furthermore, it is necessary to adopt more cost-effective materials for spinal implants and identify biologics able to extend the bony healing effects of autograft. Finally, it is desirable to introduce pharmacologic strategies able to slow down or reverse the neuronal degeneration related to DCM.

ENHANCED DIAGNOSTIC PROTOCOLS: TOWARD NEURORADIOLOGICAL AND METABOLIC BIOMARKERS

Baptiste and Fehlings[4] suggested that the demyelination and neurologic deterioration seen at later stages of DCM are due to factors such as ischemic injury caused by chronic compression of the spinal cord vasculature, glutamate-mediated excitotoxicity, and oligodendrocyte apoptosis. Therefore, many attempts have been made to develop diagnostic protocols focused on early identification of DCM, and the correlation of clinical and laboratory biomarkers.[5,6] The diagnostic protocols developed have since been adopted as predictors of disease outcome during the decision-making process for the management of patients with DCM.[5,6] For example, clinical outcome scales, such as the modified Japanese Orthopedic Association (mJOA) are sensitive to both moderate and severe DCM, but are relatively insensitive when predicting outcomes for patients with mild DCM. In an attempt to provide better clinical tools to objectively assess upper and lower extremity motor function in patients with DCM, new diagnostic tests were proposed, as shown in **Table 1**.[7–11] When examining laboratory biomarkers, as genomic and proteomic

Table 1
Recently proposed clinical tests for DCM

G&R test[a]	The test consists of counting the number of fingers' G&R cycles; it was proposed in 2 versions: 10-s and 15-s. The test identifies paradoxic wrist motion (trick motion) and lack of finger coordination in patients with DCM.	Hosono et al,[8] 2012; Hosono et al,[7] 2010
10-s step test[b]	The test consists of simply counting the number of steps patients take within 10 s. This test significantly correlates with the number of fingers G&R test in 10 s, walking grade of the mJOA score and the total mJOA score.	Yukawa et al,[11] 2009
Triangle step test[b]	The test consists of instructing patients to step on marks at each apex of a triangle. The number of steps in 10 s are counted for each foot; this test significantly correlates with the number of finger G&R test, the Nurick score, and the total JOA score.	Mihara et al,[9] 2010
Simple foot tapping test[b]	The test consists of measuring repetitive movements of the ankle joint. This test correlates with the number of finger G&R in 10 s and the total mJOA score. This test is particularly useful in assessing patients with severe CSM who are unable to walk.	Numasawa et al,[10] 2012

Abbreviations: CSM, cervical spondylotic myelopathy; DCM, degenerative cervical myelopathy; G&R test, grip and release test; JOA, Japanese Orthopedic Association; mJOA, modified JOA.

[a] This test can be used the assess the severity of motor function in upper extremities in patients with DCM preoperatively, and when performed in the early postoperative period (24 hours) can predict long-term outcome following decompressive surgery.

[b] These tests can be used to assess the severity of motor function in lower extremities in patients with DCM preoperatively, and the improvements following decompressive surgery.

methods have evolved over the past 10 years, single nucleotide polymorphisms (SNPs) have become easier to evaluate, and the function of small noncoding RNA molecules (miRNA) that negatively regulate gene expression at the post-transcriptional levels also have been highlighted.[12] Interestingly, as shown in **Table 2**, miRNA involved in the metabolism of collagen, proteoglycans, and other components of the extracellular matrix (ECM) were found to have a role in ECM disruption, cell proliferation, and inflammatory responses promoting degenerative disc disease. Conversely, a number of genetic polymorphisms have been linked with ossification of the posterior longitudinal ligament and degenerative neuropathy or myelopathy.[13–20] These findings highlight the multifactorial origin of DCM, whereby different profiles of SNPs and miRNA can spur degenerative changes that lead to spondylosis, but not necessarily to myelopathy.[21,22]

Despite the progress witnessed with identifying biomarkers of DCM, the clinical adoption of these biomarkers remains elusive due to complex acquisitions, cumbersome analysis, limited reliability, and wide ranges of normal values to compare to. Therefore, technological aids to stratify and objectively quantify these targeted biomarkers are still required to aid in the interpretation of results. For instance, although conventional T1-weighted and T2-weighted 1.5-T MR images are sensitive enough to confirm the presence of myelopathy at more advanced stages of DCM, discrepancies between the actual clinical status and imaging findings can be found in early stages. To improve the sensitivity of technological applications, 3 approaches are paving the way for further research: (1) the development and assessment of multiparameter analysis protocols of conventional and innovative 1.5-T MRI sequences, (2) the analysis of imaging data from 3.0-T MRI machines, and (3) the use of metabolic tracers in nuclear medicine investigations.

It is known that spinal application of newly designed diffusion tensor imaging (DTI) sequences allows a more sensitive evaluation of the white matter, whereas fractional anisotropy (FA), apparent diffusion coefficient (ADC), and mean diffusivity (MD) metrics are able to document and quantify the orientation changes of water molecules in the long tracts of white matter of the spinal cord.[23–25] As such, ADC was initially proposed by Sato and colleagues[26] as a reliable and predictive biomarker for patients with DCM; whereas Budzik and colleagues[23] proposed FA metrics as the most sensitive to pathologic changes in comparison with ADC and MD values. Recently, Martin and colleagues[27] demonstrated that T2*WI WM/GM (T2 weighted white matter/grey matter ratio) sequences show lower intersubject coefficient of variation compared with magnetization transfer ratio, FA, and cross-sectional area in both healthy subjects and patients with DCM.[28]

Research groups have investigated whether high-Tesla MRI machines could be more sensitive than conventional 1.5 T in identifying early change characteristics of DCM.[29–31] Using DTI on a 3.0-T MRI system, Kara and colleagues[32] found decreased FA values and increased ADC values in stenotic segments in comparison with nonstenotic ones, suggestive of myelopathic changes even without T2 signal alterations. Another recent study with 3.0-T imaging confirmed an increased MD and a decreased FA in patients with DCM

Table 2
Expression profiles of miRNA and polymorphisms associated with DCM

Association with disc degeneration	Collagen IX gene polymorphism	Wang et al,[18] 2012
	miRNA associated with dysregulation of phosphoinositide 3-kinase/Akt, mitogen-activated protein kinase, and Wnt pathways	Zhao et al,[20] 2014
	miRNA associated with dysregulation of transforming growth factor-β, platelet-derived growth factor, insulin-like growth factor, and epidermal growth factor pathways	Li et al,[14] 2008
Association with ossification of posterior longitudinal ligament	Nucleotide pyrophosphatase gene polymorphism	Tahara et al,[17] 2005
	Collagen XI gene polymorphism	Kales et al,[13] 2004
Association with degenerative neuropathy and myelopathy	Vitamin D receptor gene polymorphism	Xu et al,[19] 2012
	Apolipoprotein E gene polymorphism	Setzer et al,[15] 2008; Setzer et al,[16] 2009

Abbreviations: DCM, degenerative cervical myelopathy; miRNA, microRNA.

compared with healthy controls.[30] The investigators observed that on the receiver operating characteristic analysis, MD changes had higher sensitivity and specificity for prediction as compared with FA.[30] Arima and colleagues[33] similarly concluded that DTI might be a promising modality to predict functional recovery after surgery, whereas MD changes may reflect spinal cord condition and its reversibility.

Recent studies have suggested that a distinct metabolic pattern of the cervical cord, as assessed by PET with 2-deoxy-[(18)F]fluoro-D-glucose (^{18}F-FDG), may predict a patient's clinical outcome after decompressive surgery for DCM.[34] Focal glucose hypermetabolism at the level of cervical spinal cord compression is thought to be a functional marker of spinal cord damage in a reversible phase of DCM, and theoretically could parallel the ongoing enhanced levels of cytokine expression, microglia activation, and astrogliosis found on experimental models.[2] Floeth and colleagues[35] showed that a focally increased (18)F-FDG uptake can be demonstrated preoperatively at the level of the stenosis. This uptake remarkably decreases following surgical decompression, and significantly correlates with preoperative and postoperative changes in JOA scores.

In addition to PET, magnetic resonance spectroscopy has also demonstrated promise as a metabolic imaging modality in the DCM population.[36–39] A variety of biomarkers can be assayed using this technique that provide insight into the spinal cord cellular biochemistry and metabolic function. Of particular interest is N-acetyl aspartate (NAA), which is found almost exclusively in axons and neurons, and is an indicator of axonal integrity. Choline is a critical component of many phospholipids, and fluctuations of this marker are considered to be an indicator of cellular turnover associated with both membrane synthesis and degradation.[40] The choline-NAA ratio has been demonstrated to strongly correlate with the degree of neurologic impairment and mJOA score,[36,39] as well as outcome following surgical intervention.[37] The strength of the choline-NAA ratio as a predictor of neurologic status and outcome is because it simultaneously evaluates both the integrity of axons and neurons as well as the amount of cellular injury and turnover. At present, none of the diagnostic parameters mentioned previously have emerged as a stand-alone radiological/metabolic biomarker for DCM. Instead, a multiparameter quantitative analysis seems more promising in quantifying fine aspects of spinal cord microstructure, and eventually offering increased overall diagnostic and predictive power. Improvements to study the spinal cord could come from technological upgrades of current methods by simultaneously increasing the signal-to-noise ratio and the spatial resolution. With these improvements, it would perhaps be possible to increase the accuracy of some of the biomarkers previously proposed. For imaging methods such as PET and computed tomography, this may be obtained with improvements in detector technology. Conversely for MRI, improvements may arise from advances in radiofrequency coil design and changes in data sampling schemes (to trade off shorter data sampling periods with more sampling periods).[41] Regardless of where improvements manifest, it is clear that a better understanding of the structural and metabolic characteristics of DCM will allow for a more personalized medicine, and hopefully guide the surgical team in better deciding the timing and type of surgical approach.

EVOLUTION OF SURGICAL STRATEGIES: THE INFLUENCE OF BIOMEDICAL ENGINEERING, NEUROPHYSIOLOGICAL MONITORING, AND COMPUTER-ASSISTED NAVIGATION

The goal of surgery for DCM is to decompress the spinal cord and stabilize the cervical segment, which can be achieved either through an anterior or a posterior approach. The choice of approach is made based on imaging features of spinal cord compression, the number of levels affected, and the spinal alignment.[42] To foster innovation while ensuring safety, it is important to consider past advances, recognizing their strengths and weaknesses, and to have a vision to address future challenges.

Over the past 20 years, biomedical engineering has had an increasing role in the creation of novel strategies for biomechanically efficient spinal stabilization. From a biomechanical perspective, the likely efficacy of some devices and the potential for adverse effects is defined by how spine implants change disc stress magnitudes and distributions.[43] For example, multilevel anterior cervical discectomy and fusion (ACDF) has proven to be safe and effective in achieving neural decompression, segmental stabilization, and satisfactory clinical outcomes.[1] However, ACDF results in a loss of mobility at the treated segment and increases the stress on adjacent segments, which may cause more rapid disc degeneration.[44] To answer how the treated segment affects proximal discs, transducers for in vivo measurement of biomechanical parameters have been used. In the cervical spine, pressure sensors have been implanted into the disc nucleus in vitro and in vivo with strain gauges on vertebral bone, load cells inserted between vertebrae, and more recently through microelectromechanical (MEMS) and nanoelectromechanical (NEMS) devices.[43,45–47] Information gained from these experiments, coupled with clinical evidence of adjacent disc disease following ACDF, has since influenced the manufacturing of newer implants designed to mitigate these issues.

In patients with single-level or 2-level cervical disc disease, cervical disc arthroplasty (CDA) was developed as an alternative procedure to preserve segmental motion and theoretically prevent adjacent segment degeneration.[48] In recent years, hybrid surgery (HS), which combines CDA with fusion, was proposed as a novel treatment for patients with multilevel cervical disc disease displaying clinical features of DCM. Biomechanically, HS seems a more tailored alternative for the treatment of multilevel cervical spondylosis, as the technique accounts for different types and degrees of degeneration at each disc level. Motion cannot be restored where already lost due to collapsed intervertebral disc, facet degeneration, or bony spurs. However, with this technique, there is no need to fuse salvageable discs at other levels, allowing for large losses to range of motion to be mitigated. There is still a paucity of studies comparing the outcomes between HS and ACDF, and data from a meta-analysis on this topic are promising both in terms of clinical improvement and spinal alignment.[49] These initial results might suggest that HS warrants further investigation in the form of randomized controlled trials (RCTs).

Over the years, the posterior approach has had a similar evolution due to contributions from biomedical engineering, intraoperative neurophysiological monitoring, and computer-assisted navigation. This has led to the relatively recent introduction in clinical practice of new instruments, including scalpel-type ultrasonic bone curette for cervical laminectomies, or newly designed miniplates and hydroxyapatite spacers for laminoplasties.[50–53] In addition, the safety of the posterior approach procedure has increased for 2 main reasons. First, improved multimodal interoperative neurophysiological monitoring has achieved 100% sensitivity and 98.4% specificity for predicting postoperative deficits, and has helped to decrease the incidence of common complications, such as C5 nerve palsy.[54,55] Second, computer-assisted navigation (CAN) has made the placement of pedicular screws for instrumented fusion of the cervical spine easier and more straightforward, overcoming the difficulties related to small pedicles and reducing the incidence of damage to nerve roots and the vertebral artery.[56] However, it is important to highlight the importance of carefully assessing the value of new technologies, which may have inherent challenges when being implemented. For example, Nooh and colleagues[57] demonstrated in a recent systematic review that differences between manufacturers of CAN systems do exist. Their study reported that the accuracy of pedicle screw insertion can be affected by which navigation system is used, suggesting that future studies should focus on the technology behind these navigation systems, and attempt to determine how manufacturer differences influence the accuracy of different systems.[57]

Future studies are warranted to help determine the optimal surgical treatment for DCM: those studies should be outcome and cost-effectiveness oriented, taking into account all possible strategies able to provide a direct removal of the compressive pathology while maximizing the preservation of segmental motion of the cervical spine. To this perspective, a special consideration should be given to minimally invasive surgical approaches, which have been developed over time for both anterior and posterior procedures. Among them, the Jho procedures (Type 1–4), as well as posterior cervical foraminotomy and discectomy, perfectly describe the evolution, from microscopic-based to endoscopic-based, of the surgical techniques available for the management of degenerative pathologies affecting the cervical spine.[58–62] Nowadays, an ever growing number of patients with DCM are treated with a broad range of surgical and medical modalities; hence, the rationale for international studies, such as the CSM-S (Cervical Spondylotic Myelopathy-Surgical) RCT comparing health resource utilization for ventral and dorsal procedures, and investigating preoperative predictors (including biomechanical ones) of overall outcome.[63]

As alluded to previously, critically examining new technology is an important step in evaluating innovations that are playing a pivotal role in decreasing the need for revision surgeries and potentially reducing complication rates and negative outcomes. One last example is offered by the latest advances in fabrication of MEMS and NEMS, which has led some teams to incorporate these new materials into existing implants. Roy and colleagues[47] proposed a solution to sense implant load and strain patterns in patients undergoing instrumented cervical fusion. Furthermore, studies on MEMS and NEMS in animal models are currently being conducted to assess quality of anterior and posterior arthrodesis. Once results from MEMS and NEMS are translated to clinical practice, they will certainly be useful in reducing the risk of pullout, pseudoarthrodesis, and revision surgery. In the near future, these pressure sensors could be applied to detect an evolving pseudoarthrosis and activate the timely injection of small volumes of fusion-inducing agents, thus optimizing the chances of healing in those situations in which fusion could be otherwise unlikely.[64]

NANOMEDICINE, ADJUVANT THERAPIES, AND THE FUTURE OF DEGENERATIVE CERVICAL MYELOPATHY

The scenario described previously is becoming possible because of the numerous contributions from nanotechnology and cell therapy to spine surgery. Within the field of nanotechnology, the most exciting fields of investigation are optimizing the coatings on surfaces of spinal implants and the design of new pharmacologic therapies.

Bone integration results from the enhancement of functional activity of osteoblasts at the tissue-implant interface. To facilitate the process of bone integration, nanotechnology fabrication and coating techniques have provided functional interbody cages, screws, and rods. This new wave of biomaterials includes metals, alloys, and ceramics with nonperiodic nanostructure that enhance the interaction and activity of osteoblasts: nanoscaffolds, nanoleaves, and nanoneedles are all good examples of this type of nanofabrication. Furthermore, the architecture and immunoneutrality of those biomaterials confer them a propensity to incorporate mesenchymal stem cells, recombinant human bone morphogenetic protein, and endogenous/exogenous growth factors, thus increasing the potential for osteointegration. It is important to note that the translation of these biomaterials from laboratories to clinical use has been plagued by a wide range of adverse effects (especially in the early stages of research), as well as by issues of widespread off-label use.

The goal of using nanoassembled materials is also to achieve compression and strength properties superior to standard polymers. For instance, silicon nitride (Si_3N_4) nanoparticles have already reached the market, being used in cages for cervical spine. This new ceramic has proven to have several biomechanical advantages over polyetheretherketone (PEEK), thus receiving the CE Mark based on standard compliance and animal studies. An industry-sponsored RCT, CASCADE, comparing the new Si_3N_4 cages with a gold standard product based on PEEK, is currently ongoing.[65]

As for many other degenerative conditions, regenerative medicine is now considered as the new frontier for DCM. The use of regenerative medicine has 2 main objectives: preventing degeneration of the spine, and reversing the insult to the compressed spinal cord. Following previous studies based on injection of protein solutions and growth factors into degenerated discs to stimulate cell growth and/or anabolic responses, cell therapy was proposed for intervertebral disc repair with the goal of reversing the degenerative cascade.[66] In fact, pluripotent stem cells have been demonstrated to survive and increase the proteoglycan matrix on introduction into degenerated discs; and their propensity to stabilize the discs' inflammatory milieu supported their experimental application as cell-based therapies in models of disc disease.[67]

As described previously, much progress has been made to optimize the surgical management of the mechanical injury typically responsible for the development of DCM. Unfortunately, the secondary biological injury is frequently not addressed. Of note, the most striking success of strategies aimed to slow or reverse neuronal degeneration related to DCM come from the experimental use of drugs initially tested for other pathologic conditions, such as amyotrophic lateral sclerosis or traumatic spinal cord injury (SCI). Following administration of the US Food and Drug Administration–approved drug riluzole in a rat model of DCM, it was noticed that this treatment attenuates oxidative DNA damage in the spinal cord.[68] Mechanistic in vitro studies also demonstrated that riluzole preserves mitochondrial function and reduces oxidative damage in neurons, therefore showing potential to favor plasticity after decompression surgery. In fact, DCM rats receiving combined decompression surgery and riluzole treatment displayed long-term improvements in forelimb function associated with preservation of cervical motor neurons and corticospinal tracts, as compared with rats treated with decompression surgery alone.[69] As such, this sodium-glutamate antagonist, which was successfully tested in a phase I trial for traumatic SCI, was suggested as a promising option to optimize neurologic outcomes after surgery in patients with DCM.[70] This research question is currently examined in the CSM-Protect RCT.[71]

Similarly, regenerative technologies are on the verge of being considered for DCM. A nice example is the local application over the decompressed dura of a Rho inhibitor known as Cethrin. Activation of the Rho pathway and its downstream effector kinases represent a significant barrier to axon regeneration, whereas there is evidence that its inhibition can reverse chondroitin sulfate proteoglycan–mediated inhibition of neurite outgrowth. The regenerative properties of Rho inhibitors in animal models of SCI were reinforced by studies carried out in vitro using retinal ganglion cells.[72] Cethrin was evaluated as a therapeutic intervention for SCI in a phase I/IIa clinical trial with promising results, and a phase IIb/III RCT

(NCT02669849) is currently ongoing.[73,74] It seems likely that in the near future, a similar approach could be attempted in DCM to further augment the clinical benefits of decompressive surgery.

SUMMARY

Innovative microstructural imaging, advancements in surgical techniques, novel spinal implants, osteobiologics, and drugs have the potential to slow down the progression of DCM, to enhance fusion rates while reducing postoperative complications, and to improve overall clinical outcomes. However, as history has demonstrated, early adoption of promising technologies without proper guidance and consideration carries the risk of potential drawbacks. The future development of diagnostic and therapeutic protocols for DCM requires researchers to engage with basic scientists, equipment manufacturers, and software developers to communicate mutual needs and encourage the sharing of methods and technology. This recipe will allow innovations to become more widely accessible, especially in clinical environments, to facilitate a proper translational approach. As spine practitioners, we look forward to a bright future for our specialty due to the progress of science. However, we must continue to educate ourselves on the mechanisms of action, potential side effects, and expected outcomes related to the use of the innovative products that will soon reach the wards and operative rooms of our hospitals.

REFERENCES

1. Fehlings MG, Barry S, Kopjar B, et al. Anterior versus posterior surgical approaches to treat cervical spondylotic myelopathy: outcomes of the prospective multicenter AOSpine North America CSM study in 264 patients. Spine (Phila Pa 1976) 2013; 38(26):2247–52.
2. Vidal PM, Karadimas SK, Ulndreaj A, et al. Delayed decompression exacerbates ischemia-reperfusion injury in cervical compressive myelopathy. JCI Insight 2017;2(11). [Epub ahead of print].
3. Witiw CD, Tetreault LA, Smieliauskas F, et al. Surgery for degenerative cervical myelopathy: a patient-centered quality of life and health economic evaluation. Spine J 2017;17(1):15–25.
4. Baptiste DC, Fehlings MG. Pathophysiology of cervical myelopathy. Spine J 2006;6(6 Suppl):190S–7S.
5. Nouri A, Tetreault L, Côté P, et al. Does magnetic resonance imaging improve the predictive performance of a validated clinical prediction rule developed to evaluate surgical outcome in patients with degenerative cervical myelopathy? Spine (Phila Pa 1976) 2015;40(14):1092–100.
6. Tetreault L, Kopjar B, Côté P, et al. A clinical prediction rule for functional outcomes in patients undergoing surgery for degenerative cervical myelopathy: analysis of an international prospective multicenter data set of 757 subjects. J Bone Joint Surg Am 2015;97(24):2038–46.
7. Hosono N, Makino T, Sakaura H, et al. Myelopathy hand: new evidence of the classical sign. Spine (Phila Pa 1976) 2010;35(8):E273–7.
8. Hosono N, Takenaka S, Mukai Y, et al. Postoperative 24-hour result of 15-second grip-and-release test correlates with surgical outcome of cervical compression myelopathy. Spine (Phila Pa 1976) 2012;37(15):1283–7.
9. Mihara H, Kondo S, Murata A, et al. A new performance test for cervical myelopathy: the triangle step test. Spine (Phila Pa 1976) 2010;35(1):32–5.
10. Numasawa T, Ono A, Wada K, et al. Simple foot tapping test as a quantitative objective assessment of cervical myelopathy. Spine (Phila Pa 1976) 2012; 37(2):108–13.
11. Yukawa Y, Kato F, Ito K, et al. "Ten second step test" as a new quantifiable parameter of cervical myelopathy. Spine (Phila Pa 1976) 2009;34(1):82–6.
12. Wang C, Wang WJ, Yan YG, et al. MicroRNAs: new players in intervertebral disc degeneration. Clin Chim Acta 2015;450:333–41.
13. Kales SN, Linos A, Chatzis C, et al. The role of collagen IX tryptophan polymorphisms in symptomatic intervertebral disc disease in Southern European patients. Spine (Phila Pa 1976) 2004;29(11): 1266–70.
14. Li S, Duance VC, Blain EJ. Zonal variations in cytoskeletal element organization, mRNA and protein expression in the intervertebral disc. J Anat 2008; 213(6):725–32.
15. Setzer M, Hermann E, Seifert V, et al. Apolipoprotein E gene polymorphism and the risk of cervical myelopathy in patients with chronic spinal cord compression. Spine (Phila Pa 1976) 2008;33(5): 497–502.
16. Setzer M, Vrionis FD, Hermann EJ, et al. Effect of apolipoprotein E genotype on the outcome after anterior cervical decompression and fusion in patients with cervical spondylotic myelopathy. J Neurosurg Spine 2009;11(6):659–66.
17. Tahara M, Aiba A, Yamazaki M, et al. The extent of ossification of posterior longitudinal ligament of the spine associated with nucleotide pyrophosphatase gene and leptin receptor gene polymorphisms. Spine (Phila Pa 1976) 2005;30(8):877–81.
18. Wang ZC, Shi JG, Chen XS, et al. The role of smoking status and collagen IX polymorphisms in the susceptibility to cervical spondylotic myelopathy. Genet Mol Res 2012;11(2):1238–44.
19. Xu G, Mei Q, Zhou D, et al. Vitamin D receptor gene and aggrecan gene polymorphisms and the risk of

intervertebral disc degeneration—a meta-analysis. PLoS One 2012;7(11):e50243.
20. Zhao B, Yu Q, Li H, et al. Characterization of microRNA expression profiles in patients with intervertebral disc degeneration. Int J Mol Med 2014;33(1): 43–50.
21. Walker CT, Bonney PA, Martirosyan NL, et al. Genetics underlying an individualized approach to adult spinal disorders. Front Surg 2016;3:61.
22. Wilson JR, Patel AA, Brodt ED, et al. Genetics and heritability of cervical spondylotic myelopathy and ossification of the posterior longitudinal ligament: results of a systematic review. Spine (Phila Pa 1976) 2013;38(22 Suppl 1):S123–46.
23. Budzik JF, Balbi V, Le Thuc V, et al. Diffusion tensor imaging and fibre tracking in cervical spondylotic myelopathy. Eur Radiol 2011;21(2):426–33.
24. Cui JL, Wen CY, Hu Y, et al. Orientation entropy analysis of diffusion tensor in healthy and myelopathic spinal cord. Neuroimage 2011;58(4):1028–33.
25. Wheeler-Kingshott CA, Stroman PW, Schwab JM, et al. The current state-of-the-art of spinal cord imaging: applications. Neuroimage 2014;84:1082–93.
26. Sato T, Horikoshi T, Watanabe A, et al. Evaluation of cervical myelopathy using apparent diffusion coefficient measured by diffusion-weighted imaging. AJNR Am J Neuroradiol 2012;33(2):388–92.
27. Martin AR, De Leener B, Cohen-Adad J, et al. Clinically feasible microstructural MRI to quantify cervical spinal cord tissue injury using DTI, MT, and T2*-weighted imaging: assessment of normative data and reliability. AJNR Am J Neuroradiol 2017a; 38(6):1257–65.
28. Martin AR, De Leener B, Cohen-Adad J, et al. A novel MRI biomarker of spinal cord white matter injury: T2*-weighted white matter to gray matter signal intensity ratio. AJNR Am J Neuroradiol 2017b;38(6):1266–73.
29. Suetomi Y, Kanchiku T, Nishijima S, et al. Application of diffusion tensor imaging for the diagnosis of segmental level of dysfunction in cervical spondylotic myelopathy. Spinal Cord 2016;54(5):390–5.
30. Uda T, Takami T, Tsuyuguchi N, et al. Assessment of cervical spondylotic myelopathy using diffusion tensor magnetic resonance imaging parameter at 3.0 tesla. Spine (Phila Pa 1976) 2013;38(5):407–14.
31. Xiangshui M, Xiangjun C, Xiaoming Z, et al. 3 T magnetic resonance diffusion tensor imaging and fibre tracking in cervical myelopathy. Clin Radiol 2010; 65(6):465–73.
32. Kara B, Celik A, Karadereler S, et al. The role of DTI in early detection of cervical spondylotic myelopathy: a preliminary study with 3-T MRI. Neuroradiology 2011;53(8):609–16.
33. Arima H, Sakamoto S, Naito K, et al. Prediction of the efficacy of surgical intervention in patients with cervical myelopathy by using diffusion tensor 3T-magnetic resonance imaging parameters. J Craniovertebr Junction Spine 2015;6(3):120–4.
34. Eicker SO, Langen KJ, Galldiks N, et al. Clinical value of 2-deoxy-[18F]fluoro-D-glucose positron emission tomography in patients with cervical spondylotic myelopathy. Neurosurg Focus 2013;35(1):E2.
35. Floeth FW, Galldiks N, Eicker S, et al. Hypermetabolism in 18F-FDG PET predicts favorable outcome following decompressive surgery in patients with degenerative cervical myelopathy. J Nucl Med 2013;54(9):1577–83.
36. Ellingson BM, Salamon N, Hardy AJ, et al. Prediction of neurological impairment in cervical spondylotic myelopathy using a combination of diffusion MRI and Proton MR spectroscopy. PLoS One 2015;10: e0139451.
37. Holly LT, Ellingson BM, Salamon N. Magnetic spectroscopy as a predictor of outcome after surgery for cervical spondylotic myelopathy. Clin Spine Surg 2017;30:E615–9.
38. Holly LT, Freitas B, McArthur DL, et al. Proton magnetic resonance spectroscopy to evaluate spinal cord axonal injury in cervical spondylotic myelopathy. J Neurosurg Spine 2009;10(3):194–200.
39. Salamon N, Ellingson BM, Nagarajan R, et al. Proton magnetic resonance spectroscopy of human cervical spondylosis at 3T. Spinal Cord 2013; 51(7):558–63.
40. Carpentier A, Galanaud D, Puybasset L, et al. Early morphologic and spectroscopic magnetic resonance in severe traumatic brain injuries can detect "invisible brain stem damage" and predict "vegetative states". J Neurotrauma 2006;23(5):674–85.
41. Stroman PW, Wheeler-Kingshott C, Bacon M, et al. The current state-of-the-art of spinal cord imaging: methods. Neuroimage 2014;84:1070–81.
42. Kato S, Nouri A, Wu D, et al. Comparison of anterior and posterior surgery for degenerative cervical myelopathy: an MRI-based propensity-score-matched analysis using data from the prospective multicenter AOSpine CSM North America and international studies. J Bone Joint Surg Am 2017;99(12):1013–21.
43. Glos DL, Sauser FE, Papautsky I, et al. Implantable MEMS compressive stress sensors: design, fabrication and calibration with application to the disc annulus. J Biomech 2010;43(11):2244–8.
44. Matsunaga S, Kabayama S, Yamamoto T, et al. Strain on intervertebral discs after anterior cervical decompression and fusion. Spine (Phila Pa 1976) 1999;24(7):670–5.
45. Cripton PA, Dumas GA, Nolte LP. A minimally disruptive technique for measuring intervertebral disc pressure in vitro: application to the cervical spine. J Biomech 2001;34(4):545–9.
46. Pospiech J, Stolke D, Wilke HJ, et al. Intradiscal pressure recordings in the cervical spine. Neurosurgery 1999;44(2):379–84 [discussion: 384–5].

47. Roy S, Ferrara LA, Fleischman AJ, et al. Microelectromechanical systems and neurosurgery: a new era in a new millennium. Neurosurgery 2001;49(4): 779–97 [discussion: 797-8].
48. Pickett GE, Rouleau JP, Duggal N. Kinematic analysis of the cervical spine following implantation of an artificial cervical disc. Spine (Phila Pa 1976) 2005;30(17):1949–54.
49. Zhang J, Meng F, Ding Y, et al. Hybrid surgery versus anterior cervical discectomy and fusion in multilevel cervical disc diseases: a meta-analysis. Medicine (Baltimore) 2016;95(21):e3621.
50. Bydon M, Xu R, Papademetriou K, et al. Safety of spinal decompression using an ultrasonic bone curette compared with a high-speed drill: outcomes in 337 patients. J Neurosurg Spine 2013; 18(6):627–33.
51. Hazer DB, Yaşar B, Rosberg HE, et al. Technical aspects on the use of ultrasonic bone shaver in spine surgery: experience in 307 patients. Biomed Res Int 2016;2016:8428530.
52. Heller JG, Raich AL, Dettori JR, et al. Comparative effectiveness of different types of cervical laminoplasty. Evid Based Spine Care J 2013;4(2):105–15.
53. Tachibana T, Maruo K, Arizumi F, et al. Changing the design of hydroxyapatite spacers to improve their postoperative displacement following double-door laminoplasty. J Clin Neurosci 2017;43:185–7.
54. Eggspuehler A, Sutter MA, Grob D, et al. Multimodal intraoperative monitoring (MIOM) during cervical spine surgical procedures in 246 patients. Eur Spine J 2007;16(Suppl 2):S209–15.
55. Burke JF, Oya J, Vogel T, et al. The accuracy of multimodality intraoperative neuromonitoring to predict postoperative neurological deficits following cervical laminoplasty. Neurosurgery 2016;63(Suppl 1):168.
56. Lee GY, Massicotte EM, Rampersaud YR. Clinical accuracy of cervicothoracic pedicle screw placement: a comparison of the "open" lamino-foraminotomy and computer-assisted techniques. J Spinal Disord Tech 2007;20(1):25–32.
57. Nooh A, Lubov J, Aoude A, et al. Differences between manufacturers of computed tomography-based computer-assisted surgery symptoms do exist: A systematic literature review. Global Spine J 2017;7(1):83–94.
58. Holly LT, Moftakhar P, Khoo LT, et al. Minimally invasive 2-level posterior cervical foraminotomy: preliminary clinical results. J Spinal Disord Tech 2007;20(1):20–4.
59. Jho HD, Jho DH. Ventral uncoforaminotomy. J Neurosurg Spine 2007;7(5):533–6.
60. Lee JY, Löhr M, Impekoven P, et al. Small keyhole transuncal foraminotomy for unilateral cervical radiculopathy. Acta Neurochir (Wien) 2006;148(9):951–8.
61. O'Toole JE, Sheikh H, Eichholz KM, et al. Endoscopic posterior cervical foraminotomy and discectomy. Neurosurg Clin N Am 2006;17(4):411–22.
62. Saringer WF, Reddy B, Nöbauer-Huhmann I, et al. Endoscopic anterior cervical foraminotomy for unilateral radiculopathy: anatomical morphometric analysis and preliminary clinical experience. J Neurosurg 2003;98(2 Suppl):171–80.
63. Ghogawala Z, Benzel EC, Heary RF, et al. Cervical spondylotic myelopathy surgical trial: randomized, controlled trial design and rationale. Neurosurgery 2014;75(4):334–46.
64. Benzel E, Ferrara L, Roy S, et al. Micromachines in spine surgery. Spine (Phila Pa 1976) 2004;29(6): 601–6.
65. Arts MP, Wolfs JF, Corbin TP, et al. The CASCADE trial: effectiveness of ceramic versus PEEK cages for anterior cervical discectomy with interbody fusion; protocol of a blinded randomized controlled trial. BMC Musculoskeletal Disord 2013;14:244.
66. Dowdell J, Erwin M, Choma T, et al. Intervertebral disk degeneration and repair. Neurosurgery 2017; 80(3S):S46–54.
67. Ganey T, Hutton WC, Moseley T, et al. Intervertebral disc repair using adipose tissue-derived stem and regenerative cells: experiments in a canine model. Spine (Phila Pa 1976) 2009;34(21):2297–304.
68. Moon ES, Karadimas SK, Yu WR, et al. Riluzole attenuates neuropathic pain and enhances functional recovery in a rodent model of cervical spondylotic myelopathy. Neurobiol Dis 2014;62:394–406.
69. Karadimas SK, Laliberte AM, Tetreault L, et al. Riluzole blocks perioperative ischemia-reperfusion injury and enhances postdecompression outcomes in cervical spondylotic myelopathy. Sci Transl Med 2015;7(316):316ra194.
70. Grossman RG, Fehlings MG, Frankowski RF, et al. A prospective, multicenter, phase I matched-comparison group trial of safety, pharmacokinetics, and preliminary efficacy of riluzole in patients with traumatic spinal cord injury. J Neurotrauma 2014; 31(3):239–55.
71. Fehlings MG, Wilson JR, Karadimas SK, et al. Clinical evaluation of a neuroprotective drug in patients with cervical spondylotic myelopathy undergoing surgical treatment: design and rationale for the CSM-Protect trial. Spine (Phila Pa 1976) 2013; 38(22 Suppl 1):S68–75.
72. Forgione N, Fehlings MG. Rho-ROCK inhibition in the treatment of spinal cord injury. World Neurosurg 2014;82(3–4):e535–9.
73. Fehlings MG, Theodore N, Harrop J, et al. A phase I/IIa clinical trial of a recombinant Rho protein antagonist in acute spinal cord injury. J Neurotrauma 2011;28(5):787–96.
74. McKerracher L, Anderson KD. Analysis of recruitment and outcomes in the phase I/IIa Cethrin clinical trial for acute spinal cord injury. J Neurotrauma 2013;30(21):1795–804.

Printed and bound by CPI Group (UK) Ltd, Croydon, CR0 4YY
08/05/2025
01864708-0001